A Casebook
of Medical Ethics

A Casebook of Medical Ethics

Terrence F. Ackerman, Ph.D.
Carson Strong, Ph.D.

New York   Oxford
Oxford University Press
1989

Oxford University Press

Oxford   New York   Toronto
Delhi   Bombay   Calcutta   Madras   Karachi
Petaling Jaya   Singapore   Hong Kong   Tokyo
Nairobi   Dar es Salaam   Cape Town
Melbourne   Auckland

and associated companies in
Berlin   Ibadan

Copyright © 1989 by Oxford University Press, Inc.

Published by Oxford University Press, Inc.,
200 Madison Avenue, New York, New York 10016

Oxford is a registered trademark of Oxford University Press

All rights reserved. No part of this publication may be reproduced,
stored in a retrieval system, or transmitted, in any form or by any means,
electronic, mechanical, photocopying, recording, or otherwise,
without the prior permission of Oxford University Press.

Library of Congress Cataloging-in-Publication Data
Ackerman, Terrence F., 1949–
   A casebook of medical ethics / by Terrence F. Ackerman and Carson
Strong.
      p.   cm.
   Includes bibliographies and index.
   ISBN 0-19-503916-5   ISBN 0-19-503917-3 (paper)
   1. Medical ethics—Case studies. I. Strong, Carson. II. Title.
   [DNLM: 1. Ethics, Medical—case studies. W 50 A182c]
R725.5.A25   1989
174'.2—dc19
DNLM/DLC
for Library of Congress   89-3206
                                                                 CIP

9 8 7 6 5 4 3

Printed in the United States of America
on acid-free paper

To my mother, Marguerite F. Roberts, and the memory of my father, Merton A. Ackerman—for their gift of the security, love, and freedom in which to grow, and for their unfailing example of all that a good person should be.

T.F.A.

To my beloved parents, Ralph and Bertha Raye Strong, for nurturing me with exemplary devotion and thoughtfulness, and for teaching me the importance of ethics and reason.

C.S.

Preface

Analysis of cases plays a critical role in the study of medical ethics. Attention to case histories allows us to classify the major types of moral problems faced in the clinical practice of medicine. It permits sensitive identification of the kinds of values or obligations pertinent to the investigation of these problems. Review of cases may also suggest appropriate policies for resolving specific moral issues. Finally, application of principles or policies to case situations enables us to trace their implications, refine their content, and evaluate the degree of moral justification they possess.

Unfortunately, case histories available in the literature of medical ethics typically suffer from two major defects. First, the rich complexity of the factual dimension of most cases is rarely depicted. This shortcoming is reflected in rather superficial examination of the medical aspects of cases. Ubiquitous uncertainties related to prognosis, effectiveness of alternative treatments, risks of harm to the patient, and similar matters are rarely explored. The problem is also reflected in the failure to develop in rich detail psychosocial data regarding the patient's feelings and beliefs, relationships among family members, attitudes of staff members, and other such factors. Moreover, difficulties in interpreting the meaning of seemingly simple facts, such as a patient's stated reluctance to accept a treatment, are not often explored. As a result, the factual aspects of cases are usually portrayed as possessing a straightforwardness that misrepresents their actual complexity.

Second, failure to adequately depict the medical and psychosocial aspects of clinical situations impairs the quality of the ethical analysis in crucial ways. Important values or obligations relevant to formulation of the ethical problem may not be acknowledged. The full range of options for resolving the issue may not be identified and explored. Moreover, the assessment of how alternative policies or actions bear on the relevant values or obligations may be incomplete or superficial. As a result, the selection of a course of action or policy is frequently represented as requiring an either-or choice between two relevant values or obligations. In reality, the choice usually involves more than two values, specific actions or policies may support or thwart important values in varying degrees, and choices that partially support each of the conflicting values are often possible.

The purpose of this volume is to make available a set of case studies that accurately portrays the factual and moral dimensions of ethical issues in clinical medicine. The medical and psychosocial aspects of clinical situations are developed in substantial detail, including description of the various uncertainties they present. This development of factual detail permits identification of the numerous values or obligations that may be relevant to analysis of particular cases. Moreover, several options for resolving the case are explicitly formulated or suggested by the commentary. Finally, an attempt is made to examine in some detail the varying degrees to which particular options sustain or undercut each of the relevant values or obligations. In this manner, we hope to enrich the sophistication and usefulness of ethical analysis as applied to moral problems in clinical medicine.

None of the detailed case descriptions has appeared previously in the literature. With three exceptions, the cases derive from our clinical activities at the University of Tennessee, Memphis. One case was encountered during Dr. Ackerman's tenure as visiting professor in the School of Medicine and Dentistry at the University of Rochester; two others derive from the clinical activities of Dr. Haavi Morreim, our colleague, while a faculty member at the University of Virginia. The cases were typically encountered during clinical rounds or special consultations. In most situations, the issues generated by the cases were discussed extensively with members of the health professional staff. In many cases, we reviewed aspects of the situation with patients, family members, or other significant participants. All cases were gathered during the period from 1978 to 1987.

An early reviewer remarked that too many of the cases tottered on a razor's edge, making it extremely difficult to determine the appropriate course of action. The assumption was that features of the cases had been altered or fabricated to create especially complex dilemmas. However, with the exception of four cases which are composites of recurring clinical situations, the narratives are accurate accounts of actual cases. In all cases, the usual identifiers (names, initials, places of residence, etc.) have been altered to protect the confidentiality of patients and other participants. But other significant medical and psychosocial details bearing on the formulation and analysis of the moral problems have not been changed. On the other hand, we have refined and expanded, in some cases, the comments and views of physicians and other health professionals involved in the cases. Their reflections regarding the moral issues were often formulated within the time constraints and practical focus of case management conferences, hospital rounds, or staff meetings. There was little opportunity for extended and refined articulation of careful philosophical positions. Although we have tried to convey faithfully the substance of the views they expressed, we have added commentary that serves to identify more completely the relevant ethical views and considerations.

It is difficult to assess the degree to which the psychosocial aspects of the cases presented here are typical of therapeutic interactions. Some factors are undoubtedly common occurrences in the clinical encounter. For example, the nature of illness is such that patients undergo strong emotional reactions such as anxiety, fear, guilt, and hopelessness. Similarly, social factors such as cost-containment pressures are widely experienced phenomena. On the other hand, there may be factors operative in the cultural milieu in which these cases occurred that are more pronounced than in other subcultures. The Mid-South is notable for such features as the strong influence of religious beliefs, polite deference to authority, and skepticism about the "ideology" of using aggressive and highly sophisticated technological interventions to prolong life. Whether such factors are operative to an unusual degree in these cases and how they affect the character of the moral problems described must be considered in reading the book.

The scope of the volume is restricted to moral dilemmas arising in the clinical practice of medicine. The distribution of cases among different areas of clinical medicine is not intended to evenly represent all areas of medical specialization. To a certain extent, the sampling of cases reflects our own pattern of clinical activities and interests. However, we have selected and organized the cases in a manner intended to display in a conceptually helpful way the most important types of moral problems arising in the clinical practice of medicine. Thus, although some medical specialties may be underrepresented, we have tried to accurately portray the relative importance of various categories of moral issues.

Each chapter focuses on a particular type of clinical moral issue: conflicts between respect for patients' wishes and concern for their well-being; tensions between duties to the patient and obligations to family members; differing viewpoints concerning what is best for patients unable to choose for themselves; disputes involving the moral interests of human subjects and the goals of medical research; and clashes between obligations to patients and the interests of other persons, including physicians, specific third parties, and the general public. The cases presented illustrate the variety of ways in which each type of moral issue arises in the clinical setting. However, because many cases raise more than one type of moral problem, case descriptions frequently include a discussion of additional issues as well.

The commentaries in each chapter are intended as original contributions to the literature rather than mere analytic summaries of previous reflection and debate. Each commentary examines two conceptual approaches to the resolution of the moral issue addressed in the chapter. One type of conceptual approach involves formulating a general priority ranking of values or obligations at the level of moral principles. For cases in which a specific moral issue arises, this ranking is formulated in a policy asserting that some value(s) or obligation(s) should be assigned general priority in determining conduct. The value or obligation has priority in the sense that its requirements must be met before acting on other values or obligations. Its priority is general in the sense that it holds for all cases in which the particular issue arises. For example, the autonomy-oriented view on paternalism in chapter 1 claims that respect for autonomy has general priority over concern for the well-being of persons when these obligations require conflicting courses of action. Promotion of the well-being of persons must be constrained by respect for their wishes in all cases in which persons have the capacity to act autonomously. Similarly, the strict patient-advocacy view in chapters 2 and 5, the inviolateness-of-persons view in chapter 3, and the subject-oriented view in chapter 4 are examples of this general approach to the resolution of moral problems.

The second type of conceptual approach involves formulating a policy that acknowledges each of the major values or obligations bearing on the resolution of a moral issue. On this approach, the policy for resolving a moral problem seeks a balancing or compromise of initially conflicting values or obligations. This may involve giving priority to one value or obligation in one subset of cases while assigning priority to a different value or obligation in another subset of cases. Alternatively, it may involve formulating a policy that partially acknowledges each of the competing values or obligations in the case situations under consideration. Unlike the first conceptual approach, however, the same value or obligation is not assigned priority in all cases in which the specific moral issue is raised. The balancing view in chapter 4 illustrates this conceptual approach with regard to moral issues in human research. According to this position, it is permissible to make minor compromises in the moral interests of human subjects provided that their welfare is not significantly endangered and compromise of their interests is necessary to achieve the goals of medical research. On the other hand, compromise of the moral interests of subjects is not permitted when their welfare will be seriously endangered or the compromise is unnecessary to achieve the goals of medical research. Thus, the position formulated attempts to achieve a compromise of initially conflicting values and does not set a general priority for all cases. The holistic view in chapter 1, the modified patient-advocacy view in chapters 2 and 5, and the beneficence-centered approach in chapter 3 represent the same balancing approach to the resolution of moral problems in clinical medicine.

As illustrated in each chapter, the two conceptual approaches for resolving moral issues do not constitute specific policy proposals. Rather, each represents a general framework within which specific policy alternatives might be articulated. For example, chapter 2 examines conflicts between the interests of patients and families. The modified patient-advocacy view maintains that the physician should sometimes act in a manner that gives priority to the interests of family members. Within the framework of this approach, numerous policy alternatives might be proposed, depending on the particular interests of family claimed to have priority and the circumstances under which this priority is assigned. Similarly, the strict patient-advocacy view maintains that the moral interests of patients should always assume priority over the conflicting interests of family members. Within this general framework various policy options might be articulated, depending on how the protected moral interests of the patient are delineated. Thus, the two conceptual approaches formulated in each chapter represent general frameworks for resolving moral issues rather than specific policy proposals.

The general priority approach to the formulation of policies is most frequently encountered in the literature of medical ethics. With regard to the issues addressed in each chapter, the literature reveals various policy positions assigning general priority to a specific value or obligation. Different authors may disagree about the principles assigned priority, the interpretation of their meaning, or the consequences of their application to specific situations, but it is assumed that there is a priority ranking applicable to all relevant cases. By contrast, a balancing approach to the resolution of moral problems is more commonly utilized in the clinical practice of medicine. Physicians frequently resolve moral issues by utilizing policies that take partial account of each of the initially conflicting values or obligations. In specific cases, a course of action may be chosen that partially supports each major value. When priorities must be set, they may vary depending on perceived differences in the morally relevant features of different cases.

In each of the chapter commentaries, we compare and contrast the general priority approach to the resolution of clinical moral problems with a balancing approach. We define these distinct conceptual approaches, explore their differing implications for the treatment of individual case dilemmas, and assess their general strengths and weaknesses as basic frameworks for resolving moral problems. Insofar as the balancing approach is less frequently encountered in the literature of medical ethics, its systematic development in each chapter commentary represents an attempt to broaden the debate about how to resolve moral issues in clinical medicine. However, the frequent use of this approach in clinical practice is not sufficient to justify its use. Thus, the thoughtful reader is invited to assess the comparative merits and liabilities of these different conceptual frameworks for resolving the difficult moral dilemmas that confront the conscientious physician.

Memphis, Tenn.   T.F.A.
November 1988   C.S.

Acknowledgments

Many persons contributed to the preparation of this volume of case studies. A special debt of gratitude is owed to numerous physician colleagues at the University of Tennessee, Memphis. Without their professional trust, expressed in an open willingness to share difficult moral problems from their clinical practice, the project would not have been possible. Our colleagues were also exceedingly generous in their readiness to discuss these dilemmas and to offer advice on the drafts of particular case studies.

Colleagues elsewhere helped us to critically evaluate successive drafts of both cases and commentaries. A series of anonymous reviewers retained by Oxford University Press provided extensive comments that clarified the strengths and weaknesses of early drafts of the material. Dr. Robert Arnold of the University of Pittsburgh reviewed the entire manuscript and made numerous helpful suggestions. Dr. Robert Levine of Yale University provided excellent advice regarding the commentary to the fourth chapter, enabling us to avoid several mistakes and to resolve important ambiguities.

William Frucht, our initial editor at Oxford University Press, suggested revisions on a line-by-line basis and offered excellent advice regarding the general organization of the volume and individual chapters. The style and content of the manuscript were greatly strengthened by his assistance. In addition, he was a source of steady encouragement. Jeffrey House of Oxford completed editorial direction of the project. His critical perspective led to several major revisions in the volume which considerably strengthened the quality of the final version.

Donna Stallings, our editorial assistant and word-processing specialist, provided excellent assistance in preparing the manuscript. She cheerfully and expeditiously made countless revisions in successive drafts of the material.

Helpful contributions were also made by our wives, Christine Ackerman and

Peggy Strong, whose clinical knowledge and perspectives enabled us to explore more adequately important dimensions of a number of cases.

Lastly, we must note our special regard for the patients whose lives are encountered in these pages. Many have died, and most suffered greatly as a result of their illnesses. Empathetically, we shared their trials. It is our fond hope that this volume will, in some small way, enhance the sensitivity and knowledge with which moral problems in clinical medicine are addressed, and that the suffering of these patients will thereby gain additional meaning and significance.

Contents

1   Paternalism in the Therapeutic Relationship

1.1	Ambivalence Toward Electroconvulsive Therapy	3
1.2	Treatment Refusal in the Medical Intensive Care Unit	6
1.3	An Uncooperative Leukemia Patient	9
1.4	Rehabilitation of a Dependent Patient	12
1.5	Alternative Approaches to Informed Consent	14
1.6	Previous Refusal of Treatment by a Presently Comatose Patient	17
1.7	A Family's Refusal of Blood Transfusions for a Mother and Her Son	19
1.8	Deciding Whether to Discharge a Suicidal Patient	22
1.9	A Request for Sex-Reassignment Surgery	25
1.10	Divulging Information Concerning an Infant's Condition	28
Commentary		31
Notes		42

2   Duties to Patient and Family

2.1	A Daughter's Insistence on Aggressive Treatment	45
2.2	Parental Refusal of Cancer Treatment on Religious Grounds	48
2.3	Informed Consent and the Dying Adolescent	50
2.4	Treatment Refusal for an Infant with Possible Brain Damage	53
2.5	Venereal Disease and Adolescent Confidentiality	56
2.6	Contraceptives for an Adolescent	58
2.7	Request for Abortion for a Retarded Daughter	61
2.8	Request for Hysterectomy for a Retarded Eleven-Year-Old	64

2.9	Conflict about Maintaining a Brain-Dead Woman for the Sake of Her Fetus	68
2.10	Choosing the Method of Delivery for a Fetus with Hydrocephalus	71
Commentary		75
Notes		83

3 Deciding for Others

3.1	A Bedridden and Cognitively Impaired Elderly Patient	89
3.2	Who Should Decide for a Patient in Persistent Vegetative State?	91
3.3	Nasogastric Tube Feedings for an Elderly Stroke Patient	95
3.4	A Prolonged Stay in the Neonatal ICU	97
3.5	Deciding Treatment When the Preliminary Diagnosis Is Trisomy 18	100
3.6	Risk/Benefit Assessment of Surgery for a Child Suffering from Strokes	103
3.7	Responding to a Family's Decision for Laetrile	106
3.8	Selecting Therapy for a Mentally Retarded Teenager	109
3.9	Birth Control for a Retarded Woman	111
3.10	A Family's Lack of Commitment	114
Commentary		117
Notes		130

4 Medical Research Involving Human Subjects

4.1	Limited Consent in Alcoholism Research	135
4.2	Disclosure of Preliminary Results in a Randomized Clinical Trial	138
4.3	Constraints on Consent in a Phase I Clinical Trial	140
4.4	Proxy Consent for Incompetent Trauma Patients	143
4.5	Undue Inducement in the Recruitment of Research Subjects	146
4.6	Nontherapeutic Research Procedures Involving Children	149
4.7	Discomfort from Repeated Nontherapeutic Research Procedures Involving Competent Adults	153
4.8	Physicians' Treatment Preferences and Recruitment of Subjects for a Randomized Clinical Trial	155
4.9	Parental Preferences and a Child's Involvement in a Randomized Clinical Trial	159
4.10	Compensating Research Injuries	163
Commentary		166
Notes		179

5 Physicians, Third Parties, and Society

5.1	Request for Surgery the Physician Considers Unnecessary	187
5.2	Providing Free Care	190
5.3	Risk of Litigation as a Factor in Decision Making	194
5.4	Pressures to Provide Customary Care	197
5.5	Confidentiality and Child Abuse	200
5.6	Rejection of a Consultant's Advice	202
5.7	Abortion Resulting in a Live Birth	205
5.8	Costly Nutrition for a Terminal Patient	208
5.9	Cost Factors in the Choice of Treatment for Kidney Stone Disease	211
5.10	Artificial Insemination for a Single Woman	214
Commentary		217
Notes		233

Topical Index to Cases   239

A Casebook
of Medical Ethics

1
Paternalism in the Therapeutic Relationship

1.1 Ambivalence Toward Electroconvulsive Therapy

M.J., a sixty-year-old man, was admitted to the psychiatric ward of the Veterans Administration hospital after he threatened to kill himself and his wife with a hunting rifle. The incident followed almost two years of increasing physical and mental difficulties. The patient had suffered continually from depression and often contemplated suicide. He admitted to sleep disturbance (early-morning awakening), loss of interest in outside activities, absence of sexual interest, and problems with concentration and memory. He also had a variety of nonspecific physical complaints (such as "weakness in the legs") and considerable loss of appetite.

Formerly, the patient had been happily married for thirty-five years. He also had a good relationship with his only child, a thirty-three-year-old son who lived in the same town. He reported no special problems in childhood or adolescence and has never had a problem with alcohol or drugs. However, his mother was treated for depression and later died in a mental hospital, possibly by suicide. His brother has also been treated for depression.

The vocational history given by M.J. was unremarkable. He worked for fifteen years as a salesman and during the last twenty-one years had been an auto body repairman. He quit his job three months ago because of the weakness in his legs and his inability to concentrate on his work.

The patient was diagnosed as having endogenous depression. This term refers to depressive illness that is not a reaction to environmental stress (such as the death of a loved one), the implication being that it results from some intrinsic biological process. The case also involved other factors typical of endogenous depression, including onset at an advanced age, a previously stable personality, and the particular constellation of symptoms.

The patient was started on drug therapy, but problems developed. Tofranil was begun at 150 milligrams per day and gradually increased to the maximum dosage. But the effect on the depression was limited, and the patient developed troublesome side effects (including rapid heartbeat, nausea, and diarrhea). When the daily dosage was reduced, the limited therapeutic impact of the drug declined along with the side effects. Navane was added to the regimen to increase its effectiveness, but a severe skin allergy developed. In addition, the patient tended not to take his medication on days when the side effects were particularly troublesome. This exacerbated the difficulties in providing effective treatment. After several weeks, it was clear that drug therapy had failed.

Electroconvulsive therapy (ECT) now became the only realistic option. ECT is an effective treatment for most depressions, with several randomized trials showing it to be more effective than drug therapy for severe depressive illness. Practitioners generally begin treatment for depression with drug therapy, but ECT becomes the treatment of choice when other therapy fails and either (a) suicide becomes a real possibility, or (b) the patient risks the loss of employment, important personal relationships, or social standing if remission is not quickly achieved. Typically, depression responds to a course of six to eight electroconvulsive treatments, and there is better than a 70 percent chance of achieving a significant remission.[1] Although ECT does not prevent relapses, therapy can be repeated as the need arises.

The clinical technique involves causing an electrically induced seizure. Although the stimulus for its development was the ancient observation that mentally ill persons often improved after spontaneous seizures, it is not known how ECT works. Electrodes are applied to both temples, and approximately 70 to 130 volts of current are delivered through the electrodes for 0.1 to 0.5 seconds. Before the procedure, the patient is anesthetized with a short-acting intravenous barbiturate. A muscle relaxant is also given to prevent fractures during the convulsion. The seizure lasts for about one minute. The patient regains consciousness after a few minutes but remains in a clouded state for fifteen to thirty minutes. Headache is a frequent complaint after the procedure. Perhaps the most frequent side effect is amnesia for the treatment procedure and, after several treatments, mild loss of memory. The memory deficit usually clears within several weeks after treatment, although some studies suggest that there can be mild but permanent memory damage. The procedure does carry the slight risks of using general anesthesia and muscle relaxants (such as a temporary inability to breathe spontaneously). The frequency of death from the procedure is well below one percent.[2]

The problem in this case was M.J.'s ambivalence toward ECT. Several times he agreed to undergo ECT but then refused before therapy could be undertaken. Twice a series was initiated but stopped on his insistence. (The patient actually received four treatments, with no apparent effect.) Over several weeks in which these futile attempts to complete ECT were occurring, the patient became more reclusive, was refusing to eat, and was exhibiting exacerbated depressive symptoms and bodily complaints. The social situation was also deteriorating. His wife still cared for him, but her ability to cope was almost exhausted. When home on weekends, the patient talked openly about suicide and was extremely difficult to handle. One weekend he insisted on carrying a knife. A fight ensued during which he was slashed by his wife, creating a wound needing several stitches. (She turned herself in to the police but was released after the circumstances were explained.) Meanwhile, M.J.'s son had begun to withdraw, making only infrequent visits to the hospital and his parents' home.

The attending psychiatrist envisioned three options: (1) seek to have the patient declared incompetent to make treatment decisions; (2) threaten him with involuntary commitment to a state hospital unless he accepted ECT; or (3) continue to review the potential benefits and minimal risks of ECT with the patient.

Each option had its difficulties. To begin with, the psychiatrist was not convinced that M.J. *was* incompetent. Several lengthy discussions about ECT with the patient failed to yield clear and recurring reasons why he refused treatment, although he once mentioned a fear that ECT might kill him and that it was causing his eyesight to deteriorate. (There is no association between ECT and impairment of eyesight. However, the procedure carries the very slight risk of mortality associated with anesthesia.) He also had very poor insight into the seriousness of his condition. Although despondent and tearful about his situation, his extreme ambivalence about ECT was unshakable. These factors raised questions about the adequacy of his understanding of the situation. On the other hand, the procedures, benefits, and risks of ECT were explained on several occasions, and M.J. seemed to comprehend the information. This was suggested by his tendency to frequently consent to ECT before later withdrawing.

The psychiatrist thought that the patient might have an unarticulated fear of ECT. This phenomenon is frequent among recipients of ECT. Some psychiatrists ascribe this fear to the bad press that "shock treatment" has received in popular literature and movies. Another explanation is that the fear derives from the patient's unpleasant experience of waking up after ECT and temporarily not knowing who or where he is. This "loss of identity" is rarely mentioned by patients but would explain why many refuse treatment only after a week or two, when the amnesia for the first treatment is wearing off, the events are being recalled, and their emotional impact is being felt. But it would be difficult to request an incompetency determination based on an unarticulated, hypothesized fear.

Another possibility involved applying pressure to the patient to persist in completing ECT. On a couple of previous occasions, the psychiatrist had mentioned that involuntary commitment might become necessary if the patient continued to deteriorate. M.J. had reacted very negatively and expressed a commitment to avoid this eventuality. If the psychiatrist pointedly threatened to have M.J. committed whenever he refused ECT, it might be possible to complete therapy. But it would be necessary to use this strategy as a constant coercive lever. The psychiatrist was concerned that a power play of this sort might exacerbate the patient's low self-esteem and sense of helplessness and in the short term could be risky. But it might permit resolution of the depression by ECT. Besides, the threat was not idle. State law permits involuntary commitment when a person's mental illness renders him "dangerous" to himself or others. The patient's suicidal ideation and his occasional threatened aggressions placed him in this category.

The other option involved continued negotiation in a noncoercive way. The psychiatrist recognized that this would respect the patient's freedom of choice. It might also preserve the therapeutic alliance with the patient and avoid the negative impact of a coercive strategy on his self-esteem and sense of control. But from a risk/benefit standpoint, this option was much less attractive. Continuing failure to complete the treatment could end with the patient's suicide. Even apart from this outcome, he would continue to suffer severely without a remission of the disease, and his remaining social supports might crumble. There was also an excellent chance of a significant remission if ECT could be completed. These considerations weighed heavily in light of the psychiatrist's belief that the patient would continue to be ambivalent about ECT.

1.2 Treatment Refusal in the Medical Intensive Care Unit

E.P., a thirty-five-year-old man, came to the hospital after experiencing a fifty-pound weight loss over several months as well as night sweats, shortness of breath, and chronic general fatigue. A chest X ray revealed a diffuse disease process in both lungs, and the diagnostic workup confirmed that the patient suffered from tuberculosis. The physician prescribed two antibiotics, isoniazid and ethambutol, which are usually effective in treating tuberculosis of the lung.

E.P. had little formal education and was functionally illiterate. Until his illness, he was a migrant farm worker. He was socially isolated, being unmarried and having few, if any, friends. His only surviving family member, a brother, was killed in an auto accident while driving to the hospital to visit E.P. The patient had not taken care of his health, having been both a moderately heavy drinker (eight to ten cans of beer per day) and a heavy cigarette smoker (two packs per day) for a number of years.

About eight weeks after the start of therapy, serious complications developed. The patient began to suffer from loss of appetite, nausea, vomiting, and recurrent fevers. Diagnostic evaluation determined that these symptoms were partly the result of an inflamed liver, a serious side effect sometimes caused by isoniazid (more frequently in heavy drinkers). The drug was stopped to avoid lethal liver damage, and a new regimen of rifampin, streptomycin, and capreomycin was initiated. E.P. also had peritonitis (an infection of the membranous lining of the abdominal wall), as well as infective microorganisms in his bloodstream. Additional drug therapy with vancomycin, amycacin, and metronidazole was initiated to resolve these infections. However, a few days later, E.P. experienced severe shortness of breath and rapid heartbeat. A chest X ray revealed fluid congestion in his lungs. When his condition quickly deteriorated, he was trans-

Paternalism in the Therapeutic Relationship 7

ferred to the medical intensive care unit (MICU) and placed on an artificial respirator.

A diagnosis of congestive heart failure was made, and the condition was treated in the MICU with the drugs digitalis and lasix. Within one week, E.P. was weaned from the respirator and returned to the general medical floor. But three weeks later he returned to the MICU, again requiring ventilatory support to deal with the fluid in his lungs.

The second episode in the MICU proved more lengthy. Troubles persisted in relieving the congestive heart failure and weaning the patient from the respirator. Repeated infections plagued his progress. After three weeks in the unit, E.P.'s behavior began to change markedly. On several occasions, he refused medications or pulled out his intravenous line. When able to eat, he usually refused. When asked questions or given encouragement, he was typically unresponsive. On one occasion when he had improved enough to be off the respirator, an attendant in the unit tried to encourage him. But he responded, "What do I have to live for? I have no home, no family, no job."

At this point malnutrition was becoming a serious, perhaps life-threatening problem. The medical staff decided that treatment could be facilitated by use of a Hickman-Broviac catheter. The catheter would be inserted through the chest wall into the right cephalic vein, which requires a minor surgical procedure. It would provide "permanent" access to the patient's bloodstream through which complete nutrition could be administered in liquid form (parenteral hyperalimentation). It would also provide an access route for taking blood samples and for administering medications. Thus, not only would the catheter provide a way to improve E.P.'s nutritional status, but it would also increase his comfort by eliminating the need for constant venipunctures to administer drugs or to remove blood samples. However, the Hickman-Broviac device is not without problems. Studies suggest that approximately 10 percent of patients develop blood clots in the catheter or in nearby blood vessels. This difficulty can usually be resolved by administering clot-dissolving drugs. Development of catheter-related infections is another problem, which studies indicate may occur in 13 to 42 percent of patients. This problem can also be effectively handled using antibiotics or other drugs.

The attending physician sought the patient's consent for insertion of the catheter. At the time, E.P. was on the artificial respirator and unable to talk. The physician discussed how the line is inserted and explained how its use could benefit him. After each portion of his explanation, he asked whether E.P. understood what he was being told. But each question was answered by either a shrug or a blank stare. At the end of his explanation, when the physician asked if E.P. would consent, he shook his head no in an animated fashion. Further discussion ensued. When the physician asked E.P. if he wanted to die, he again shook his head. However, when he asked if E.P. was willing to undergo treatment needed to stay alive, he only shrugged. Despite assurance that the line would make treatment easier for him, E.P.'s refusal remained firm.

At their daily patient care conference, the medical team discussed E.P.'s competency to refuse insertion of the catheter. First, there were some doubts about whether he understood the procedure and its purposes. Because he was illiterate, it was not possible to provide E.P. with a written explanation. Effective conversation was ruled out by the respirator. His general unresponsiveness compounded the problem of assessing his understanding, because it was very difficult to distinguish behaviorally between unwillingness to respond to questions and genuine confusion about what was being proposed.

Again, E.P.'s unresponsiveness might also be a result of a reactive depression following the death of his brother and his own recent medical complications. Or it might be the only way E.P. could find to assert control over his situation. Unfortunately, his refusal to answer questions made it impossible for the staff psychiatrist to draw any useful conclusions about whether he was depressed.

A third factor was the ambivalent character of E.P.'s wishes. Although he had refused insertion of the catheter and various other treatments, he had also said that he did not want to die. One staff member noted that although disruptive behavior was increasing, the patient had *not* tried to pull out his respirator tube. Thus, it was not clear that he intended to refuse further medical treatment.

Finally, another staff member expressed concern about the stress that the unit itself might be causing the patient. Lack of sleep from the brightly lighted and busy environment of the MICU room, the sounds and sights of strange equipment, and the constant monitoring of his own situation might be causing a disabling emotional reaction. Perhaps it would be better to proceed with aggressive therapy until the patient returned to the general ward. At that point, it might be easier to assess the validity of his refusal.

The attending physician viewed the refusal with great concern. From a medical standpoint, E.P.'s situation was critical but not hopeless. The damage to his liver had apparently been contained. The congestive heart failure would necessitate permanent use of medications but could be controlled. Cultures for active tuberculosis had become negative, indicating that his disease was in remission. Although the extent of lung damage suggested that E.P. would be permanently disabled and might be unable to work, the lesions were not incompatible with life. A difficult challenge was to prevent and treat opportunistic infections attacking the patient in his weakened condition. But the attending physician believed that if E.P.'s malnutrition was relieved, these other problems would become easier to resolve.

If the patient were judged incompetent and the Hickman line inserted over his objection, then the staff would face additional problems. One was the risk that E.P. might pull apart the Hickman line, causing serious bleeding from the tube inserted into his cephalic vein. This risk brought up the issue of restraints. Arm restraints or sedative medications could reduce the likelihood of the patient pulling out his lines or otherwise disrupting treatment. However, this approach represented a substantial and perhaps long-lasting coercive intervention.

The physician delayed his decision in order to further assess the patient's refusal. Another attempt was made to investigate the patient's understanding of the proposal and his current emotional state. But E.P. simply ignored the physician. Indeed, over the next forty-eight hours his behavior became more disruptive and combative. He refused all medications and tried to swing at nurses when they approached him.

1.3 An Uncooperative Leukemia Patient

The patient was an eighteen-year-old male in a locked ward undergoing a psychiatric evaluation of his competence to refuse treatment. He had been convicted twice of criminal offenses, once for burglary and assault and more recently for attempted rape. He had a ninth-grade education and a history of frequent fights and drug use. After his last conviction he had undergone psychiatric evaluation to determine his suitability for a special rehabilitation program for rape offenders. The conclusion was that he lacked sufficient motivation and that he was borderline mentally retarded. He was subsequently sentenced to a juvenile detention center.

At the detention center he was sniffing cobbler's glue and collapsed. The infirmary physician discovered that he was anemic and that his lymph nodes were enlarged and firm. These findings suggested that there was another medical problem, so the patient was taken to a hospital for a more thorough workup. Although the patient was somewhat uncooperative, additional tests were performed, including a bone marrow biopsy, because leukemia was suspected. In that test some bone marrow was removed and examined under a microscope. Cancer cells were visible, and a diagnosis of acute myelomonoblastic leukemia was established.

The remainder of his sentence (two months) was commuted so that he could return home to receive treatment at a regional medical center. After being admitted to the hospital, the young man was again a "difficult" patient. Not only was his behavior toward the staff obnoxious, but he would consent to procedures necessary to treat his leukemia until they were about to be performed, and then he would refuse them. This difficulty caused him to be discharged, but he soon returned to the hospital because of an abscess on his left upper arm which he said was caused by an injection he had received at the hospital near the detention center. The abscess was treated by an incision and drainage. Treatment of the abscess also required a ten-day course of antibiotics, but the patient continued to be uncooperative. He violently pulled out his intravenous line, and his abusive behavior toward the nurses frightened them.

A psychiatric commitment was instituted under a state law permitting temporary commitment to evaluate whether a person is a danger to self or others. The patient agreed to take antibiotic pills while the psychiatric assessment was being conducted. The psychiatrist was asked by the oncologist to also address the question of whether the patient was competent to consent to treatment of his leukemia.

Acute myelomonoblastic leukemia is a cancer of white blood cells characterized by rapid proliferation of granulocytes, one type of white blood cells. The cancerous cells are abnormal in structure and do not properly perform the function of protecting against infection. As the disease progresses, an overaccumulation of abnormal cells occurs throughout the body, interfering with the function of various organs. Treatment consists of several components, the first of which aims at inducing remission within four weeks by chemotherapy. Remission consists of the disappearance of leukemic cells and the regeneration of normal cells in the bone marrow. The drugs most often used include cytosine arabinoside, daunomycin, 6-thioguanine, and prednisone. If remission is achieved, then continuation chemotherapy using other drugs is begun in an attempt to prevent relapse.

There is no cure for acute myelomonoblastic leukemia. Without treatment, death may occur within days or weeks. With drug treatment, remission occurs in approximately two-thirds of cases. Even if remission is achieved, the average survival time after the disease is discovered is about one year, although some patients may live two years or longer.

There are serious risks and discomforts associated with treatment. Approximately 25 percent of patients die during the initial phase of chemotherapy. The major cause is infection resulting from a reduced number of normal white blood cells, a side effect of the drugs. Some deaths follow bleeding caused by a reduced number of platelets[3] in the blood, another side effect. Additional side effects can occur, including nausea, vomiting, mouth ulcers, heart damage, and hypertension. Numerous tests involving some discomfort would be needed to monitor the patient's condition, including blood samples, bone marrow aspirations, and lumbar punctures to obtain samples of cerebrospinal fluid.

During the psychiatric evaluations, the patient was relatively cooperative. Discussion with the psychiatrist revealed that the patient knew he had leukemia and that he needed treatment. He was found to have an IQ of 79, which is borderline dull-normal but not low enough to be classified as mentally retarded.[4] He was also considered to have normal contact with reality. In the psychiatrist's view, the patient had the mental capacity to understand his medical situation and the proposed treatment. However, the patient would not explain why he was refusing treatment, and the psychiatrist reported that it was impossible to reason with him. The patient was also considered to have an antisocial personality. Based on his previous aggressive behavior and impulsiveness, he was considered potentially a danger to others. However, the psychiatrist did not consider long-term commitment on this basis appropriate, because the patient's antisocial behavior was not caused by a treatable psychiatric pathology.

Several options were possible, including (1) to release the patient; (2) to seek to have his mother appointed legal guardian for the purpose of consenting to treatment and then proceed with treatment, forcibly if necessary; (3) to continue the involuntary commitment in an effort to determine why the patient is refusing treatment; or (4) to release the patient and continue efforts to persuade him to accept treatment.

Various considerations were relevant in deciding what to do. One was the autonomy of the patient. If he were indeed competent to make his own decisions, then respect for his autonomy would favor options such as 1 or 4. However, one issue in this context concerns what criterion of competence should be used. One view is that a standard definition used in legal determinations of competence is the appropriate one. According to this definition, persons are competent if they are capable of understanding the nature and consequences of the proposed medical procedures. In the psychiatrist's view, the patient would be considered competent according to this criterion.

Another view is that the criteria of competence should vary, depending on the patient's decision and the balance of risks and benefits of the proposed treatment. According to this view, if a patient refuses treatment that involves high benefit and low risk, then relatively stringent criteria are appropriate in order to ascertain whether the patient has made a considered, informed decision. An example might be a Jehovah's Witness who refuses a lifesaving blood transfusion. One might require, rather than the capacity to understand, evidence of actual understanding. One could require evidence that the patient understands not only the medical facts but also the implications his decision has for his life. Furthermore, one might require patients to give reasons showing that they have carefully thought through the pros and cons of treatment. On the other hand, if treatment offers potential benefit but there are substantial risks and the outcome of treatment is relatively uncertain, then criteria that are moderate in degree of stringency are appropriate. Although it may not be necessary for patients to defend their decisions in an articulate manner, one might require evidence that they understand the medical aspects of the various options and the consequences of treatment decisions for their lives. This approach to competence represents, in effect, an attempt to balance respect for autonomy and concern for the patient's well-being. The more patients' decisions appear contrary to their objective well-being, the greater the evidence required that patients are making informed, considered decisions.

According to the latter approach, in the case at hand, the stringency of the criteria of competence to be used would be decided by weighing the risks and benefits of the proposed chemotherapy. Several considerations would enter into this assessment. On one hand, treatment might provide the patient an added year of life, perhaps two years. On the other hand, the treatment involved significant discomforts such as nausea, vomiting, and susceptibility to infection, which could adversely affect the patient's quality of life. Moreover, there was a significant risk of death from the treatment itself. It was possible that these discomforts or risks would materialize and that the treatment would not be effective in extending life. In that event, treatment might be contrary to the patient's best interests. It could be argued, however, that the discomforts would be transient and, in all likelihood, outweighed by the extension of life, so that treatment would promote the patient's well-being. Thus, judging the competence of the patient involved difficult decisions concerning selection of criteria of competence applicable to the particular case.

Another issue concerned how far health professionals should go in trying to promote the well-being of an uncooperative patient. Attempts to treat the patient against his will or, if he were released, to keep in touch with him and try to persuade him to seek treatment would probably involve considerable effort. If the patient was considered competent, then with regard to option 4 it could be argued that there is no obligation to expend great effort in trying to maintain ongoing contact. If the patient seemed to be incompetent, on the other hand, it could be argued that there is an obligation to try to promote the patient's well-being, perhaps by pursuing options 2 or 3.

1.4 Rehabilitation of a Dependent Patient

L.R., a seventy-year-old woman, was admitted to the rehabilitation center to gain improved facility in walking and self-care. In recent years, she had suffered from numerous medical problems. Fifteen years ago she was diagnosed as having adult-onset diabetes, which had been well controlled with a rigid diet. Six years ago she had a serious heart attack and underwent coronary bypass surgery. Within the last year, she had suffered from blocked arteries in her left leg and underwent a graft procedure in which a vein was inserted to circumvent the blocked artery. After the surgery, she had substantial edema in her lower left leg, which compressed the peroneal nerve. Although the pressure was surgically relieved, the damage to the nerve was permanent. As a result, her left foot did not lift properly when she attempted to walk, and she needed a leg brace and a walker to get around.

She recently had several episodes in which she became too weak to return to her bed after going into the bathroom. During these incidents, L.R. had no pain, dizziness, loss of consciousness, or heart palpitations. Rather, her inability to walk farther seemed to involve decreased strength and balance. After a general diagnostic evaluation for new disease proved negative, she was admitted for physical therapy to improve her strength and balance while walking.

Her daughter reported that L.R. had rapidly declined during the past eighteen months. She had become progressively less active and ambulatory. She spent most of her time in bed, only walking back and forth to the bathroom. L.R.'s husband, who was seventy-six years old and in good health, bathed her and assisted her in dressing. In addition, he did all the shopping, housework, and cooking. He said that those responsibilities were very tiring, and he wished that his wife could assist with the cooking and cleaning. L.R.'s daughter, who lived out of town, claimed that her mother was able to get around and help with household chores but expected her husband to do all the work. She also said that her father seemed all too willing to submit to her mother's persistent demands.

L.R. was assessed by the occupational and physical therapists. The occupational therapist determined that she was still sufficiently dexterous and ambulatory to work in the kitchen and perform other simple household tasks. The physical therapist found that her leg strength had declined through lack of use and that the previous nerve damage caused her left foot to drop and drag when she lifted it while walking. But it was clear after a few therapy sessions, as her strength improved, that she was able to get around quite effectively using her walker when she gave deliberate attention to the placement of her left foot. The most salient feature of both assessments concerned L.R.'s attitude. She was unwilling to take any initiative in performing the occupational tasks or walking exercises. She repeatedly said that she was unable to perform tasks that she would later complete satisfactorily. It usually required two or three requests from the therapists before she would begin each activity. L.R. also constantly complained about being too tired and sore to continue the sessions.

The attending physician found no physical basis for L.R.'s self-perceived inability to undertake various activities or for her discomfort. In addition, there were no clinical signs of reactive depression, such as melancholy, loss of appetite, or sleep disturbance. The patient simply seemed satisfied to be entirely dependent on her husband in dealing with her personal needs.

Tensions were rising in the family. The daughter had investigated several nursing homes and made tentative arrangements for her mother's entry following discharge from the hospital. She insisted that her father had reached the limit of his ability to care for her mother. In discussions with the staff, he had not expressed any definitive opinion about the nursing home option and seemed willing to let his daughter make the final decision. But L.R. had said on three separate occasions that she was looking forward to returning home.

The situation placed the attending physician in a difficult dilemma. On one hand, L.R. preferred to be dependent on others for the satisfaction of her basic needs. In the hospital, she had tenaciously held to this regressive style of coping and had refused to discuss the matter with staff members. The physician believed she had made a conscious decision to handle her physical problems in this way and would have to live with the consequences. In addition, interference with her habitual dependence would undoubtedly cause anxiety and annoyance for the patient. It might also undermine their therapeutic rapport, inclining the patient to avoid contact with the attending physician when future medical problems arose. If the physician accepted this reasoning, it would now be time to discharge the patient. He should explain to the family and the patient what she was capable of doing but should leave it up to them to determine what would be done following discharge.

On the other hand, there are good reasons for a more active stance. The patient's well-being would probably not be served by entry into a nursing home as long as she remained physically capable of living independently. If she were placed in a nursing home, the physician feared that her decline into permanent physical incapacitation would be much more rapid. Moreover, she clearly would rather remain at home with her husband. If the physician did not intervene, she probably would be pressured to accept the nursing home option. Unfortunately, she refused to recognize that her desire to remain dependent on her husband conflicted with her desire to remain at home. In light of these considerations, it may be appropriate to keep her in the hospital and aggressively address her attitudinal problems. This would involve pointed discussions with her about her need to assume responsibility for self-care and housework if she wishes to avoid exhausting her husband and being sent to a nursing home. A similar aggressive stance could be taken by the therapists in their sessions with her. At the same time, attempts could be made to alter the behavior of the family. Discussions with L.R.'s husband might emphasize the importance of refusing to do things she is able to do for herself. In conversations with the daughter and the husband, the physician might also strongly insist that it would be inappropriate to place L.R. in a nursing home.

But the physician knew that this approach would create considerable friction. The patient may angrily resist any attempt to change her dependence. After all, her needs were being met and her responsibilities minimized, and she could easily manipulate her husband to provide assistance. Given her behavior in previous therapy sessions, it would require a good deal of pressure to goad the patient into more appropriate behavior. Similar difficulties could be expected in attempting to neutralize the daughter's role in the discharge plans.

1.5 Alternative Approaches to Informed Consent

W.L. was a twenty-two-year-old man who worked as a farm laborer. He was married with one child.

The patient first noticed a swelling on his left hip about fifteen months earlier. It was tender but caused no serious impediment in his daily work. It remained relatively stable in size for ten months. At that time, W.L. began to experience pain in his left leg and some restriction in its use. Soon thereafter he noticed a lump in his abdomen. He consulted a general practitioner in a nearby town and was referred to a cancer center 275 miles from his home.

Diagnostic evaluation established that W.L. suffered from a bone cancer (osteosarcoma) arising in the ridge of the left hip (the iliac crest). The cancer was extended along the pelvic bone and across the middle of the abdomen. Workup for tumor elsewhere in the body (metastases) was negative. Extension of the tumor across the middle of the abdomen and its position around key anatomic structures precluded surgical treatment, such as a hemipelvectomy (removal of half of the pelvis and the adjoining leg). The patient was placed on a chemotherapy regimen of vincristine, cyclophosphamide, and adriamycin, which was a front-line experimental protocol. But within two months there was documented progression of the tumor. With the failure of this regimen, it was no longer realistic to hope that he could be cured. However, alternative chemotherapies might achieve temporary remissions of the disease. The patient was switched to a regimen involving escalating doses of methotrexate, which had shown positive preliminary results in treating osteosarcoma.

At this time, the management of pain was becoming a significant problem. The patient was requiring very high doses of morphine and dilaudid to relieve his pain. These were not sufficient to provide adequate pain control yet often caused him to slip into a clouded state of consciousness. The problem was complicated by the fact that W.L. had not developed lung metastases characteristic of osteosarcoma, even though his disease had been present for at least a year before therapy. This fact, conjoined with clinical observation that the tumor was growing slowly, suggested that he might remain alive for as long as a year. Given this prospect, there was deep concern about the adequacy of the narcotics in providing pain relief. Being in relatively constant and often severe pain, W.L. began to press the staff for more adequate management of his pain.

There were essentially three alternatives for improving control of the severe pain in the patient's hip, abdomen, and left leg. One was to amputate his left leg by performing a hemipelvectomy. This would remove the leg in which intense pain was occurring and reduce the amount of tumor in the abdomen. Substantial pain relief (following postsurgical recovery) could be expected, although pain might recur with further spread of the disease. Some rehabilitation would also be necessary, such as learning to use crutches.

Two other options were outlined by a consulting neurosurgeon. One was to control pain through nerve-block procedures. This would require a series of procedures in which specific nerve roots are exposed to chemicals that impair their ability to conduct pain impulses. The results of each procedure would be used to determine what additional nerve roots might be blocked to achieve additional pain relief. Completion of this process might require several weeks. Although nerve-block procedures carry less than a 10 percent risk of urinary bladder and bowel incontinence, there may be motor weakness in the affected limb. The neurosurgeon thought it unlikely that W.L.'s pain could be completely controlled in this way, but it was reasonable to expect a very substantial reduction in the need for analgesics.

The other neurosurgical approach involved performance of a cordotomy. In this procedure, nerve tracts responsible for pain conduction are surgically severed. The neurosurgeon believed that the procedure would need to be performed at the level of the twelfth thoracic (T12) vertebra. He was virtually certain that it would produce complete pain relief. The patient would also be able to leave the hospital within a few days after the operation. However, there are side effects. Although sensation of touch, vibration, and position are preserved in the denervated area, sensation of temperature is eliminated. More importantly, the neurosurgeon estimated an 80 percent chance that a cordotomy at T12 would cause urinary bladder incontinence and sexual impotence.

An important problem facing W.L.'s physician concerned how he should manage the informed-consent process. On one hand, he recognized that there were significant trade-offs among the treatment options. How the patient might assess these options would depend on his reaction to the specific benefits and problems associated with each treatment. For example, if complete pain relief were his overriding and exclusive concern, the cordotomy would be the obvious choice. By contrast, if he were hesitant to risk the loss of bladder function and impotence and willing to accept an extended hospitalization away from his family, he might choose to have the nerve blocks.

The importance of the patient's preferences in evaluating the options supported an open-ended approach to the consent process. On this model, the physician would lay out, as completely as possible, each procedure and its associated risks and benefits. He would help the patient compare the three alternatives. But he would remain neutral, leaving it up to W.L. to make a final choice.

On the other hand, several factors inclined the physician to be more directive. First, W.L. had shown a clear proclivity toward surgical removal of his tumor. Although the uselessness of surgical resection for curing his disease had been explained before initiation of chemotherapy, he continued to ask frequently about surgery. This persistent interest in surgery appeared to have a couple of components. The patient seemed to view it as a decisive, one-shot approach to the removal of the tumor and the relief of his pain, which did not carry the chronic suffering (nausea, vomiting, etc.) associated with chemotherapy. W.L. also seemed to have difficulty understanding how chemotherapy works. Although he had a commonsense understanding of cutting a tumor out, the idea of "melting" it away with drugs was confusing, and he had little confidence in this mode of treatment. In some preliminary discussions about management of his pain, he seemed to lean toward the hemipelvectomy for these inappropriate reasons, despite its mutilative impact and temporary results for pain control.

A second concern was that W.L.'s preference seemed to vary with the intensity of his pain. On a couple of occasions when his pain was especially severe and had persisted for several hours, W.L. said that a cordotomy would probably be the best step to take. However, on several occasions when he had achieved moderate relief of his pain, he expressed much deeper concern about being rendered impotent and incontinent by the cordotomy. At these times he was also much less inclined to undergo the hemipelvectomy. As a result, he would lean toward a series of nerve blocks. Thus, there was a legitimate worry that the patient's choice might reflect how tolerable his pain was on a given day, rather than being determined by a careful weighing of the risks and benefits of each option.

Third, the physician was very concerned about the patient's needs in the coming months before his death and about W.L.'s ability to genuinely appreciate these needs at the present time. The physician believed that his most serious need would be for relief of his pain. It could be expected to worsen with time. Only the cordotomy would ensure complete pain control without moderate-to-heavy use of analgesics. If performed, it would reduce the physical drain of pain-related suffering and allow him more quality time to share with his family.

The patient's other major need was to be reunited with his family. They had little money, and his wife could not afford to visit him. After nearly three months away from home, he was very lonely. The remaining period before death was quite limited, so spending time back home was quite important. Moreover, the physician felt that the patient's degree of suffering might decline if he could be with his wife, child, and extended family. Again, either alternative to the cordotomy would require an additional hospitalization of several weeks. With the cordotomy, he could return home within a few days.

The physician appreciated the importance of respecting the patient's choice and knew that this treatment decision involved numerous value considerations.

Paternalism in the Therapeutic Relationship

But he was also very concerned about these various impairments of the patient's capacity to make a decision based on his own values and interests. Whereas the former considerations inclined him to leave the decision entirely to the patient, the latter factors prompted him to be very directive and persuasive in recommending the cordotomy. Because W.L. was typically very quiet, cooperative, and deeply respectful of the authority of the nurses and physicians, his doctor felt confident he could be persuaded to undergo the cordotomy.

1.6 Previous Refusal of Treatment by a Presently Comatose Patient

The patient was a fifty-nine-year-old man brought to the emergency room by his wife. He had experienced the onset of frequent headaches approximately five weeks earlier. These had increased in severity during recent days. In addition, he had suffered from mental confusion and left-sided weakness during the two days before hospitalization. At the time of admission, he was very disoriented, hostile, and combative. He also had bilateral papilledema, a swelling of the optic disks frequently caused by increased pressure within the skull. An emergency CT scan showed a large mass near the right lateral ventricle of the brain, with some surrounding edema. Based on the CT scan, it was diagnosed as a high-grade astrocytoma, a highly malignant brain tumor.

The development of a bowel obstruction caused by fecal impaction delayed neurosurgical evaluation. During this period, the patient was treated with a high-dose steroid (Decadron) to relieve the cerebral edema. He became oriented with respect to person, time, and place. However, his behavior remained rather hostile and combative.

Ten days after admission, the neurosurgeon met with the patient. He said that the tumor was probably malignant, although confirmation was only possible after inspection of surgical specimens. Without surgery, the patient was likely to die within six months. With surgery, radiation, and chemotherapy, there was a 10 to 60 percent chance of surviving five or more years with a malignant tumor, depending on the precise makeup (grade) of the tumor. The neurosurgeon also pointed out that the operation carried a 5 to 10 percent risk of mortality or serious disability. But without it, there was no hope for survival. Therefore, he recommended further diagnostic testing (useful in planning the operation) and surgery to remove the tumor. The patient was completely opposed to undergoing both the tests and the surgery.

The patient's mental status was usually impaired during the initial two months of hospitalization. He remained oriented to person, time, and place. But he was often hostile and combative, refusing to answer questions, grabbing at family members, and acting very jumpy when touched. He was frequently restless and would wander about. He engaged in rambling and incoherent conversations about friends, family, and religious convictions. At times, he discussed imaginary business transactions with the staff. He exhibited emotional lability, changing suddenly from states of anxiety and sadness to moods of cheerfulness and elation. Sometimes he claimed not to know why he was hospitalized. These periods were interspersed with briefer periods of more appropriate behavior. The family insisted that the behavioral problems were entirely out of character.

During this time the attending physician also had several conversations with the patient about the need for further diagnostic evaluation and treatment. Although the patient steadfastly refused, he did accept symptomatic treatment for the cerebral edema. After weeks of stalemate and periods in which the patient's behavior was aberrant, the attending physician requested neuropsychological and psychiatric assessments of his competence.

These assessments occurred during a week when the patient's behavior was relatively normal. The psychiatrist found his behavior socially appropriate, and the patient expressed appreciation for the care he had received. He talked sadly about his sister-in-law's long terminal illness after brain surgery and about his desire to avoid such a course. He said that he feared complications of the arteriogram and of surgery. He hoped that God would provide a miracle cure. The psychiatrist's judgment was that the patient had not come to grips with the seriousness of his condition but that he was competent to decide regarding treatment. The neuropsychologist also judged the patient to be competent based on a battery of mental tests but noted some socially inappropriate behaviors.

Following these assessments, the attending physician appealed to the wife and the son to change the patient's mind. After several discussions with them, the patient consented to the arteriogram. He also agreed to enter a research study calling for radiation and chemotherapy followed by neurosurgery. But during his first radiation treatment, the patient told the radiotherapist that he signed the consent form only to obtain the chemotherapy and radiation. He had no intention to permit the surgery.

Within four weeks, radiation therapy had to be stopped because the patient had become nearly comatose. It was assumed that the new neurological problems were again the result of cerebral edema, and intravenous steroid treatment was stepped up. The patient improved somewhat over the next three days, but he had a mild left-sided hemiparesis (paralysis) and could converse only in disjointed statements. Within one week, there was a progression of the neurological symptoms, and he lapsed into a coma.

At this point, a repeat CT scan was performed to determine the status of the tumor. The radiologist reading this scan questioned the diagnostic assessment made earlier. Although the tumor had a very low density on the CT scan similar to an astrocytoma, it lacked pockets of intratumor hemorrhage usually exhibited by this tumor. Its homogeneous appearance led him to suspect a meningioma, usually a benign tumor. This would clearly change the likelihood of survival. Sixty percent of patients with meningioma survive at least ten years, whether or not complete removal of the tumor is achieved at surgery. This contrasts with 10 percent ten-year survival rates for patients with malignant astrocytomas. Although the risks of surgery remained, they would be offset by this much brighter prospect for long-term survival.

The new information placed the attending neurosurgeon in a considerable dilemma. On one hand, he doubted that any improvement in the patient's neurological status would now occur without surgery, and delay would only exacerbate the damage of intracranial pressure. In addition, the only hope for long-term survival hinged on surgical removal of the tumor, whether partial or complete. The patient's wife and son were now deeply upset by the patient's deterioration into a comatose state and were very solicitous about further treatment. The neurosurgeon was confident that they would accept a strong recommendation for surgery. The surgery would confirm the diagnosis, remove as much tumor as possible, and relieve the cerebral pressure. On the other hand, the patient had consistently refused surgery, even though he knew his life was in danger.

There were reasons to question the relevance of his wishes. The circumstances under which treatment was refused had changed. The patient believed he had a malignant tumor. There was now strong evidence that the tumor was benign. If so, the chance of long-term survival was much greater than the patient had assumed when he refused surgery. Moreover, the patient had refused surgery when his condition was less critical. Had he remained competent as his deterioration progressed, perhaps he would have had a change of heart. Finally, cerebral tumors may cause changes in mood and behavior, and the patient's refusal of surgery might be related to these physical effects. Certainly, the increase in intracranial pressure had contributed to his aberrant behavior during the past several weeks.

But some factors made it difficult to attribute the refusal of surgery to the effects of the tumor. Although the use of steroids had at times relieved the patient's mental confusion, his attitude toward surgery remained steadfast. The psychiatrist thought his refusal was based on his sister-in-law's difficult death and his fear of the neurological sequelae of surgery. Even if the probability of survival following surgery was now much brighter, and even though the patient was now much closer to death, he might still refuse surgery.

1.7 A Family's Refusal of Blood Transfusions for a Mother and Her Son

At eleven forty-five on a Saturday evening a mother and her son were brought to the hospital emergency room by ambulance. Their car had been struck head-on by a drunken driver who had entered the expressway on the wrong side. The father and his sister, who had been riding in a car behind the two victims and were not involved in the accident, accompanied the mother and the son to the hospital in the ambulance.

The victims were examined by a medical and a surgical resident in the emergency room. The mother, who was fifty-two years old, showed signs of serious hemorrhagic shock. Her pulse rate was moderately fast (111 beats per minute), and her systolic blood pressure had fallen to 98 mmHg. Her initial hematocrit, a test measuring the percentage of red blood cells in whole blood, was 36. (Although this is within normal limits, the hematocrit may not immediately reflect serious bleeding.) She had heavily labored breathing and cool, moist skin. She gave no response to verbal requests and reacted only to deeply painful stimuli, although she occasionally moved her arms. Physical examination revealed a fracture of the bone in her upper right leg (femur) and a fracture of a bone in her lower left leg (tibia), as well as several serious contusions of the skin and muscles of her legs. A CT scan showed no abnormalities of her skull, but there was a serious hemorrhagic lesion within the left rear portion of her brain. The physical exam and vital signs suggested that she had already lost 25 to 35 percent of her total blood volume.

An intravenous line was placed in each arm and rapid infusion of 2000 ml of lactated Ringer's solution (a bloodstream volume expander used to reduce the effects of hemorrhagic shock) was initiated. She was also given Decadron to relieve the swelling of her brain, and she was placed on a heart monitor. She was intubated with an endotracheal tube and placed on an artificial respirator. Blood typing was begun in preparation for transfusions.

Her sixteen-year-old son also appeared to be in serious shock. His pulse rate was 99 beats per minute, and his systolic blood pressure 108 mmHg. His skin was cool and moist, and he responded only to deeply painful stimuli. He had several contusions on his face. Although his extremities were intact, there were physical signs of blunt trauma to his abdomen. A catheter was inserted into his abdominal cavity (lavage) in order to determine whether internal hemorrhage was occurring. The 128,000 red blood cells noted in the lavage were a clear sign of serious internal bleeding. On admission his lungs were clear. Because he had also lost nearly 25 percent of his total blood volume, rapid intravenous infusion of lactated Ringer's solution was begun, and preparation for transfusions was initiated.

After the initial assessment, the surgical resident went to the waiting area to speak with the father and his sister. He quickly explained that the injuries were very serious and that the first step was to control the effects of the hemorrhagic shock. This would require blood transfusions for both patients. After they were stabilized, surgery would be necessary. At this point, the father's sister stated that they were lifelong, devout Jehovah's Witnesses and that their religious beliefs did not permit blood transfusions. The father, distraught and in tears, said very little. However, he did quietly confirm that they were Jehovah's Witnesses and could not permit transfusions. The surgical resident responded that he did not think that either the mother or the son could survive without transfusions. But the sister adamantly insisted that they must not have them.

Jehovah's Witnesses are fundamentalist New Testament Christians. Their belief regarding transfusions derives from the Acts of the Apostles, chapter 15, verses 28–29, in which Christians are urged to "keep abstaining from things sacrificed to idols and from blood and from things strangled and from fornication." Similar passages in the Old Testament appear to describe only a dietary restriction against eating meat that has not been bled and cooked. However, in Hebrew doctrine, blood is identified with the soul of living things, and respect for life has fundamental importance. Thus, Jehovah's Witnesses view not "eating blood" as an obligation dictated by respect for life. They believe that the importance of this rule is confirmed by its mention in conjunction with other essential Christian obligations, such as the duties not to worship false gods and

Paternalism in the Therapeutic Relationship

to avoid fornication. Because blood transfusions involve nourishment with the blood of other living things, they believe that the biblical injunction against "eating blood" applies to blood transfusions as well as the blood of raw animal meat. Moreover, since the injunction is discussed in the context of other obligations whose violation may result in the loss of one's soul, Jehovah's Witnesses hold that acceptance of blood transfusions will result in eternal damnation.

After initial efforts to stabilize the patients, things began to go badly for both mother and son. Within four hours, the mother's hematocrit had dropped to 24, confirming a massive blood loss. Her blood pressure was falling despite the massive intravenous administration of fluids. Initially, her son responded to the intravenous therapy, and at one point he was able to grunt in response to his name. However, by two A.M. his lungs had developed congestion, and his breathing became rapid and shallow. An endotracheal tube was placed to assist his breathing. At this point it was noted that he had contusions in both lungs, and he soon began to hemorrhage fresh blood from both lungs. His blood pressure also began to fall.

The medical staff knew that time was running out and that the survival of both patients required immediate blood transfusions. The emergency room staff physician and the attending residents had several heated discussions. The staff physician said he had encountered other Jehovah's Witnesses and that they routinely refused transfusions. There was no reason to doubt that the family members were devout Jehovah's Witnesses. Based on this commitment, they could assume that the mother and her son would not permit the transfusions if conscious and able to state their wishes. He wasn't comfortable with allowing them to die but felt they had no choice.

But the surgical resident insisted on giving the blood transfusions. He said that no one, not even a father or husband, has a moral right to refuse lifesaving treatment for a family member. The fact that both patients might recover gave added weight to this point. He also said that the inference regarding what the mother and son would want was mere conjecture. Even if they were devout Jehovah's Witnesses, they had never been close to death and in need of transfusions. Faced with this situation, they might decide contrary to their religious beliefs. He insisted that if they had any doubts about what the patients would want, they should err on the side of life and administer the transfusions.

The medical resident had points of disagreement with both lines of reasoning. She was willing to withhold transfusions for the mother, since she was a lifelong church member and at some point in her life must have seriously considered the implications of her religious belief. Surely she must know members of the congregation who had faced similar decisions, yet she had maintained her religious commitments. But the medical resident was much more uneasy about allowing the death of the boy. How many sixteen-year-olds, she asked, have seriously considered such life-and-death issues? Even if he were regularly involved in church activities, this might be better evidence of an authoritarian family than of his own religious commitments. Besides, many children reject the religious beliefs of their parents upon reaching adulthood. How could they reasonably allow him to die for a religious belief that he might think utterly foolish in four or five years? Parents, she insisted, should never be allowed to make a decision based on their own religious beliefs to permit a child's death—especially since there was a good chance of the boy's full recovery.

The surgical resident spoke again with the father and his sister. They were sitting quietly in the waiting room, holding hands. The father appeared dazed and said little. Despite the resident's intense report of how critical the situation had become, they would not permit the transfusions. Again, it was the sister who firmly stated that their religious beliefs would not allow the transfusions. The father nodded his agreement.

1.8 Deciding Whether to Discharge a Suicidal Patient

The patient was a fifty-six-year-old man who came to the Veterans Administration hospital seeking psychiatric help. At first he was somewhat belligerent and verbally abusive toward the staff. When asked why he had come, he complained of loss of employment and family stresses. It was soon evident that the patient was quite depressed. He revealed that he had been thinking about committing suicide. When asked why, the patient became tearful.

He was admitted voluntarily to the psychiatric unit for treatment of his depression. Further discussions revealed a number of factors that had apparently contributed to his depression. For several years he had suffered from peripheral vascular disease, in which the blood vessels in the legs and arms become narrowed or occluded. This resulted in a diminished supply of oxygen to his extremities, producing serious problems. One was the occurrence of severe pain in the feet whenever he engaged in moderate exercise, such as walking. Another was "dry gangrene," or dead, blackened flesh resulting from loss of circulation. Both of the patient's legs had been amputated because of gangrene. In fact, he had undergone multiple amputations on his legs and fifteen skin grafts during the previous two years. He had been confined to a wheelchair during the past year.

There are several varieties of peripheral vascular disease, and his doctors were not certain concerning the specific diagnosis. It was possible that the patient had Buerger's disease, a disorder of unknown cause in which blood clots block the arteries. On the other hand, he could have had arteriosclerosis obliterans, in which hardening of the arteries and a buildup of fat deposits inside the arteries occlude them. Both are progressive degenerative diseases for which there is no cure. Progression of the patient's disease might be slowed or prevented by eating less fat, increasing exercise, and stopping smoking. Although the last was perhaps the most important, the patient had been unable to stop smoking. Recently he had been experiencing tingling and numbness in his right arm, indicating a loss of circulation. He was also beginning to have kidney problems. The uncertainty concerning his medical prognosis was reflected in the varied opinions he had received. One physician had told him that his arm might not have to be amputated; another said that it probably would need to be amputated within six months to a year. (If the loss of circulation continued to progress, it would probably produce pain in his hands and eventually more gangrene, which is itself painful.) One doctor had informed him that he might live another twenty years or more in his present condition; another had counseled that it was likely he would not survive long.

The patient had also experienced a number of social and family difficulties. He used to be an affluent restaurant manager, but his physical illness forced him to quit his job several years ago, and he had since been unemployed. Because of his illness and financial problems, his wife became depressed and required hospitalization. As a result, she lost her job, for which the patient blamed himself. Their only income now consisted of social security benefits. The patient had five children, including a fifteen-year-old boy with Down's syndrome residing in a private out-of-state institution. The patient wanted to spend more time with his son, but he had been unable to visit the boy since the onset of his own illness. He talked to him on the phone occasionally, but the boy did not seem to understand why his father did not visit. This added to the patient's anguish. He also had an unmarried eighteen-year-old daughter who had recently given birth to a child. She gave the child up for adoption, in opposition to the patient's wishes, and he felt much resentment toward her. Also, he had attempted to persuade a stepson to assume the role of head of the family, believing he himself could no longer function in that role. However, the stepson refused to accept those responsibilities. These various problems caused considerable tension in the family. He said that having to be cared for by others had made him feel a loss of dignity. He also felt guilty about losing his role of leadership in the family.

The patient was preoccupied with suicide. He began to talk about it constantly and said that he had read extensively about it. Although he had only an eighth-grade education, he appeared to be well-read and quiet intelligent. He was a devout Orthodox Jew and had discussed suicide with his rabbi, who emphasized that their religion strictly forbids it. The patient felt guilty at the thought of violating this religious rule.

The patient's psychiatric treatment consisted primarily of psychotherapy. The only drugs he was being given were Aldomet and Dyazide, both to control his high blood pressure. He made a pact with his therapist that he would not try to kill himself in the hospital. In spite of the pact, two weeks after admission the patient attempted to commit suicide by hanging, using a macramé cord tied to the trapeze bar across his hospital bed. An attendant, however, quickly discovered the double amputee suspended above his bed.

After this failed effort, the patient at first denied that he had tried to kill himself. He said it was an "accident." Several days later he acknowledged the attempt and called it a stupid mistake. He said he had failed to consider the emotional suffering his death would bring to his wife and children. He also said that he had not thought about the financial harm this would cause them. He was heavily insured, but his family would get nothing if he committed suicide.

After the suicide attempt the patient became more optimistic about his life. He felt he could contribute to society by working as a volunteer for charitable organizations. (He had previously been a volunteer for United Cerebral Palsy and several other community service organizations.) The psychiatric staff, however, was suspicious of this rapid turnaround in attitude. They feared it might mean he had definitely decided to kill himself. Several were rather pessimistic about his psychiatric prognosis, because of the previous suicide attempt and the physical and social factors that were diminishing his quality of life.

Several days later the patient informed his psychiatrist that he wanted to be discharged. He felt that he was not benefiting from being in the hospital and wanted to go home. The next morning his request was discussed in a staff meeting, and there was considerable disagreement about it. One psychiatrist was strongly opposed to discharging the patient. The risk of suicide, she argued, would be considerably greater outside the hospital. As an inpatient he would be closely observed by the staff, who could intervene in any suicide attempt. She emphasized that the staff members had a professional obligation to prevent harm to their patients. She recommended that, if necessary, the patient be involuntarily committed. A state law authorized such commitment whenever there is reasonable evidence that a person is likely to cause serious harm to himself.

Another psychiatrist argued that the patient's wishes should be respected, since he was mentally competent to decide whether to stay or leave the hospital. To incarcerate him in the hospital would be an unwarranted violation of his liberty. It should not be assumed, he asserted, that suicide is always unreasonable. In this case, the patient had a serious physical illness likely to lead to further debilitation and suffering. The increased debility would only exacerbate his loss of dignity. The illness and its treatment would probably continue to interfere with the patient's ability to resume work and to regain his role in the family. He would continue to be deprived of those activities he cherished most. The quality of his future life might not, according to the patient's own values, be worth the suffering his illness was likely to impose on him. The psychiatrist added that many people would accept suicide if the patient were a terminally ill cancer victim. Why not recognize it as reasonable in this case as well? Furthermore, he stated, there was little that could be done for the patient in the hospital. Previous psychotherapy had failed, and antidepressant drugs were not considered effective in treating depression caused by catastrophic life events. Moreover, psychotherapy had failed before, so it was unlikely to be successful if administered under coercive conditions.

A third psychiatrist supported keeping the patient in the hospital. He believed that the patient was grieving for his losses and might eventually resolve the current emotional crisis. He argued that psychotherapy and occupational therapy might prove effective. Treatment should focus on helping the patient regain control of his life. The staff should reinforce his beliefs about the value of community volunteer work and help him to see that there was still something to live for.

A chaplain who occasionally attended the staff meetings reminded the group that many people, including those of the Jewish faith, believe that life is a gift from God. On this view, whoever takes his own life commits a sin. The chaplain suggested that there is an obligation to prevent people from doing what is wrong.

One of the nurses suggested that attempts be made to persuade the patient to stay in the hospital a while longer. If he insisted on going home, however, she believed he should be permitted to leave.

1.9 A Request for Sex-Reassignment Surgery

Ro was a twenty-eight-year-old woman who visited a gynecologist at the medical college and requested a sex-change operation. She was accompanied by Sharon, an attractive, nicely dressed woman who was also twenty-eight years old. Ro was a large-framed, wide-shouldered 232-pound woman. She was dressed in jeans and a man's sport shirt, and her mannerisms were rather masculine. The couple stated that they were currently living together and had known each other for about ten years. Sharon was asked how she felt about Ro's request. She replied that they had been thinking about it for a long time and she wanted to do what would make Ro happy. The patient was asked about her current life-style, and she said that outside the home she had not tried to pass as a man. On the other hand, she did not own any women's clothes and intended to have her status legally changed to male after the sex-change operation.

Sex-change surgery is considered by some to be an appropriate procedure for transsexuals. One of the main characteristics of transsexualism is a persistent feeling that one is a member of the opposite sex. There is a sense of being a man in a woman's body or a woman in a man's body. According to the *Diagnostic and Statistical Manual of Mental Disorders* (DSM-III), the diagnosis is based on the presence of all of the following criteria: (1) a sense of discomfort and inappropriateness about one's anatomic sex; (2) a wish to be rid of one's own genitals and to live as a member of the opposite sex; (3) disturbance that has been continuous (not limited to periods of stress) for at least two years; (4) absence of physical intersex (a condition in which the body contains tissue of both male and female reproductive organs, as a result of a flaw in embryonic development) or genetic abnormality; and (5) disturbance not caused by another mental disorder, such as schizophrenia.

The gynecologist explained that there was no local physician who performed sex-change surgery. He said that he could give hormone injections and refer her to someone who did the surgery. However, before making any decision, he wanted to obtain more information.

Hormone injections (androgen) would stop Ro's monthly periods and cause the growth of hair in the beard zone of the face, on the chest, and on the body generally. In addition, androgen lowers the voice to a masculine level, causes clitoral growth (to an inch or more), and increases the sex drive. These effects are generally reversible, with the exception of lowered pitch of voice.

Ro agreed to meet with a psychologist, who found her history to be consistent with transsexualism and without signs of any major psychiatric disorders. The patient stated that she had consistently felt like a male for as long as she could remember, even in her preteen years. As a child, her activities were masculine. For example, she played "uncle" with her nieces and nephews. She remembered trying to deny these feelings, thinking that there was something wrong with them, but they persisted.

She was raised in a middle-class family, the youngest of six children. It was an intact home, and she reported a good relationship with both parents. She described her childhood as "terrific," with no traumatic events or significant physical or psychiatric problems. She was a high school graduate, had attended college for three years, and had a stable work history.

She said that her first sexual experience occurred at the age of thirteen and involved kissing another girl and fondling her breasts. At fifteen she had a more intimate experience with another female. Since then, she had engaged in sexual activities with approximately twenty-five females. In her sexual fantasies she was a male. She felt that she was well-adjusted socially and did not find it very difficult to relate to others. She had a poor body image, however, because she felt uncomfortable about her biological gender.

Transsexuals usually have sex partners of the same anatomical sex, yet they often deny that their behavior is homosexual, because their gender identity—their sense of masculinity or femininity—is opposite their biological sex. True homosexuals, on the other hand, are typically satisfied with their anatomical status. The girlfriends and wives of female-to-male transsexuals usually regard themselves, similarly, as heterosexual. The girlfriend is often a woman who has been married, has children, and responds to the patient as if she were a man without a penis rather than a homosexual.

Sharon had, in fact, been married and divorced twice. She had two daughters, ages three and thirteen, who were living with her and the patient. Sharon, Ro, and the older daughter had lived together before Sharon's second marriage. Ro had never been married.

It was explained to Ro that the achievable results in female-to-male sex-reassignment surgery (SRS) leave much to be desired. It is not presently possible to give a female functioning testes or a penis that can attain an erection. To produce an erection, a splint must be inserted. The skin grafts used in constructing the phallus do not allow any sexual sensation; they lack the necessary network of nerves. However, the nerves at the base of the phallus, where it apposes the clitoris, would remain intact and could be stimulated by friction. It is possible to construct the phallus so that the patient can urinate through its end while standing. A scrotum can be simulated by inserting prosthetic testes into the labial skin folds. Although Ro seemed somewhat disappointed upon learning these limitations, she still desired surgery. Other surgical procedures that can be performed include bilateral mastectomy and hysterectomy.

In some cases psychotherapy permits one to avoid the more invasive surgical and hormonal approach. Judgments about its potential effectiveness in a particular case are usually based on a distinction between primary and secondary transsexualism. The primary transsexual is one who has always felt like a member of the opposite sex, even from the earliest times remembered in childhood. Such a girl typically is "tomboyish" and plays male roles in games with other children but, unlike most "tomboys," retains a masculine identity following puberty. Even the earliest sexual desires are directed toward females. The secondary transsexual exhibits transsexual symptoms but does not fit the pattern of the primary transsexual. Such persons, who often have a normal gender identity in childhood, are a diverse group. One example would be a behaviorally masculine female homosexual who, because of family attitudes or social stigma, feels uncomfortable about her sexual behavior. The request to become a man might be based on a desire to achieve a state in which her preferred sexual behavior is more socially acceptable. A psychotherapeutic approach toward such secondary transsexuals, which attempts to resolve the inner conflicts leading to the request for a sex change, has been successful in some cases. However, psychotherapy has proven unsuccessful with adult female-to-male primary transsexuals.

The categories of primary and secondary, however, may not always be accurately diagnosed. One reason is that patients sometimes misrepresent the facts, because they may view psychotherapy as an obstacle to obtaining the desired sex change. Furthermore, the patients frequently know exactly what to tell the physician in order to get their way. The characteristics of primary transsexualism have been discussed in several popular books written for the lay public, and the patient is often familiar with these writings.

Sometimes patients are disappointed with the cosmetic results of the surgery. Occasionally there is postoperative depression or severe anxiety. Patients sometimes regret having SRS and request surgical reversal. In order to avoid such bad outcomes, some physicians advocate careful screening before surgery. Some will perform SRS only for primary transsexuals and require the successful completion of a trial period of one to two years in which the patient receives androgen injections and lives as a man. Others doubt the usefulness of the distinction between primary and secondary and screen only on the basis of the successful completion of a trial period.

The gynecologist had to decide how to respond to Ro's request. The alternatives included the following: (1) refer her to a physician who does the surgery; (2) insist on a trial period of a year or more on androgen injections before referral; (3) insist on an attempt at psychotherapy; or (4) decline to proceed any farther. He thought it would be paternalistic to insist on a trial period involving androgen injections. However, he did not want to refer her unless it seemed likely that surgery was right for her, and a trial period could help ascertain this. He also wondered whether even the less invasive approach of providing hormones would be ethical itself, in light of its irreversible effect on the voice, assuming the patient would agree to it.

In addition, he was concerned about the impact on the two children in the household. He asked the couple whether they had thought about what they would tell the children if Ro started living as a man. They had talked about this and felt that the three-year-old was young enough that there would be no problems in her adjustment. They would discuss their plans with the thirteen-year-old before any medical treatment. Sharon said that the thirteen-year-old was glad to be living with Ro, already regards Ro as a father figure, and would be able to adjust.

There is little information available concerning the impact of being raised by a transsexual. One question is whether the child's own gender identity would be affected. Green studied the gender identity of nine children raised by female-to-male transsexuals and seven raised by male-to-female transsexuals, using measures found in previous research to best predict ultimate sexual identity.[5] These included toy and game preferences, peer-group composition, roles played in fantasy games, and clothing preferences. All were found to be heterosexually oriented.

The physician was also concerned about the patient's own well-being. He had asked Ro what she planned to do for a living if she were to present herself as a man, and she said that she didn't know. She believed that she would be pressured to leave her job in the credit department of a local company. Sharon, however, was not as pessimistic about Ro's losing her job. In addition, Ro had previously been employed in a warehouse doing work typically done by men, and she believed that Ro could probably find other work.

The physician was also aware that surgery does not "cure" transsexualism, nor is it even a treatment, strictly speaking. Some have even claimed that the surgery mutilates the body in order to satisfy the cravings of a disordered mind. Those who defend SRS point out that it often helps reduce suffering and produce peace of mind. Although most patients have a favorable subjective response after SRS, some researchers have claimed that objective measures of well-being, such as job and educational levels and need for psychiatric treatment, show no more long-term improvement following SRS than for patients not selected for SRS.[6] Such results, however, have been disputed.[7] Unfortunately, the current literature leaves many questions unanswered.

1.10 Divulging Information Concerning an Infant's Condition

A twenty-six-year-old woman began to labor prematurely and was taken to a community hospital, where she gave birth to a one-and-one-half-pound girl by vaginal delivery. At birth the infant had low Apgar scores[8] and difficulty breathing because of lung immaturity associated with her premature birth. The obstetrician's initial assessment was that she was too premature to survive. This judgment was based on the infant's small size and the fact that her gestational age, based on the mother's report of her last menstrual period, was estimated to be twenty-one weeks, which is below the age of viability. It was believed that respiratory support would be futile, so it was not provided.[9] After about twenty minutes, the infant was still alive, at which point the obstetrician reconsidered and began to provide respiratory support. Arrangements were made to transport the infant to a regional neonatal intensive care unit (NICU).

At the NICU the infant's medical condition was found to be relatively poor. Her blood pH was much lower than normal, indicating severe oxygen deprivation. Such asphyxia is associated with a relatively high incidence of brain damage, but it was not yet known whether there was brain damage in this case. The infant also required rather high respirator settings—high oxygen concentration

Paternalism in the Therapeutic Relationship

and pressure—in order to maintain an adequate level of oxygen in her blood. A physical examination indicated that the infant's stage of development corresponded to a gestational age of approximately twenty-six weeks, considerably greater than the obstetrician's estimate. Although some infants born at twenty-six weeks gestational age who receive intensive care survive, it was believed that this infant's chance of surviving was very low, based on her poor clinical condition.

The resident caring for the infant discussed her condition with the mother, informing her that the infant's chance of surviving was very small. She told the mother that she did not believe that heroic efforts would be effective in keeping the infant alive. She recommended that the respirator settings controlling oxygen concentration and pressure not be increased. The current settings would be maintained, however, as long as needed. The mother agreed with this approach. (The child's parents were separated, and the father was not available for discussion.)

The mother was very upset about her infant's poor prognosis. Learning that one's newborn is seriously ill produces serious emotional distress. Typical reactions include shock at first hearing the bad news. Sometimes this is followed by anger, with parents asking themselves, "Why did this happen to *me*?" Denial of what is happening is a frequently exhibited psychological mechanism for dealing with the situation. These reactions are sometimes referred to as anticipatory grieving because they are caused by the expectation of a grave loss. Although the ability to deal with the situation varies, depending on the infant's medical course and the individual parent's coping abilities, coping is usually difficult. Emotional support from compassionate and understanding NICU staff can often be helpful to parents. Although it is a difficult process, the mother in this case appeared to be coping fairly well. When the resident saw her the next day, the mother appeared to have accepted the reality of the infant's impending death.

The following day, however, the infant's condition was slightly improved. The fact that there had not been further deterioration of her condition was viewed by the physicians as a hopeful sign, suggesting that this might be one of the few infants of such small size and relatively poor condition who survive. It was decided on rounds that the best interests of the infant called for an increased level of support if it were needed. This decision recognized that there was still considerable uncertainty concerning the infant's outcome.

Once this decision had been made, the resident raised the question of what to tell the mother. One view was that the mother should be told about the slight improvement and the plans to increase the level of support if needed. Several reasons can be given in support of keeping parents informed of their child's condition and the treatment plans. First, information helps provide emotional support to parents during this time of stress. It helps reduce fear and anxiety associated with the unknown. Also, it helps prepare parents to cope with any bad news that may come later. Second, information enables parents to participate in decisions concerning how aggressive to be in treating the neonate. Third, being kept informed enables parents to start making any plans for the future care of the child. Fourth, it is reasonable to think that parents have a right to such information, quite apart from its utility.

Another physician in the group argued that emotional support for the mother could best be provided by not divulging at that time the change in outlook and plans. There was still a high probability that the infant would die. The concern was that telling her would raise her hopes only to have them shattered if the infant died. The mother was adjusting well, and it was argued that her physician should avoid putting her on an "emotional roller coaster."

In support of the latter view, it could be argued that NICU doctors and nurses have a duty to provide emotional support to help parents cope with such difficult situations. This is a role-specific duty arising from the need parents typically have for such support and the ability of NICU staff to provide it. It could be argued that withholding the information in question is necessary in order to fulfill this duty to the mother. This does not imply, however, that the staff should lie to the mother. In the health professional-client relationship there may be morally relevant differences between lying and withholding information which must be considered in any attempt to justify lying. In the absence of such a justification, it can be argued that the information concerning the prognosis and treatment plans should be provided if it is requested.

Another neonatologist challenged the idea that the mother should be informed so that she could participate in treatment decisions. His argument was based on the view that the interests of the infant should always be given priority. He claimed that there is a very limited role for the mother in decisions about treatment, based on two considerations. First, at that time it could not reasonably be concluded that survival would be a fate worse than death for the infant. If she survived, the infant might have normal cognitive and physical abilities; and even if she were handicapped, that would not necessarily mean that survival was worse than death. Second, the potential for survival with handicaps meant that there was a conflict of interest between the infant and the family, since raising an impaired child can involve significant sacrifices as well as disruptions to family life. Because of this conflict, someone other than the mother should make the decisions concerning how aggressively to treat.

Others would claim that it is permissible to allow the interests of the family to take priority if it is reasonable to believe that raising the child would cause serious harm to the family. On this view it would be permissible to withhold treatment, however, only if the family were likely to be seriously harmed. It was too early to determine whether the infant would be impaired if she survived; therefore, it was uncertain that survival would cause harm to the mother and her family. Thus, even on this view a parental decision to withhold lifesaving treatment would be unwarranted at this time.

In opposition to withholding the information, it could be pointed out that it would be paternalistic to do so; the mother's right to information would be violated in order to prevent harm to her. Several reasons can be given against such paternalistic behavior. It is difficult to predict how the mother would respond to the information. Perhaps her hopes would not be unduly raised. One should not violate her right to information unless doing so is clearly necessary to prevent harm. Another consideration is that she might subsequently learn that the information had been withheld. That could undermine her trust in the NICU staff and hamper their ability to provide further emotional support. It could also be argued that condoning paternalism in such cases might encourage more widespread paternalism violative of liberty and freedom of information.

Commentary

Paternalism involves taking action to benefit persons without regard to their wishes.[10] The question of when it is morally justified has been a major focus of discussions of rights and responsibilities in the therapeutic relationship. The prominence of the issue reflects concerns about the excessive use of life-prolonging treatments, demands for expanded personal rights in therapeutic exchanges, and doubts about the sensitivity of physicians to the values and wishes of patients.

The conceptual and clinical focus of the paternalism debate involves situations in which the patient's exercise of autonomous self-direction may be impaired and regard for his or her wishes may result in harm to the patient. Autonomous behavior involves four major components: awareness of a set of values and interests within the framework of which one makes decisions; understanding the facts of the situation that are relevant to protecting or promoting one's values and interests; rational deliberation about these facts in order to form an appreciation of the impact of various options (e.g., treatment options) on one's values and interests; and undertaking action based on the results of such deliberation about one's own values and interests. Autonomous behavior can be impaired in various ways. Persons may lack a stable and clear conception of their own values and interests, such as a patient who has recently suffered a permanent disability. They may suffer from physical problems that limit their understanding or rational assessment of important information, such as persons with senile dementia. Emotional factors, such as serious depression or denial, may also impair the ability to retain information and deliberate rationally about it. Finally, undue influence of other persons may cause individuals to make decisions that do not reflect their own values and interests.[11]

The cases in this chapter explore three types of situations representing differences in the patient's degree of decision-making impairment. In some situations, it is questionable whether patients possess minimal decision-making capacity— that is, competence—as illustrated in cases 1.1 through 1.3. In other circumstances, represented in cases 1.4 through 1.7, patients are competent but suffer from more limited decision-making impairments. Finally, there are cases in which it is not clear whether persons are suffering from any decision-making impairments, although in such circumstances impairments are frequently operative. This situation is illustrated in cases 1.8 through 1.10. In each type of case, the focal question is whether the physician should undertake actions to protect the welfare of patients without regard to their wishes.

One approach to this issue was captured in the traditional Hippocratic ethic. As reflected in the professional codes of medicine, this view held that the primary obligation of the physician is to protect the patient's well-being. The clear implication was that the patient's wishes should not be respected when doing so negatively affects his or her welfare. Recent scholarly analysis has focused attention on the failure of this ethic to even consider the moral importance of respect for the patient's wishes. This shortcoming undermined its acceptability.

A major alternative to the Hippocratic ethic has emerged within the framework of liberal moral theory. This approach assigns the obligation to respect the capacity of persons for autonomous behavior a greater weight than the duty to protect and enhance their well-being. Efforts to benefit persons must be channeled within constraints set by the duty to respect them as decision makers. The only exception to this requirement occurs when persons lack minimal ability to promote their own welfare because of serious encumbrances upon their decision-making capacities. In this instance alone, the duty to respect personal autonomy becomes less stringent, because the rational capacities for whose protection the principle is formulated have waned.[12] Moreover, respect for personal autonomy is so important that paternalistic behavior should be contemplated only when persons may cause substantial harm to themselves. Thus, the core liberal position on paternalism considers it morally justified only when (1) persons suffer from some serious encumbrance in their capacity for autonomous behavior, and (2) failing to act paternalistically may result in substantial net harm to them.[13] We call this the *autonomy-oriented* approach.

This core position formulates necessary conditions for justified paternalism, and there is a variety of views about what further conditions must be satisfied. However, one important implication is that protection of patients from serious harm is never a sufficient reason in itself to justify the failure to respect their autonomy. The preeminent importance of personal autonomy requires that persons with at least minimal decision-making capacity be allowed to deliberate and act on their own choices, even if these decisions are foolish and seriously compromise their well-being. This approach has strayed little from John Stuart Mill's century-old formulation of the harm principle, which restricted interference with the autonomous behavior of competent individuals to situations where their actions may harm others.[14]

But there is also a third approach to the paternalism issue which occupies the conceptual middle ground between the Hippocratic ethic and the autonomy-oriented approach. It requires a genuine balancing of respect for personal autonomy and concern for the welfare of patients. The permissibility of paternalistic behavior does not require that the patient lack minimal capacity for autonomous behavior. Rather, this approach requires that the degree of decision-making adequacy be weighed against the seriousness of the net harm to be prevented. As the degree of decision-making quality declines and the probability and magnitude of the harm to be prevented increases, the justification for paternalism gains strength. Conversely, as the adequacy of autonomous behavior increases and the probability and magnitude of the harm to be avoided declines, the justification for paternalistic intervention wanes. Thus, this approach considers paternalistic behavior to be morally justified only if the seriousness of the harm to be prevented clearly outweighs the quality of the decision making that informs the patient's choice. This approach seeks a balance between the autonomy and needs of persons, and we call it the *holistic* approach. In examining the differences between the autonomy-oriented and holistic approaches, we explore their implications for the types of clinical situations representing differing degrees of impairment in patient decision making. Having examined the implications of both views for clinical decision making, we assess the general theoretical grounds supporting these distinct approaches.

The first area of clinical controversy involves cases in which there are serious questions about whether the patient possesses minimally adequate decision-making capacity, that is, competence. Although the general features of autonomous decision making are clear, clinical determination of whether patients are incompetent raises difficult epistemological and moral issues.[15] The epistemological problem is that evidence supporting a clear judgment of incompetence is frequently not forthcoming. First, patients hold many beliefs regarding treatment options, some of which may be false. Consequently, it is difficult to determine whether they are able to satisfactorily understand their medical situation. For example, in case 1.1, the patient was continually ambivalent about receiving electroconvulsive treatments. On several occasions, the psychiatrist explained in detail the low risk of the treatment, its high rate of effectiveness, and the lack of therapeutic alternatives. The patient seemed to understand the need for ECT. However, on one occasion when he refused ECT, he mentioned the concern that therapy might cause blindness or death. The presence of this belief raised doubts about his ability to adequately appreciate his situation.

Second, patients are often unable or refuse to fully articulate the reasons for their decisions regarding treatment. In case 1.2, a patient on a respirator refused placement of a central venous catheter needed to provide adequate nutrition. Attempts to determine the basis for his refusal through pointed questions were not successful; he made little effort to respond. In case 1.3, a leukemia patient was extremely uncooperative with the medical and nursing staffs, consistent with his history of violent antisocial behavior. The psychiatrist judged that he understood his medical circumstances, but the patient vehemently refused to explain his lack of cooperation. In both cases, it was unclear whether the patient had weighed the advantages and disadvantages of treatment.

A third problem is the possible impact of affective states on the patient's appreciation of the clinical situation. Strong emotional reactions such as fear and depression can cause patients to focus too narrowly on specific features of their situation. In case 1.2, the patient refusing placement of a central venous catheter had previously said that he had nothing to live for. His only sibling had recently died. He had also experienced a difficult and long illness. These problems may have clouded appreciation of the chances for a limited recovery. In case 1.1, the patient was inconsistent in the statement of reasons for refusing ECT. One possible explanation was the unarticulated fear that patients often have regarding this therapy. But again, it was extremely difficult to determine whether this factor seriously limited his recognition that the depression was worsening and that no reasonable therapeutic alternatives remained.

These problems illustrate epistemological difficulties in determining competence. They lead directly to the moral issue of how to deal with "borderline cases." Since the autonomy-oriented view assigns to respect for liberty a general priority over concern for the welfare of persons, it is claimed that we should approach clinical situations with a presumption of competence, which must subsequently be overruled by available evidence.[16] Thus, where there is mixed evidence about the competence of patients, the presumption should hold and paternalistic intervention should be ruled out. Moreover, since the presumption is based on the principle of respect for personal liberty rather than concern for the patient's welfare, the determination of competence must not be influenced by consideration of the harmful consequences of the patient's choice.

But other theorists question the claim that this presumption should hold in all clinical circumstances.[17] Rather, they would adjust its weight to the seriousness of the patient's choice for his or her welfare. If the proposed treatment represents a high-benefit/low-risk proposition for the patient, then the presumption of competence can be overruled by relatively weak evidence of decision-making incapacity. For example, the patient who refused electroconvulsive therapy for his depression (case 1.1) had exhausted other therapeutic alternatives and faced complete incapacitation. But ECT produces effective relief of depressive illness in more than 70 percent of cases with little risk of harm. By contrast, when the risk/benefit ratio of treatment is significantly less favorable, then the presumption of competence should be overruled only by relatively strong evidence. For example, treatment for the patient with acute myelomonoblastic leukemia carried high risk for substantial discomforts and potentially fatal side effects. Moreover, successful treatment would only briefly prolong his life. Thus, the presumption of competence could be more easily overridden by clinical evidence in the former case than in the latter. This holistic approach requires a balancing of the principles of respect for the patient's decision-making capacity and concern for his or her welfare. Unlike the autonomy-oriented approach, it assigns to concern for the welfare of patients a role in determining how physicians ought to act toward patients whose capacity for competent decision making is not clear-cut.

A second area of clinical controversy involves patients who suffer from limited decision-making impairments, even though their wishes are competent expressions of their preferences. In one case, the patient was referred to a geriatric rehabilitation unit to gain improved facility in walking and self-care (case 1.4). She refused to cooperate in her rehabilitation program and seemed inclined to remain highly dependent on her husband for her personal needs. Nevertheless, she wanted to remain living at home. Thus, her physician and therapists faced the issue of whether they should goad her into better conformity with the rehabilitative regimen. In another case, the patient faced a decision about surgery to relieve severe pain from an incurable osteosarcoma of the pelvis (case 1.5). The staff was convinced that a cordotomy would offer the greatest net benefit among therapeutic alternatives, providing complete pain relief and enabling him to spend much of his remaining time at home. The patient's opinion frequently changed, depending on the severity of his pain. The staff was concerned about how to secure consent. On one hand, if they simply presented the options, the patient's choice might not represent a settled view concerning his preferences. On the other hand, they were confident that if they were highly insistent in making a recommendation, the patient would accept the cordotomy.

In each of these cases, the patient's decision-making capacity was above the minimal threshold necessary for the attribution of competence. Nevertheless, these patients exhibited inadequacies in the quality of their decision making that might impair their ability to promote their own welfare. These inadequacies resulted from various physical, cognitive, affective, or social factors, such as intense physical suffering and excessive dependence on others. Finally, in each case paternalistic behavior by the physician might prevent certain harms from befalling the patient.

The autonomy-oriented view involves two claims about these situations. First, because these persons are not incompetent, their wishes should be respected. The elderly rehabilitation patient should be allowed to not participate in her rehabilitation exercises when she declines and should not be forced to talk about the matter. Similarly, the staff should help the osteosarcoma patient to clarify his priorities, rather than urging acceptance of their own treatment preferences. Second, attempts to ameliorate impairments in their capacities as autonomous decision makers should address these patients as rational beings. For example, staff members should carefully explain to the elderly woman the critical importance of conscientiously performing her rehabilitation exercises if she wishes to achieve an optimal recovery. Likewise, the staff should help the osteosarcoma patient to gain a clear understanding of the positive and negative consequences of the alternative approaches that might be used to control his pain. In both cases, interventions involving undue pressure or persuasion should be avoided.

The holistic view involves two major points. The first is that illness unavoidably impairs the ability of competent persons to deliberate about and act on their own values and interests. Without appropriate interventions by health professionals, these impairments frequently result in the failure of patients to achieve adaptive outcomes that comport with their own values and goals.

These impairments in decision making fall into several categories. To begin with, illness may require revisions in the goals and activities that have previously formed the framework for personal decision making. For example, like most persons, the osteosarcoma patient in case 1.5 has not previously thought out his priorities for living with a terminal illness. As a result, there may be considerable confusion and uncertainty. In addition, illness can tax the deliberative capacity of persons. One aspect of this problem is that many patients have very limited knowledge of basic anatomy and physiology, making genuine appreciation of their situation difficult. The osteosarcoma patient had a clear concept of surgical removal of a tumor but found the notion of "melting" the tumor with drugs much more difficult. Another aspect of the deliberative problem is that powerful physical and affective states can prevent a balanced appreciation of the situation. For example, stress experienced by the osteosarcoma patient in dealing with severe bone pain might incline him to choose a "definitive" solution for his pain (e.g., the cordotomy) without carefully considering its negative consequences. Finally, affective and social factors can make it difficult to act on previous decisions reflecting one's values and interests. For example, the patient undergoing rehabilitation expressed the desire to continue living at home, but extreme dependence on her husband resulted in a lack of resolve to complete her rehabilitation. Also, patients undergoing rehabilitation after disabling illnesses (such as strokes) are often inordinately pessimistic about regaining functional capacities.

The second element in the holistic view is the observation that interventions capable of ameliorating these impairments may often require more than appeal to the rational capacities of patients. For example, helping the osteosarcoma patient to deal with his serious ambivalence and limited understanding of his future needs might require being highly directive in discussing options for controlling his pain. Another example is the need of many disabled patients to be pushed and goaded into achieving rehabilitative goals. Patricia Neal's words reflect this point:

> Oh, what a mess I was. I wanted to give up. I was tired. I felt certain I was as good as I would ever be. But Roald, that slave-driving husband of mine, said no. And today, I cannot thank him enough. That is why it is so important for a stroke victim to have someone around who cares enough to force him into doing whatever must be done, regardless of how cruel it may seem at the time. When a person has had a stroke, he doesn't feel like doing anything. . . . [H]ad it been left up to me, I would still be the idiot I was after that terrible ordeal in California.[18]

Similarly, helping the elderly woman to achieve satisfactory rehabilitation might require continuous urging of additional effort on her part, even when she asks not to be bothered.

Based on these considerations, the holistic view requires that the degree of decision-making adequacy exhibited by the patient be weighed against the probability and magnitude of the harm to be prevented in determining the permissibility of paternalistic behavior. For example, the rehabilitation patient may lose the opportunity to remain living at home with her husband and may be forced into a living situation that precipitates further incapacity. Prevention of this harm might be considered more important than acceptance of decision-making behavior that reflects extreme dependency on her husband. If this is correct, then a limited paternalistic intervention (such as discussing the matter with her when she does not want to talk about it) may be morally permissible. By contrast, the osteosarcoma patient faces a choice between options (particularly the nerve-block procedure and the cordotomy) whose net impact on his well-being may not be determinable apart from his own preferences related to the prospect of lengthy hospitalization versus the risk of losing bladder function and sexual potency. Moreover, his ambivalence may reflect the difficulty of the choice. Perhaps the level of harm to be prevented by highly directive counseling does not clearly outweigh the degree of decision-making impairment present. A paternalistic intervention is therefore much less defensible than in the former case.

There is another important species of cases in which the patient's choices are competently made but exhibit some degree of decision-making impairment. This involves patients who are currently incompetent, although their choices regarding treatment can be inferred from previously stated wishes or behaviors assumed to reflect competent choices. As in the previous two cases, the moral rub is evidence of some decision-making impairment, as well as the prospect of serious harm if the patient's choice is accepted. However, unlike the other cases, nothing can currently be done to assess or ameliorate the impairments affecting their choices. For example, in case 1.6, a patient repeatedly refused neurosurgery for a brain tumor thought to be malignant. A consulting psychiatrist believed that the basis of his refusal included a component of denial, as well as a wish to avoid the catastrophic complications experienced by his sister-in-law after another type of brain surgery. Nevertheless, the psychiatrist considered the patient competent to decide regarding treatment. After he became comatose, additional X rays suggested that his tumor might be a benign meningioma, carrying a much better prognosis for long-term survival after surgery. Although his previous refusal of treatment had not been directly tied to his prognosis, the improved chance for survival heightened concern about the adequacy of the decision making that had informed his choice.

In another situation, only the previous behaviors of the patients could be used as the basis for drawing inferences regarding the autonomous character of their choices. A mother and her sixteen-year-old son sustained serious injuries in an automobile accident, and both required immediate blood transfusions to avoid death (case 1.7). Both became unconscious soon after arriving at the hospital. The husband and his sister refused to permit transfusions because the patients were practicing Jehovah's Witnesses. Although the mother had been a Jehovah's Witness for many years, it was uncertain that she would have affirmed the prohibition against blood transfusions in the immediate face of death. The quality of the young man's religious commitment was even less clear; many children withdraw from their family's religious practices as adults. This young man's past behavior might not represent a knowledgeable and settled commitment to the tenets of the Jehovah's Witness faith.

The autonomy-oriented view regarding these situations seems clear. Respect for persons as decision makers has priority unless they suffer from serious decision-making encumbrances, that is, incompetence. Moreover, the previously stated wishes or behaviors of presently incompetent persons should be given the same moral weight if competently formulated. This priority should be maintained even if their choices are contrary to their interests but reflect only limited decision-making impairment. For example, although the tumor patient may not have made an entirely sound analogy between his own circumstances and his sister-in-law's postsurgical course, his wishes should be respected. Similarly, although the mother's previous inexperience with a potentially fatal illness may have limited her appreciation of the gravest consequences of her religious faith, her lifelong commitment should be accepted as a basis for inferring a wish to not receive blood transfusions.

The holistic view would again require a genuine balancing of respect for the patient's autonomy and concern for his or her welfare. The proper course of action would depend on the level of decision-making adequacy and the degree of net harm that observing the patient's wishes will cause. In situations where the decision making of patients may have been impaired and there is a high risk of serious and irreversible harm, it is permissible to violate their wishes. For example, it is very uncertain whether the adolescent Jehovah's Witness patient embraced his religious faith with the knowledge and commitment of a lifelong church member. Moreover, without transfusions he is sure to die. Similarly, the tumor patient's refusal of neurosurgery seemed to reflect denial of the inevitable outcome of nonintervention and a preoccupation with the postsurgical complications endured by his sister-in-law. Yet his current prospects for long-term survival after surgery appeared quite good. Thus, intervening against the wishes of these patients would be morally permissible. On the other hand, where the patient's decision-making impairments are more limited or the dangers less serious, respect for their wishes should take precedence. Thus, if adequate evidence exists that the mother has maintained a lifelong commitment to the Jehovah's Witness faith, her wishes should be respected. Again, this approach yields conclusions different from the autonomy-oriented view.

A final category of controversial cases involves situations in which it is unclear whether competent patients are suffering from some degree of decision-making impairment, and a paternalistic intervention is contemplated which may forestall or prevent any harmful effects. In case 1.8, a severely depressed patient desired to leave the hospital. He maintained that the acute crisis had passed and that he was not gaining anything from remaining in the hospital. Staff members did not doubt his competence, but some believed that he was still at high risk for another suicide attempt and could profit from close observation and further psychotherapy. In case 1.9, a woman requested performance of sex-reassignment surgery after years of persistent desire to be a man. The physician believed that she should initially receive androgen injections for one year. These injections cause a reversible masculinization, allowing experience of secondary male sexual characteristics such as growth of a beard. This trial period might also involve psychotherapy to ensure that the patient did not suffer from a remediable psychological problem. Finally, in case 1.10, a newborn's clinical condition and extreme prematurity suggested that survival was very unlikely. Her mother, although deeply upset, agreed that more aggressive care should not be used if the child's condition deteriorated. The next day the child unexpectedly improved, and more aggressive treatment became appropriate, but staff members disagreed about informing the mother. Some feared that she might be placed on an "emotional roller coaster," subjected to the stress of alternating between hopefulness and grief. With the child's survival still unlikely, it might facilitate the mother's emotional adjustment to forestall further discussions.

In each case, the person's decision-making capacity was above the minimal threshold necessary for the attribution of competence. Nevertheless, each patient might be suffering from an affective impairment—serious depression, stress associated with sexual expression, or the emotional trauma of having a seriously ill newborn. If present, these impairments could compromise the ability of each to pursue his or her own values and interests. Finally, an intervention might be helpful in preventing the harmful effects of these impairments if they were operative.

The popular liberal view regarding these situations derives from John Stuart Mill's famous example of the man about to cross an unsafe bridge, perhaps unaware of the risk.[19] Mill allows that he may be forcibly restrained until he is fully apprised of the condition of the bridge. A temporary paternalistic intervention is morally permitted until it is clear that the competent person does not lack understanding of the possible dangers. However, once this information is provided, the paternalistic intervention must cease. Thus, in the case of the depressed patient, it would be permissible to keep him in the hospital until the need for further observation and psychotherapy is carefully explained to him. Similarly, the request for sex-reassignment surgery may be denied until the patient is properly informed about the usefulness of preliminary androgen therapy and psychotherapy in ensuring a settled desire to proceed with a sex change. Likewise, the new mother might be asked if she wishes to be involved in regular discussions of the child's care, and the possible emotional dangers might be carefully explained. However, if, after being fully informed, competent persons insist that their wishes be respected, it is not permissible to disregard them for paternalistic reasons.[20]

The holistic view requires that the possible extent of decision-making inadequacy be weighed against the seriousness of the net harm that might be prevented by paternalistic intervention. In the case of the depressed patient, there is a serious risk that he may try again to take his own life. Moreover, staff members are very uncertain that he has recovered from his acute emotional crisis. Consequently, it is permissible to keep him in the hospital until it is more certain that his intense depression has passed and that the risk of another suicide attempt has abated. Similarly, the female patient is requesting an extensive surgical procedure, which may result in a substantial net harm if it fails to relieve her emotional suffering. In addition, some patients find after preliminary androgen therapy and psychotherapy that their request for sex-reassignment surgery has been ill advised. On these grounds, it is permissible to require preliminary therapy. Finally, in the last case, the initial interaction with the mother suggested that she was adjusting appropriately to an enormously stressful situation. Moreover, there was a serious risk that discussing the recent changes in the child's condition would cause unrealistic hopefulness about the child's chances for survival and thereby intensify the trauma if the child later deteriorated. As a result, further discussion about changes in the baby's medical care might be appropriately delayed until the probable clinical course became clearer. Thus, although the holistic view also permits temporary paternalistic interventions, these need not be restricted to interventions designed to better inform competent persons of the risks associated with their decisions.

From our review of clinical situations involving various types of impaired decision making, there emerge two radically different positions. One is the autonomy-oriented approach, which requires respect for the wishes of persons unless the presumption of decision-making competence can be overruled by clinical evidence. On this view, respect for persons as autonomous decision makers absolutely constrains actions to benefit them as long as this presumption holds. Concern for their welfare overrides respect for the wishes of patients only when the presumption is clearly refuted.

The holistic view, however, requires a balancing of respect for patients' wishes and concern for their welfare. Paternalistic intervention must be assessed along two dimensions. One is the seriousness of the net harm the patient will incur if the intervention is withheld. The second is the extent of the patient's decision-making impairments. As the seriousness of the harm and extent of decision-making incapacity increases, the justification for a paternalistic intervention gains strength. By contrast, as the seriousness of the harm and decision-making inadequacy decline, the justification for paternalistic behavior wanes. Thus, paternalistic intervention is permissible when the adequacy of the decision making that might be respected is clearly outweighed by the seriousness of the net harm to be prevented.

The traditional Hippocratic ethic proved unacceptable because it ignored the status of persons as autonomous decision makers, and determination of the moral importance of this capacity weighs heavily in assessing the merits of these other approaches to the paternalism issue. Arguments by proponents of the autonomy-oriented view, which assigns preeminent moral weight to personal autonomy, have taken two basic forms, depending on whether personal autonomy is considered valuable in itself or valuable as a means to other human goods. Many recent proponents hold that the capacity to deliberate and act on one's own choices is valuable in its own right. They maintain that this capacity for rational self-direction is the distinctive property of persons, which makes them special objects of moral respect. Paternalistic suppression of this capacity violates the essential characteristic that defines them as persons.[21] As a result, paternalism toward competent persons is never morally permissible.

The problem with this line of argument is that the intuitive weight assigned to respect for personal autonomy is countered—in the context of concrete clinical situations—by the equally respectable intuition that special moral weight must be given to the status of persons as potential bearers of physical and emotional suffering. Persons do have a special capacity for rational self-direction, but they also have a special capacity for pain and suffering (especially emotional suffering) not present in other animal species.[22] Paternalistic intervention involves the recognition of this special property in terms of which persons are special objects of moral concern. Thus, the moral weight assigned to personal autonomy as intrinsically valuable must be balanced by the moral weight of potential suffering, disvaluable in itself, which persons may endure as a result of their choices. From this perspective, the dispute between opposing views regarding paternalism appears to be a standoff.

However, other liberal philosophers, such as John Stuart Mill, defend the moral priority of personal autonomy based on its status as a means to other human goods. These goods have been variously identified as individuality, happiness, or personal growth. Once the status of personal autonomy as a means to other human goods is accepted as the basis for the liberal argument against paternalism, its proponents must show that respect for the choices of competent persons is always the most effective means for ensuring that they maximize the realization of other human goods. In defending this proposition, they appeal to two descriptive claims about human behavior. First, they claim that persons themselves are best able to identify and realize these other human goods. One reason is that the concrete content of such ends as individuality, happiness, or personal growth depends on the special character, desires, and social circumstances of individual persons, and they are in the best position to understand their own unique characteristics. Another reason is that the very opportunity to choose and experiment allows persons to refine their values and interests more effectively than when their choices are disregarded or regulated by others. Second, proponents of the autonomy-oriented view maintain that interference by other individuals in the affairs of competent persons is likely to result in a net detriment in their ability to pursue their plans. In part, this is because other individuals have less interest than persons themselves in matters pertaining to their own welfare. Moreover, the interference of others must, as Mill asserts, "be grounded on general presumptions; which may be altogether wrong, and even if right, are as likely as not to be misapplied to individual cases."[23] If these descriptive claims about human behavior are correct, then the capacity for intelligent self-direction should be afforded maximum protection in social relationships.

The crucial question is whether these generalizations apply in all circumstances of therapeutic interaction involving competent persons who are ill. The first descriptive claim holds that patients themselves are in the best position to maximally utilize their capacity to deliberate about and implement their life plans. However, the impairments that illness generates for patient decision making raise doubts about the accuracy of this assumption. The disabilities of illness may require drastic revision in life plans, creating confusion and uncertainty. The limited medical knowledge of patients and affective reactions to illness may limit their deliberative capacity. Affective and social factors may also weaken resolve to act on their cherished values and interests. Moreover, these impairments often operate in situations where the choices of patients may have serious and irreversible consequences for their own welfare which preclude the potential role of their decisions as "learning experiences."

Even if the first assumption underlying the autonomy-oriented view is suspect, the prohibition against paternalism toward competent adults retains its attractiveness if other persons are less likely than patients themselves to ensure realization of their life plans in the context of illness. Defenders of the autonomy-oriented view maintain that the net impact of intervention by other persons is to decrease the likelihood that patients will achieve the other human goods to which personal freedom is a means. One factor they emphasize is the increasingly impersonal nature of medical care which undermines the formation of ongoing therapeutic relationships. The continuing fragmentation of care caused by specialization, as well as the development of group practices (such as health maintenance organizations) requiring contact with numerous primary-care physicians, are examples of factors that decrease personalized care. Some commentators maintain that these trends in medical practice require that all decision-making power be relegated to the individual patient. If physicians do not know their patients, they can hardly be expected to sensitively balance their needs and wishes in making decisions about their care.[24]

Another factor is the increasingly technical character of medical training. The explosion of medical knowledge has crowded the medical curriculum with an extensive smorgasbord of scientific facts and technical procedures. Admissions standards and board examinations focus heavily on the scientific acumen of candidates. As a result, humanistic and social science subject matter is pushed to the periphery of the medical school curriculum, and hard-pressed students are forced to devote their attention to core scientific material. Again, liberal critics charge that if physicians are not trained to deal sensitively with the values, goals, and emotional needs of patients, then decision-making prerogatives of the patient must be zealously guarded.

These factors support the autonomy-oriented view regarding paternalism. But other factors favor the holistic approach. One is the unique existential crisis that illness often precipitates for the patient.[25] Illness frequently impairs the ability of persons to achieve optimal adaptive responses. These cognitive, affective, and social disabilities often cannot be adequately resolved without the sensitive assistance of others. Thus, on this view, the challenge in medical care is not to ensure that patients' wishes are rigidly respected, whatever the quality of the decision making that informs them. Rather, it is to reform the context of medical education and practice in ways that produce caring physicians who are able to sensitively balance the needs and wishes of their patients in morally ambiguous circumstances.

Thus, in large measure, it is the problems and prospects of medicine as a social enterprise that weigh heavily in assessing the attractiveness of alternative views regarding the limits and justified practice of medical paternalism.

Notes

1. In a review of 153 studies, Wechsler and colleagues found that ECT produced remission of depressive illness more frequently than drug therapies. See H. Wechsler

et al., "Research Evaluating Antidepressant Medications on Hospitalized Patients: A Survey of Published Reports during a Five Year Period," *Journal of Nervous and Mental Diseases* 141 (1965): 231–39.
2. For a thorough review of the techniques, results, and side effects of ECT, see Thomas Hurwitz, "Electroconvulsive Therapy: A Review," *Comprehensive Psychiatry* 15 (July–August 1974): 303–14.
3. Platelets are small disk-shaped cells in the blood which have an important role in blood coagulation. When a blood vessel is injured, platelets adhere to the edge of the injury and to each other and form a plug which covers the hole. This is the first stage in the blood-clotting process. Chemical substances in the blood then assist in forming a clot that seals the wound.
4. According to a widely used classification, mild mental retardation corresponds to an IQ between 50 and 70.
5. Richard Green, "Sexual Identity of 37 Children Raised by Homosexual or Transsexual Parents," *American Journal of Psychiatry* 135 (1978): 692–97.
6. Jon Meyer and Donna Reter, "Sex Reassignment: Follow-up," *Archives of General Psychiatry* 36 (1979): 1010–15.
7. Leslie Lothstein, "Sex Reassignment Surgery: Historical, Bioethical, and Theoretical Issues," *American Journal of Psychiatry* 13 (1982): 417–26.
8. The Apgar score is a method of assessing the status of an infant's cardiorespiratory system at birth by scoring the heart rate, degree of respiratory effort, muscle tone, cry response, and skin color. Each item is rated from 0 to 2, the highest possible total score being 10. A total score of 0 to 3 indicates severe distress; 4 to 6 represents moderate problems.
9. Initial respiratory support usually consists of inserting an endotracheal tube through the infant's mouth, attaching it to a squeeze bag and oxygen supply, then squeezing the bag periodically in order to pump oxygen into the infant's lungs.
10. See James F. Childress, *Who Should Decide? Paternalism in Health Care* (New York: Oxford University Press, 1982), pp. 12–13.
11. For a discussion of factors causing reduced autonomy, see Tom Beauchamp and Laurence McCullough, *Medical Ethics: The Moral Responsibilities of Physicians* (Englewood Cliffs, N.J.: Prentice-Hall, 1984), pp. 114–17.
12. The duty becomes "less stringent," rather than lapsing completely, because other duties derived from the principle of respect for persons as decision makers continue to hold. For example, interference with the wishes of the patient should be limited to the minimum level necessary to protect his or her welfare.
13. The term *net harm* refers to the comparison between the harm that will result if the patient's wishes are accepted and the consequences that will follow a paternalistic intervention. In some cases, a paternalistic action might result in a greater harm to the patient than nonintervention.
14. John Stuart Mill, *On Liberty* (Indianapolis: Bobbs-Merrill, 1956), p. 13.
15. It was Jeffrie Murphy who recognized the theoretical importance of "borderline cases." See "Incompetence and Paternalism," in Jeffrie Murphy, *Retribution, Justice and Therapy* (Boston: Reidel, 1979), pp. 165–82.
16. For example, see Childress, *Who Should Decide?* pp. 104–5.
17. Loren Roth, Alan Meisel and Charles Lidz, "Tests of Competency to Consent to Treatment," *American Journal of Psychiatry* 134 (1977): 279–84.
18. This passage is quoted from Miriam Siegler and Humphry Osmond, *Patienthood: The Art of Being a Responsible Patient* (New York: Macmillan, 1979), p. 165.

19. Mill, *On Liberty*, p. 117.
20. Two additional points may forestall misunderstanding of this interpretation of the autonomy-oriented view. First, we are not claiming that it permits paternalistic interventions only for reasons involving cognitive decision-making impairments. This approach permits paternalistic behavior when persons lack minimal decision-making capacity, which may result from cognitive, affective, or social impairments. Rather, the present discussion concerns cases in which persons do possess minimal decision-making capacity, even though they may be suffering from some degree of decision-making impairment. The autonomy-oriented view permits paternalistic behavior in this circumstance only on a temporary basis and only to ensure that persons understand the facts relevant to their choices. This is the point that Mill's example is intended to establish. Second, we are not claiming that the autonomy-oriented view requires the physician to acquiesce in the patient's request for positive assistance (e.g., performance of sex-reassignment surgery). Physicians also have rights to exercise personal autonomy, and they may choose not to assist patients in achieving their goals. However, we maintain that the autonomy-oriented view does not permit failure to acquiesce in the competent patient's wishes for paternalistic reasons.
21. For example, Childress writes that paternalism "is insulting because it treats the patient as a child, that is, as one who has not yet freely and competently, and with adequate information, formed a conception of good and evil, of benefits and harms, or is not able to act on that conception" (*Who Should Decide?* p. 69).
22. Philosophers are given to arguing that the capacity for intelligent self-direction is unique to human persons, whereas the capacity for suffering is a property shared with other animal species. The results of modern zoological investigations simply do not sustain this claim. Higher species of animals show increasingly sophisticated capacities for intelligent self-direction, where the latter is properly operationalized to various forms of behavior (abstraction, memory, self-perception, learning, adherence to social rules, etc.) associated with rationality. Similarly, higher species of animals exhibit increasingly sophisticated capacities for various forms of suffering, especially emotional suffering. Thus, one cannot move from the assertion that the capacity for intelligent self-direction is unique to human persons to the claim that it deserves preeminent moral weight in our social interactions, without allowing a similar argument based on a special capacity for pain and suffering.
23. Mill, *On Liberty*, p. 93.
24. Robert Veatch, "The Physician as Stranger: The Ethics of the Anonymous Patient-Physician Relationship," in Earl Shelp, ed., *The Clinical Encounter* (Boston: Reidel, 1983), pp. 187–207.
25. Edmund Pellegrino, "Toward a Reconstruction of Medical Morality: The Primacy of the Act of Profession and the Fact of Illness," *Journal of Medicine and Philosophy* 4 (1979): 32–56.

2
Duties to Patient and Family

2.1 A Daughter's Insistence on Aggressive Treatment

D.M., a seventy-four-year-old woman, had lived alone in her own home for six years following the death of her husband. The physician first encountered her when she was brought to the clinic by her daughter after several days of a flulike illness. A routine blood-pressure check revealed that she had severe hypertension (207/137 mmHg), and she was admitted to the hospital for diagnostic assessment. Careful evaluation suggested that she had essential hypertension, or hypertension that cannot be ascribed to a determinate organic cause such as kidney disease. Because she had not been to a physician in many years, it was uncertain whether the hypertension was a long-standing problem or a recent development.

D.M.'s past medical history was generally unremarkable, although her daughter reported that she had been a scotch drinker for many years and that her drinking had become somewhat heavier since her husband's death. In the hospital, D.M. was extremely cantankerous and apprehensive, and she complained constantly to the medical and nursing staffs that she did not want to be there. Her daughter, who lived in the same city and often saw her mother, was very concerned about her mother's health. She was highly instrumental in mollifying D.M. sufficiently to allow the diagnostic evaluation to be completed. At the time of discharge, the physician prescribed a regimen of three antihypertensive medications, including chlorothiazide, propanolol, and hydrazaline. He explained that, if not controlled, her hypertension might lead to grave medical consequences, such as heart attack or stroke. He said that she should moderate her use of alcohol and follow a low-sodium diet.

Little progress was made in controlling D.M.'s hypertension. She missed several appointments for clinic checkups and complied poorly with the treatment plan. About three months after the hospitalization, D.M.'s daughter called the physician to report that her mother was taking the antihypertensive medications only occasionally and that she had not altered her drinking habits. The physician asked her to bring her mother to the office.

He spoke with the patient alone for about 40 minutes. He told her that no progress had been made in controlling her hypertension. He reiterated the grave dangers to her health and reemphasized the importance of using the medications. When asked why she did not take the medications, D.M. was characteristically blunt. She said that, although the medications did not bother her, she had never been keen about going to doctors or taking medicines. In fact, she had come to his office only to satisfy her daughter. When told about the medical consequences of noncompliance, she only said that she never wanted to be "hooked up to machines" in the hospital should she become gravely ill. Her physician specifically asked if she would want such care if there were a chance of improving her health. But she replied, "I mean *never*. I've gotten this far without doctors, and I intend to go the rest of the way without them." He carefully noted her wishes in the chart.

About five months later he was called to the emergency room. D.M. had apparently suffered a stroke.[1] She had spoken with her daughter earlier in the morning and said that she had a severe headache and had vomited. Her daughter insisted that they see a doctor as soon as she could get away from work. However, when she arrived at her mother's home about three hours later, she found D.M. slumped on the floor, unresponsive, and "not breathing right." In the emergency room, physical examination revealed that she was paralyzed on the right side of her body. Her eyes were deviated toward the left side of her body, and her pupils were only minimally responsive to light. Stiffness was noted in her neck. She appeared to be comatose, and her breathing was labored. Her systolic blood pressure was 211 mmHg. An emergency CT scan revealed a large lesion, more than 3.5 cm in diameter, on the left side of her brain in the vicinity of the lenticular nucleus. The diagnosis was that she had suffered an extensive cerebral hemorrhage.

After the initial assessment, the physician met with D.M.'s daughter in a private waiting room. The daughter was deeply shaken. The physician explained what had happened and told her that her mother had less than a 10 percent chance of surviving the next several days. He also said that there was little hope for improvement in her mother's neurologic status even if she did survive. He told her that surgery was not effective in such cases and that they could do little more than offer supportive care. Finally, he related the earlier conversation with her mother in which D.M. had insisted that she not be hooked up to any machines, and he expressed his willingness to observe her mother's wishes.

But the daughter was completely opposed to anything other than aggressive treatment. She said that the Lord would choose the time of her mother's death. In the interim, the doctors should do everything possible. She also expressed a deep concern about having delayed in getting to her mother's house that morning. But the physician assured her that bringing her mother to the hospital earlier would not have prevented the hemorrhage or altered the degree of its severity.

By the next morning, the patient's condition had worsened. She was paralyzed and her reflexes seriously disrupted (positive Babinski sign) on both sides of her body. She was deeply comatose, and her pupils were less responsive to light than previously. Her respirations were becoming highly irregular. The physician assumed that swelling from the lesion was beginning to compress the vital function control centers in her brain stem. He ordered respirator support and intravenous Decadron to relieve cerebral swelling.

He spoke again that afternoon with D.M.'s daughter. He explained that hope for her survival had dimmed even further. He again raised the issue of observing her mother's wishes and said that he felt very uncomfortable in ordering ventilatory support. But again the daughter insisted that the matter be left in the Lord's hands. They again discussed the previous day's events, and the daughter required fresh reassurance that she bore no responsibility for what had happened.

The physician was very upset by the situation. On one hand, D.M. had been very explicit about the use of life-prolonging intensive care procedures. Although there might be a remote chance for survival, she had pointedly said "never." Moreover, her behavior had been entirely consistent with this expression of her wishes. She had insisted on being released from the hospital during the initial evaluation, had been generally noncompliant with treatment, and had usually resisted suggestions that she see the doctor. The physician had little doubt that she had made a competent and consistent choice to avoid any contact with physicians.

On the other hand, the physician was also sensitive to the needs of D.M.'s daughter. He believed that she was not yet resigned to her mother's death and perhaps needed more time to accept the probable outcome. Her own emotional needs seemed to require assurance that "everything possible" was being done. Related to this was her apparent guilt regarding the delay in going to her mother's house the morning of her stroke. It appeared that she could not tolerate any further "responsibility" for the death of her mother. The physician feared that if treatment were discontinued, the daughter might suffer serious emotional strain after her mother's death if she continued to misinterpret what had happened.

Of course, he could not assume that the daughter's needs were related to the immediate event of her mother's stroke. The daughter might have long-standing dependency needs or guilt about neglecting her mother which had only been exacerbated by her mother's illness. In that case, it was doubtful that any orchestrating by the physician of the events leading to her mother's death would significantly reduce the mental anguish of the daughter. Since he had not known the family for long, however, it was not possible to make any well-grounded observations about their ongoing relationship.

There were other reasons favoring the continuation of treatment. It might be supposed that D.M.'s wishes would also include acting in a way that served her daughter's well-being. On at least two occasions, she had been willing to accede to her daughter's desire that she seek medical assistance. If D.M. were now competent, she might (grudgingly perhaps) consider the course of action that relieved her daughter's anxieties to be more important than her own reluctance to have any further involvement with doctors. Unfortunately, the physician had not previously discussed this matter with D.M.

It was also true that aggressive therapy was causing D.M. no apparent distress. Since she had become deeply comatose, it was very unlikely that she was having any significant experience of "suffering." As long as she remained comatose, her own well-being would not be compromised by continued aggressive therapy.

The physician was also aware that discontinuation of treatment contrary to the daughter's wishes might have serious legal ramifications. It was conceivable that the daughter might bring criminal charges against him or later sue for damages related to her mother's death. Although he believed his course of action would be upheld, discontinuing treatment would place his own interests in serious jeopardy.

He envisioned several options: (1) drop further discussion of the matter and aggressively treat the patient; (2) continue to discuss with the daughter the reasons for withdrawing life-prolonging treatment; (3) surreptitiously reduce the levels of aggressive support sufficiently to hasten D.M.'s death; (4) insist in a forceful manner that aggressive supportive therapy be discontinued; or (5) seek court permission to have further treatment stopped.

2.2 Parental Refusal of Cancer Treatment on Religious Grounds

At eighteen months of age, K.S. was taken by her mother to a family physician after several days of a flulike illness. The mother reported that the child had been lethargic, irritable, and without much appetite for about ten days. She also said that the infant had frequent diarrhea, a low-grade fever, and episodes of sweating and chills. During his physical examination, the doctor discovered a large mass in the child's liver. He referred the family to a pediatric hospital about fifty miles from their home.

The child spent a week in the hospital and underwent a battery of diagnostic tests, including CT scans, bone scans, X rays, an intravenous pyelogram (an X ray of the kidneys and ureters enhanced by the injection of radiopaque material into the veins that perfuse the area), and various tests on blood and urine specimens. These tests revealed a large tumor in the abdomen, arising from the left adrenal gland. The tumor was extended into the liver and some abdominal lymph nodes. The urine tests detected elevated levels of chemical substances called catecholamines, which certain tumor cells may secrete in large amounts. Based on the patient's age, the location of the primary mass, its pattern of dissemination, and the urine tests, it was concluded that the child suffered from neuroblastoma, a common form of childhood cancer.

The family lived in a small farmhouse about one hour's drive from the medical center. The child's father was a small engine repairman. The mother stayed at home with K.S., their only child. Neither the father nor the mother was a high school graduate. During the week that the diagnostic tests were performed, the parents appeared extremely apprehensive and were very quiet. They were sometimes joined in the waiting room areas by the minister from their church. They belonged to a small fundamentalist religious sect and were very involved in church activities.

On Friday morning, the pediatric oncologist met with the parents. They were very upset by the results of the diagnostic assessment. The oncologist outlined the extent of their child's disease, the likelihood that she would achieve a disease-free outcome, and the features of the experimental treatment program. She explained that in neuroblastoma, prognosis correlates with the extent of disease at diagnosis and the age of the patient. Widespread dissemination of the tumor beyond its site of origin decreases the chance for long-term, disease-free survival. Unfortunately, their child's disease had already spread beyond its original site in the abdomen, affecting both abdominal lymph nodes and the liver. In addition, she said that children with disseminated disease older than one year, as K.S. was, have a much poorer prognosis than children less than one year of age. In one large series of patients with disseminated disease at diagnosis, nearly 40 percent of patients less than one year of age survived disease-free after treatment, compared with only 15 percent older than one year.

She also outlined the difficult treatment process. First, surgery is performed to remove operable tumor in the abdomen and to sample various tissues in the abdominal cavity (through biopsies) to determine the extent of the disease. This is followed by four months of treatment with cancer drugs to eliminate remaining pockets of tumor. At this point, a "second-look" surgery is performed to determine if complete remission has occurred. If no remaining tumor cells are found, then patients receive three months of chemotherapy before the treatment is discontinued.

The oncologist warned that the chemotherapies employed can produce serious side effects. In this study, the drugs employed were cyclophosphamide, adriamycin, and cis-platinum. All three drugs may cause substantial nausea and vomiting for several days during each course of treatment. (In the first four months, patients receive an eight-day course of chemotherapy five times.) The drugs also impair various types of blood cells, increasing the risk of serious life-threatening infections and hemorrhages. Cyclophosphamide frequently causes irritation of the urinary bladder, resulting in bloody and painful urination. Nor are all side effects temporary. For example, cis-platinum causes serious, permanent loss of hearing in some patients, and adriamycin can result in congestive heart failure.

Nevertheless, the oncologist recommended immediate treatment. The parents appeared somewhat dazed and asked very few questions, but they signed the consent form.

But on Monday, the mother called to say that they would not return for treatment. They had been reassured by their minister that their child would be cured by God if they showed faith in his power. The mother said that their interpretation of the Bible required them to rely on the "medicine" of the Lord rather than that of physicians. She and her husband had searched their souls, and they were now sure that God would reward their strong faith. The physician implored the mother to return to the hospital for further discussions, but to no avail. Two conversations with the mother later in the week produced no change in the family's commitment to forgo therapy.

The attending physician and her colleagues considered seeking a court order for treatment. Without therapy, the child would likely die within six months. (Neuroblastoma sometimes matures into ganglioneuroma, a benign tumor that may not be life-threatening. But this is a very rare occurrence.) But several considerations weighed against this course of action. The treatment regimen was long and arduous, and various side effects of therapy were possible. Even with treatment, the child's chances for achieving long-term survival free of disease were quite poor. Thus, considerable suffering would result from the therapy, but the child's life would probably not be saved. Nontreatment would at least not add to the suffering caused by progression of the disease itself.

Another concern was that a close working relationship between physician and family would be unlikely to develop. In the setting of pediatric cancer treatment, parents usually depend heavily on the physician—the one person who can save their child. Moreover, the parents are often isolated from their usual sources of emotional support; they must spend long periods of time at a distant hospital. Thus, staff members must be available to offer sensitive counseling and support during intensive therapy and to help make difficult decisions if treatment begins to fail. A court order for treatment would surely preclude the mutual trust necessary for such close cooperation. To the parents' already considerable suffering would be added the insult of having their child's care taken out of their hands. Yet there was an 85 percent probability that the child would die anyway.

One final factor was discussed among the staff physicians. Some maintained that the status of the facility as a research hospital and the treatment plan as an investigative study were decisive considerations. They suggested that research facilities exist primarily to generate improved medical knowledge. Persons do not have obligations to participate in this work. Families should be no less free than competent adults to decline involvement in experimental treatment programs. In cases such as this, where no "conventional" therapy for the disease yet exists, families should be able to forgo therapy altogether. These staff members favored interventions to provide conventional lifesaving therapies, but they viewed research therapies as falling in a different moral category.

Still, the treatment seemed to offer the child's only chance to survive beyond her second birthday, and a court order seemed to offer the only means of providing it.

2.3 Informed Consent and the Dying Adolescent

L.T. was fifteen years old and one of four children. Her mother was a registered nurse and her father a machine operator in a local factory. She was admitted to the hospital with a two-day history of nausea, vomiting, and persistent abdominal pain. A gastrointestinal X-ray series and a gastroscopy confirmed an obstruction in the initial portion of the small intestine. Exploratory surgery revealed a large tumor which appeared to arise in the pancreas and had penetrated the

Duties to Patient and Family

intestine. The tumor had also spread to regional lymph nodes, the liver, and one kidney. Pathological examination of specimens removed at surgery confirmed the diagnosis of carcinoma of the pancreas.

Within two weeks after surgery, an intensive six-week course of chemotherapy with three drugs was undertaken. After this course, there was a marked regression of the tumor in the pancreas. All other tumor had disappeared entirely. A second six-week cycle of treatment was initiated, but by the end of this course, X-ray and physical examination revealed that the tumor was again growing rapidly and metastases were appearing.

Throughout the early period of treatment, the patient was very interested in how treatment was going. She was also very cooperative through a series of difficult procedures. She often expressed to the nurses a concern about the impact of her illness on her parents and siblings. However, she was also usually very reserved in interchanges with hospital staff members, and she never initiated discussions of her condition. In addition, the patient's mother was very protective of the child and, as the health professional in the family, assumed the decision-making role. At all times, the family, particularly the mother and the patient, appeared to be very close-knit and loving.

After failure of the first regimen of chemotherapy, a different anticancer drug therapy was attempted. However, two weeks later the patient was admitted to the hospital with acute gastrointestinal bleeding. Endoscopic examination (a procedure allowing direct visual inspection of the digestive tract) revealed bleeding in three sites in the initial portion of the small intestine, suggesting that tumor was eroding blood vessels. Over the next three days the gastric bleeding continued, and the patient occasionally vomited large clots of blood. The patient's blood volume was kept stable by daily administration of red cells. Generalized abdominal pain was controlled with a moderate dose of intravenous morphine.

The physician visited the room each day to discuss the patient's condition with the family. These discussions were held at the bedside and were focused on day-to-day changes in her condition. The patient remained awake and alert during this period, but she was always very quiet. She usually closed her eyes during the conversations. She did not ask whether she might soon die, and the issue was not raised with her. On a couple of occasions, the mother expressed a concern outside the room about conducting discussions of her daily condition in the patient's presence. But in private conversations with the nurse-practitioner, the child said that she was aware that she might not become well enough to return home, although she would like to do so. She expressed further concern about her parents. She also said she believed God would make her well again.

One week after hospitalization the patient's prognosis was discussed privately with her mother. The mother inquired about the availability of other chemotherapeutic agents. She was told that no other drugs with established dosages or effectiveness were available for the treatment of pancreatic cancer, although some experimental agents might be tried. It was emphasized that the chance for regression of the tumor was slight, and at best life could be prolonged only briefly. At any rate, chemotherapy could not be administered until the bleeding abated, and the physician said that it would probably not be possible to stop the bleeding. He suggested that it might be appropriate not to send the patient to the intensive care unit should her condition worsen; doing so might subject her to needless discomfort. He also raised the possibility of discontinuing the blood transfusions. However, the mother was unprepared to accept either suggestion, asked that the transfusions be continued at their present rate, and held out the hope that additional chemotherapy might be possible. Finally, the question was raised about involving the patient in the decision-making process. But the mother also firmly resisted this possibility, indicating that she did not wish to intensify the anxiety and suffering of her daughter.

This interchange placed the physician in a considerable quandary. On one hand, he was inclined to respect the wishes of the mother to continue treatment and avoid involvement of the patient in the decision making. The mother had, after all, assumed decision-making responsibilities throughout her daughter's illness. Moreover, even if the mother's desire to continue aggressive treatment was ill advised, he recognized that her well-being and the well-being of her husband would continue to be affected even after their daughter's death by decisions made at this crucial time. Possibly they needed further assurance that everything possible had been done, and failure to provide such assurance might lead to considerable guilt in the grieving period following the child's death. On the other hand, he was concerned not to block the patient's possible contribution; he considered her competent to participate in the decision making. She had been involved in discussions of her therapy and had been particularly interested in developments during the early phase of her treatment. He was confident of her ability to comprehend the information relevant to the decision, and he knew (from the nurse's report) that the patient understood that she might soon die. He did, however, have reservations about her emotional capabilities to handle such decision making, because she had seemed willing to defer to her mother's wishes throughout her treatment. At the same time, securing some understanding of the patient's feelings might help determine whether continued aggressive therapy was enhancing her well-being or intensifying her suffering.

The physician had several options: (1) Accept as final the mother's decisions to continue aggressive treatment and to not involve the daughter. (2) Tentatively accept the mother's decision, but spend the next several days (should the patient survive) attempting to change her mind on both counts—possibly by helping her to accept her daughter's impending death. (3) Accept the mother's wishes not to involve the child in the decision making, but taper off various supportive measures (such as blood transfusions) to hasten the child's death and relieve her of further suffering. Reduction of aggressive efforts would be accomplished without the mother's knowledge. (4) Interview the patient without her mother's knowledge. Sensitively ask her to clarify her feelings about continuing aggressive support measures. This approach would necessitate open acknowledgment and discussion of the likelihood that she would soon die. (5) Interview the patient without her mother's knowledge. However, make an attempt to "feel out" the patient about her desire to discuss the situation. Introduce the specifics of the

Duties to Patient and Family

decision only if the patient "opens up." (6) Wait until the next day, and sensitively introduce the whole issue of further aggressive therapy when the family members are gathered together in the patient's room.

2.4 Treatment Refusal for an Infant with Possible Brain Damage

A three-pound, thirteen-ounce male infant with a gestational age of approximately thirty-three weeks[2] was delivered by emergency cesarean section for placenta previa.[3] The infant apparently had suffered asphyxia as a result of bleeding associated with the placenta previa. Resuscitation with oxygen was necessary, and the infant was transferred to a regional neonatal intensive care unit in another city.

In the ambulance, the infant's condition worsened. His heart rate fell to 40 beats per minute. Epinephrine was given, and in response the heart rate rose to a near-normal level.[4] On arrival at the regional center, the infant was lethargic and cyanotic (having bluish-colored skin), and his blood pH was acidotic, all indicating significant asphyxia. He had difficulty breathing, occasionally gasping, and a diagnosis of hyaline membrane disease was made.[5] An umbilical artery catheter had been inserted to administer fluids and take blood samples, and intravenous water and dextrose (sugar) were being provided. Respirator therapy was begun in an attempt to prevent death from the lung disease. Other life-preserving measures would soon be needed. First, a blood transfusion would be required to correct a low hematocrit[6] possibly caused by bleeding associated with the placenta previa. Second, levels of oxygen and carbon dioxide in the blood would be monitored so that appropriate adjustments could be made to the pressure and oxygen levels of air delivered by the respirator. Third, levels of electrolytes in the blood, such as sodium and potassium, would be monitored so that safe levels could be maintained.

The physician in the NICU contacted the patient's family by telephone. He spoke with the mother and maternal grandmother, describing the infant's condition and explaining what was being done. They replied that they were aware that the baby had suffered a lack of oxygen during labor. Moreover, they stated firmly that they did not want "heroic" efforts carried out to sustain life, such as respirator treatment or blood transfusions. The family was concerned about the child being seriously handicapped if he survived. In response, the physician pointed out that withdrawal of the respirator would almost certainly result in the child's death. However, the mother and grandmother expressed a belief that death would be better than survival with severe handicaps.

In fact, several medical conditions that can cause handicaps were present or foreseeable in this case. First, asphyxia during labor and delivery may have already caused handicaps ranging in severity from relatively mild learning disabilities to extreme mental retardation with an inability to walk or communicate. Second, the child's lung disease might cause continued poor oxygenation, resulting in further brain injury. A particularly worrisome complication would be an intraventricular hemorrhage, caused when cerebral blood vessels weaken as a result of the death of vessel tissue from a lack of oxygen. Such bleeding can deprive brain tissue of oxygen, thereby causing brain damage. Depending on severity, the outcome could be death or handicap in varying degrees. Third, the infant might survive with respiratory support but develop bronchopulmonary dysplasia, a chronic lung disease caused by the respirator therapy which is sometimes severely debilitating.

Clinically, there was considerable uncertainty concerning the outcome of continued aggressive treatment. The survival rate for infants with comparable birth weight was more than 90 percent. When pronounced asphyxia occurs, as in this case, a considerably lower survival rate would be expected. However, it was not clear how much lower it would be. There were similar problems in predicting degree of handicap if survival were to occur. Several published studies had attempted to correlate the clinical condition of asphyxiated newborns with long-term outcome.[7] However, conclusions about this patient could not yet be drawn from those studies because the effects of birth asphyxia are sometimes reversible, and it was too soon after birth to ascertain whether there would be a recovery in this case. Because neonatology is a new and evolving field, often it is not possible to make reliable predictions near the time of birth about survival and degree of handicap.

The physician was concerned that the family might be assuming that handicaps were a certainty if the child survived. He continued the telephone conversation, therefore, by discussing the uncertainties concerning survival and permanent handicap. Although the mother and the grandmother acknowledged his statement that the child might survive and be normal, they seemed to remain quite skeptical. They again stated their opposition to transfusions and respirator treatment. At that point the physician felt the pressure of conflicting ethical demands. On one hand, he recognized that parents ordinarily have the right to give or withhold consent concerning proposed treatments for infants. On the other hand, he believed that there are limits to that right and that parental wishes should sometimes be overridden when contrary to the infant's interests. He wondered whether treatment would be in the infant's best interests in this case. The mother and the grandmother, still on the phone, were waiting for his reply.

The physician's options included the following: (1) Seek a court order authorizing treatment, and continue all life-sustaining measures regardless of the family's wishes. (2) Discontinue respiratory therapy and withhold transfusions, as requested by the family. (3) Continue all life-support measures while pursuing further discussions with the family, providing them information and an opportunity to reconsider their decision. After a period of deliberation by the family, perhaps a couple of days, do what the family wants.

At the time of this case, there were no federal regulations concerning provision of lifesaving treatment to newborns.[8] Thus, the decision would not be constrained by such guidelines. Several other considerations were highly pertinent, however, including the well-being of the infant. In spite of the uncertainty concerning prognosis, it could be argued that the infant's interests would best be served by aggressive treatment, at least in the near term. It was possible that with vigorous treatment the infant would survive to be a normal, healthy child. If, on the other hand, the infant's condition later deteriorated and it became clear that treatment was not beneficial to him, life-sustaining efforts could be withheld at that time. This strategy would give the infant a chance for a normal life while attempting to avoid treatment that inflicted harm. Considerations such as these supported option 1.

Another concern was the potential harms to the family if faced with the task of raising an impaired child. Such harms have been widely documented[9] and occur in part because of inadequate community resources to help families cope with the demands of raising a handicapped child. The harms can include marital disharmony and divorce, as well as behavioral problems of siblings. There can be a serious compromise of careers, education, and other valued activities due to the large commitment of time, energy, and finances sometimes required in the care of a handicapped child. Of course, the degree of harm varies considerably, depending on factors such as parental attitudes toward the disabled child, the degree of support from other family members, and the parents' financial situation. Unfortunately, it was difficult to predict how well this family might cope with the task of raising an impaired child, in part because the physician knew little about the family. It can be argued that the physician has an obligation to avoid causing harm to the family and that pursuing aggressive treatment against the family's wishes can result in a violation of this obligation. These considerations supported option 2.

An additional factor was the ability of the family members to make a well-considered decision. Although the response to news that their baby is seriously ill varies among families, certain reactions are typical. Situations in which their infant might die are usually experienced by parents as a crisis. Grief reactions can arise from the loss of the normal baby that was expected. Such grieving can express itself in various ways. Emotional shock can be followed by anger, denial, or sadness. Parents often become irritable, have difficulty sleeping, and suffer loss of appetite. They may feel a sense of failure or guilt because they did not produce a healthy baby.[10] These reactions can sometimes encumber the ability of parents to assimilate information about the infant's condition and participate in treatment decisions. Some physicians maintain that most parents are incapable of making decisions during this period of crisis. Others believe that support and counseling by health professionals can help parents to actively participate in decisions. Such support would include doctors and nurses repeatedly meeting and discussing the basic facts with family members. This process might take several days or even weeks. The physician wondered whether this family understood the basic facts, including the uncertainty about prognosis. The telephone conversation suggested to him that the mother and the grandmother did not appreciate the extent of uncertainty. Thus, he wondered whether the parents' role as proxy decision makers would truly be respected in following their wishes at that time. The possibility that it would not supported option 3. Since the infant's condition was critical, the physician would soon have to make a decision.

2.5 Venereal Disease and Adolescent Confidentiality

T.S., a thirteen-year-old girl, was brought to the emergency room after four days of fever, abdominal pain, and occasional vomiting. Her seventeen-year-old sister, who cared for her and two other siblings in the evenings when their mother worked, brought her to the hospital after her mother became concerned about T.S.'s continuing illness.

When she was examined by the pediatric resident, her fever was 101.4 degrees. She had tenderness and pain across her entire pelvic region. Because the symptoms suggested an infection of the female organs, the doctor performed a pelvic examination. The exam revealed a purulent vaginal discharge. When the resident palpated her uterine tubes and ovaries, T.S. felt significant discomfort, especially on the right side, and the resident noted some swelling in this area. Movement of her cervix caused pain. The patient also said that she had experienced pain when urinating for several days. A urine culture, urinalysis, and culture of the cervix were performed to identify the organism causing the infection. During the entire examination, T.S. was extremely apprehensive.

The resident told T.S. and her sister that she had a bad infection and would need antibiotic therapy. Privately, he was concerned that she might also have an abscess in the right uterine tube or ovary. Given his impression that the girl's mother was away from home much of the time, he was also concerned about satisfactory compliance with a ten-day course of antibiotic therapy. For these reasons, he decided to admit her to the hospital for intravenous antibiotics. It would take about forty-eight hours for the cervical culture to incubate sufficiently to determine the organism causing the infection.

The following afternoon, the girl's mother came to the hospital. She spoke briefly with the resident, who explained that her daughter had an infection of the female organs and needed intensive antibiotic therapy to prevent serious complications. Although it was likely that T.S. had a sexually transmitted infection, the resident decided not to broach the subject until the culture results were available. The girl's mother did not seem aware of this possibility.

On the second afternoon of her hospitalization, the lab results came back indicating that T.S. had gonorrhea. Afterward, the resident and the attending physician visited with T.S. in her room. They told T.S. that she had an infection caused by sexual contact and explained that the law required them to report such cases to the health department, along with the names of her sexual partners so that they could be notified. T.S. became tearful. She said that she had had sexual relations with only one boy, a sixteen-year-old who attended the same public school. T.S. also said that she did not want her mother to know that she had engaged in sexual relations. The attending physician said that sexual activity is a very serious step, and that perhaps she needed to talk with her mother about it. However, T.S. said that her mother would react angrily if told and would just "hold it against her." She said that her mother was usually not home and that she rarely talked with the children about personal matters. She and her brother and sisters were pretty much on their own. So she just didn't want to talk to her

Duties to Patient and Family

mother about it. In fact, she pleaded with the physicians not to tell her mother. The attending physician said that he wanted to think about it and would talk with her again.

State law regarding treatment of venereal disease in minors did not settle the matter. According to the statute, "any physician may examine, diagnose and treat minors infected with venereal diseases without the knowledge or consent of the parents of the minors and shall incur no civil or criminal liability . . . except for negligence." Nearly all states have similar statutes. Thus, the physician was legally permitted to treat the girl confidentially or to discuss the diagnosis and treatment with the girl's mother.

There were several factors to consider. The attending physician believed that mature adolescents deserve confidential treatment if they desire it. Some health professionals maintain that adolescents who are sexually active and who seek treatment for sex-related problems are, ipso facto, mature enough to deserve confidential treatment. However, the attending physician had mixed feelings about the maturity of this patient. On one hand, she had become sexually active, and, from all appearances, she and her siblings were pretty much left to fend for themselves. On the other hand, her attitudes toward her mother appeared typical of "rebellious" adolescents, and he knew from his conversations with her that she had not taken any contraceptive precautions.

He also had to consider her physical well-being. He wanted to be sure that she completed the antibiotic therapy and understood its importance. If gonorrhea is not properly treated, it can result in deformities of the uterine tubes and ovaries which cause sterility and chronic abdominal pain. He considered it important that she not be hesitant in seeking treatment for venereal disease in the future. She also required some frank counseling about the dangers of pregnancy and about appropriate contraception. It might be difficult to accomplish these goals if he acted contrary to her wishes and informed her mother. She might "turn off" the hospital staff, no longer trusting or listening to any of them.

He was also concerned that unless physicians treat adolescents confidentially, the epidemic of venereal disease in this age group will continue to grow. In this regard, he was worried not only about T.S.'s failure to seek treatment in the future but also about her sharing with friends the experience of being "betrayed" by a physician, thereby leading other young persons not to seek timely treatment. Indeed, this was one of the concerns that led to state laws allowing physicians to provide confidential treatment to minors for venereal disease.

But a number of factors inclined the pediatrician to fully inform the girl's mother. He did not believe that there is an implicit promise of confidentiality in the relationship between doctors and children. When children receive medical care, they typically expect their parents to be informed about their diagnosis and treatment. Consequently, any promise of confidentiality must be negotiated with particular teenage patients. He had not made any promises to T.S., saying only that he would think about the matter and talk with her again. Thus, he was not constrained by the duty of promise keeping in deciding whether to inform her mother.

He was very concerned about obstructing the ability of the mother to protect the well-being of her daughter. He believed that parents are usually in the best position to meet the needs of their children and often do their best to fulfill these obligations. He was also painfully aware that this girl was only thirteen years old and in need of considerable guidance from a trusted adult. However, he was less certain about whether this mother was providing adequate parental nurturing. She apparently worked long hours as a waitress to provide very modest financial support for her four children. But conversations with T.S. and her older sister suggested that the mother did not pay much attention to the children even when not at work, often being away from the apartment with friends. The seventeen-year-old daughter was usually left in charge, and, with the mother working evenings, the children were very often out after dark in the vicinity of the public housing project where they lived. There was also no permanent male figure in their lives to provide parental supervision. Nevertheless, the physician could not assume that the mother would neglect the child's needs in this difficult situation. Moreover, the hospital staff would have only brief contact with T.S., so the mother was the only person in a position to provide continuous guidance.

In addition, the physician felt strongly that parents have a right, which is independent of their role in promoting the well-being of their children, to inculcate special values, moral norms, and religious beliefs of their own choosing. The parent-child bond is an especially intimate relationship, and persons should be free to mold and nurture these relationships in uniquely personal ways. Undoubtedly, attitudes about sexual behavior and personal relationships are among the most important value beliefs which parents might share with their children. If the physician failed to disclose his knowledge of T.S.'s sexual activity to her mother, he might foreclose an opportunity for her to mold the attitudes and values of her daughter.

Finally, he had no illusions about the negative consequences that early sexual activity might have for T.S.'s personal development. Although he knew that sexual experimentation is one way in which adolescents learn who they are and what values they will cherish, premature sexual activity can also have serious negative consequences for the fragile and emerging self-concept of young persons. Moreover, pregnancy and child-care responsibilities in adolescence can thwart educational opportunities and lead to difficult personal problems. Perhaps informing T.S.'s mother might help avoid these problems.

2.6 Contraceptives for an Adolescent

A sixteen-year-old girl went to her physician, whose specialty was internal medicine, to request birth control pills. The patient's parents had also been under his care for several years. The father had abdominal surgery two years earlier and currently had hypertension. The mother also had hypertension and required vascular surgery approximately one year earlier. Because of these medical problems, the family and the physician had numerous contacts and had developed a close association. In addition, the daughter had recently come to the physician complaining of dizziness and tightness in the chest, symptoms he believed were related to stress caused by pressure from her parents to achieve at school. The physician suspected that this pressure was an attempt by the parents, perhaps not a fully conscious one, to compensate for recent setbacks to the family. The major setback had occurred when the father lost his job as a middle-level executive. Because of his medical problems, he was no longer able to perform satisfactorily and had to settle, at middle age, for another job with lower status and salary. The resulting financial difficulties forced the mother to resume work in a job that was highly stressful. The daughter attended an expensive private school, where she was an honor student. The dominant interest of the parents was their daughter and their ambitions for her. After determining that the daughter's symptoms were probably caused by stress, the physician had referred her to a counselor at school to help her cope with these pressures.

The daughter had a boyfriend and had a close relationship with him. She said that she had not had intercourse with him but that she planned to. She said that she had read the pros and cons of the various methods of contraception and preferred the pill. She also said that she did not want her parents to be informed about the contraceptives. She was currently living at home with her parents.

The physician felt that he was placed in a difficult situation by her request. Through his established relationship with the parents, he was confident that they would want to know that their daughter was requesting contraceptives. He believed that as parents they had a responsibility to provide counseling to foster the personal development of the girl and that in order to carry out that responsibility they needed this information. On the other hand, he was aware that to reveal this information would violate the patient's confidentiality.

He was aware that adolescents sometimes choose to be sexually active as a way of getting even with parents for being too restrictive. He therefore decided to ask a few probing questions in an attempt to ascertain how she was getting along with her parents and whether such attitudes were motivating her request. The response suggested, however, that they had a relatively good relationship, even though there were differences of opinion on matters such as sexual behavior and the girl's social activities. She said that she did not want to have a confrontation with them.

State law allows that any minor "who requests and is in need of birth control procedures, supplies or information" may receive them without parental consent. There are no statutes or regulations requiring or prohibiting parental notification of the request for contraceptives.

The physician had four options: (1) contact the parents; (2) refer the girl to a family planning agency and do nothing else himself; (3) provide the contraceptives along with standard medical information and not inform the parents; and (4) provide the contraceptives, together with standard medical information *and* advice about her sexual conduct, and not inform the parents.

The physician believed that referring her to a family planning agency would be ducking his responsibility. For one thing, it would not eliminate the problem of whether to inform the parents that their daughter was seeking contraceptives. Nor would it eliminate the questions of whether he should counsel the patient and what form the counseling should take. On the other hand, he was concerned about what would happen if he provided contraceptives and the parents later discovered that he had done so. Perhaps they would discover the girl's pills at home. That outcome might undermine his relationship with them. (Although the information might be upsetting for the parents, he did not think that it would be especially harmful with regard to their hypertension.)

Another concern was that if the girl did not obtain contraceptives she might engage in sexual activity anyway as a result of peer pressure. That such peer pressure exists is supported by recent data indicating that a relatively high percentage of adolescents engage in sexual activity. Zelnick and Kantner reported that the proportion of American women aged fifteen to nineteen years having had premarital sexual intercourse increased from 30 percent in 1971 to 50 percent in 1979. The proportions of sixteen-, seventeen-, and eighteen-year-old single women who had experienced intercourse were 38 percent, 49 percent, and 57 percent, respectively, according to the 1979 study.[11] Thus, a failure to provide contraceptives might result in an unwanted pregnancy, which could have an adverse effect on the girl and her parents. He also wondered what would happen to the offspring if pregnancy occurred.

The question of whether to give advice to the patient was worrisome. On one view, physicians in such situations should restrict themselves to providing information, attempting to be as value-neutral as possible. According to another view, if the teenager could benefit from the advice of a more mature adult and if such advice by her parents was precluded, then perhaps there was a need that could be fulfilled by the physician. This could involve an attempt to help the patient consider the various aspects of the situation and make an informed, considered decision based on her own values. By showing that he regarded her as a mature young adult, the physician might be able to establish a rapport that would encourage the patient to speak openly. She might appreciate having someone she could talk to concerning her personal decisions. The physician might explore, for example, whether sexual activity with her boyfriend was what she really wanted or whether she was being pressured by her boyfriend and peers. He might ask if she had considered the possible consequences of her parents' discovering the birth control pills, including the impact on her relationship with her boyfriend.

The physician also considered a closely related issue; namely whether to tell the patient about a correlation between coitus at an early age and the subsequent occurrence of cervical cancer. For example, Rotkin found that 82 percent of a study group with cervical cancer had experienced first coitus before age twenty; the proportion was 54 percent for a control group without cervical cancer. The percentage of the study group who had intercourse before age seventeen was 51, compared to 28 percent among the controls.[12] In support of discussing this information is the fact that it appears relevant to an informed decision concerning whether to engage in sexual activity. Nevertheless, several reasons can be given against discussing this information. First, its significance is not clear, since the

Duties to Patient and Family 61

question of how much the risk is increased by early intercourse is not answered by the available data. Second, the information is not directly relevant to informed consent for contraceptives. What is required for such consent is a comparison of the risks and benefits of the various methods of contraception. Although the information in question may be relevant to the decision about whether to have intercourse, that decision, it can be argued, has already been made by the patient. Third, it could be argued that the information would probably not make a difference in the adolescent's decision about sexual activity. These decisions appear to be based on psychological needs of the teenager which may be far more compelling than the relatively abstract notion of a possible future harm. Fourth, this information could be perceived as an attempt by the physician to persuade the patient not to become sexually active, even if that is not the intent.

2.7 Request for Abortion for a Retarded Daughter

S.P. was a twenty-one-year-old severely mentally retarded woman brought to the obstetrics clinic by her mother because she appeared to be pregnant. The mother said it had been about thirteen weeks since the last menstrual period. The patient was totally blind, unable to converse, confined to a wheelchair, and slightly hydrocephalic.[13] Her handicaps were caused by a brain tumor which had been surgically removed at eight months of age. The mother said that the patient was unable to perform most of the everyday activities involved in taking care of herself. She was on a waiting list to be admitted to a nearby residential institution for the mentally retarded. She had never been pregnant before.

Severely retarded patients are often uncooperative during pelvic exams, and this patient was no exception. She screamed and moved throughout the exam, apparently from fright because she did not understand what was happening. Fetal heart tones were heard, confirming pregnancy. An ultrasound revealed a single fetus with a size corresponding to fifteen weeks.

The mother was noticeably upset by her daughter's pregnancy. She suspected that it had resulted from incest with the patient's brother, but the boy had denied it. She said she had been the sole caretaker of the daughter and would have to take care of any children her daughter might have, since the daughter was unable to do so. She was particularly upset at the prospect of having to raise another child. She requested an abortion for her daughter, pointing out that she was fifty-six years old and "too old to start raising another child."

The family's income was relatively low. The mother received welfare checks, and the patient's medical bills were paid by Medicaid. The physician explained that Medicaid would pay for an abortion only if the life of the mother would be endangered by carrying the fetus to term or if the pregnancy was the result of rape or incest.[14] The physician's exam had indicated that the life-endangerment grounds would not be applicable. In the case of rape or incest, Medicaid would pay only if the incident were reported within sixty days to a law enforcement agency or public health office.[15] A report had not been made, so Medicaid would not pay in this case. The mother was disappointed to hear this, saying that she could not afford an abortion.

Another problem would be obtaining legally valid informed consent. There was no state statute explicitly permitting abortions for incompetent persons. Since the patient was twenty-one, the legal principle that parents can consent to medical procedures carried out on minors was not applicable. Although the next of kin can consent to medical procedures for incompetent adults, such proxy consent is most clearly valid for necessary treatment of illness. It was uncertain whether proxy consent would be legally valid for an elective abortion. Therefore, it would be advisable to seek the appointment of a guardian for the purpose of giving consent. It was unclear, however, whether the local court would grant such authorization.

The physician mentioned the possibility of carrying the fetus to term and putting the child up for adoption. The mother was opposed to this, however. She said that if her daughter had a child, she would never "give it away." It was apparent that she considered her responsibilities to a newborn grandchild to be considerably different from any responsibility she might have to a fifteen-week fetus.

The physician's options included the following: (1) refuse to perform the abortion; (2) attempt to persuade the hospital administrators to permit an abortion at no charge, and if they agree, perform it; (3) pursue option 2, but seek the appointment of the mother as legal guardian for the purpose of consenting to an abortion; or (4) try to identify an abortion clinic willing to do the abortion for a reduced fee, and refer the patient.

One issue is whether it would be ethically permissible to perform the abortion. The right of women to determine what happens to their bodies would not be directly applicable in this case since the patient was clearly incompetent to make decisions. However, an important factor was her well-being. An abortion involves risks, which vary with the method used. At sixteen weeks gestational age, the safest method would be dilatation and evacuation.[16] The mortality rate for this method is approximately 9.5 deaths per 100,000 procedures.[17] On the other hand, the mortality rate resulting from the complications of pregnancy and childbirth (excluding abortion and adjusted for this patient's race) is about 20.2 deaths per 100,000 live births, more than twice as high as that of the abortion.[18] The patient's emotional well-being could also be affected by the decision. If the pregnancy continued, she would probably not understand what was happening to her body, and this could cause anxiety. Although an abortion procedure could itself cause fear and anxiety, such reactions would presumably be minimized by the heavy sedation, perhaps even general anesthesia, that would be needed to control the patient. Although the abortion might cause some pain, there are also some typical discomforts of pregnancy, such as morning sickness, indigestion, heartburn, and fatigue. The well-being of the patient would also be affected by the ability of her mother to provide care. The task of raising a newborn might substantially reduce the time and energy the mother could spend caring for the patient.

The reproductive rights of the patient were another concern. It could be argued that all persons, including the mentally retarded, have a right to reproduce and that an abortion without the patient's consent would be a violation of that right. On the other hand, it could be questioned whether this patient had a moral interest in carrying the fetus to term. There was no evidence that she understood what procreation is, or that she desired to procreate. Because she would be unable to care for a child, the various psychological and emotional benefits of parenting were also not realizable. The fact that she was pregnant as a result of nonvoluntary intercourse raised further doubts about her moral interest in continuing the pregnancy.

The well-being of the patient's mother was another important factor. The task of raising a child would involve a significant expenditure of effort and finances for her. With advancing age, the demands of child rearing can be increasingly fatiguing. Although the patient was on a waiting list for institutionalization, it was unclear how long it would be until such placement would occur. The mother might have to continue taking care of the patient for a considerable time. The difficulties for families in caring for handicapped children have been widely documented.[19] It appeared, then, that raising another child would augment what were already considerable demands on the mother.

The mother's autonomy was another consideration. It could be argued that her wishes should be respected, given the significant impact the abortion decision would have on her. It could also be argued that her desire not to give up a grandchild for adoption is defensible. The bonds of kinship can be strong. She might have deep affection and sense of responsibility toward a grandchild.

The moral status of the fetus was, of course, another important consideration. According to one view, only sentient creatures can have interests. If the ability to have sensations, such as feeling pain, develops at a later time, then the fifteen-week fetus does not have interests. Another view is that the fetus's potential to become a conscious, thinking individual is relevant to its moral status. One version of this view is that fetuses have a right to life based on this potential. Even if the fetus in this case has interests, the question remains whether they are outweighed by the other moral considerations.

If the pregnancy were continued, the interests of the future child would be another consideration. If the grandmother became less able to care for the child because of advancing age or illness, there would be a diminution in the quality of care the child received. If the grandmother became incapacitated, some other caretaker would have to be identified. Separation from the grandmother could be emotionally traumatic for the child. Also, there was an increased risk of genetic impairment if the pregnancy was in fact due to incest. On the other hand, it could be argued that the child's life would itself be of value and that continuing the pregnancy would therefore probably benefit the child who would be born.

If an abortion is ethically permissible, another issue concerned how much effort should be devoted by the physician in helping obtain one. Options 3 and 4 could involve considerable effort. It could be argued that since an abortion would not be a treatment of an illness, there is no obligation either to perform the procedure or to refer the patient to someone who will. On the other hand, it can be argued that laws preventing the poor from having access to abortions constitute a violation of the right to health care. The need to redress that inequity, on this view, provides the physician a reason to help the patient obtain an abortion.

Additional considerations were pertinent to the question of whether to seek a court order. For one thing, the legal risks of performing the abortion without court authorization were unclear. A civil suit by the mother on behalf of her daughter for assault and battery was unlikely, since she would be a party to the putative offense. However, it was possible that someone (perhaps an antiabortionist) would bring the matter to the attention of the district attorney. Basis for a criminal charge could be found in the state abortion statute, which stated, "An abortion otherwise permitted by law shall be performed or induced only with the informed written consent of the pregnant woman." Seeking a court order would protect against this risk but would involve legal fees the mother might have difficulty paying. Also, if the physician decided to help the mother obtain an abortion but the court refused the authorization, then their plans would be thwarted.

2.8 Request for Hysterectomy for a Retarded Eleven-Year-Old

The patient was an eleven-year-old girl with congenital impairments including mental retardation, total blindness, deafness, and microcephaly (small head size). It was believed that her handicaps may have been caused by a viral infection during her mother's pregnancy. The patient was being raised at home by her parents and attended a municipal school for handicapped children. Initial assessments of the child's capabilities had indicated that she was severely to profoundly retarded. However, a more recent evaluation showed that she was only mildly retarded. The improvement was believed to be the result of active teaching through tactile stimulation during her five years at the school.

The parents brought the girl to the physician and requested a hysterectomy for her. There were two main reasons why they wanted this procedure. First, she had recently begun her menstrual cycle, and her menstrual hygiene was creating problems for the family. Although she could manage her toilet hygiene with assistance, she was not able to manage her menstrual hygiene. Not only was this an added burden to the parents, who had two other children to care for, but the task of caring for her menstrual hygiene in the afternoons fell upon those other children, daughters aged ten and thirteen. Both parents worked and could not be at home in the afternoons. Previously a great-grandmother had taken care of the handicapped girl, but she had renal disease which had recently worsened. She had to be dialyzed frequently and was no longer available.

Second, the parents feared the possibility of pregnancy. They were aware that retarded girls sometimes invite, and often do not know how to resist, sexual advances. The parents could not be at home all the time to protect her, and male friends of the two other daughters might be at the house on occasion. They were happy to raise their own children, but they did not want to raise children of the retarded daughter.

The physician discussed the physical risks associated with hysterectomy, which include infection, excessive bleeding, and the risks of general anesthesia. He also suggested that there were several other options the parents might want to consider. One was to seek professional assistance in training the child to handle her personal hygiene. There was a nearby residential institution for mentally retarded individuals offering such training. Staff members would conduct the training in the patient's home, and such efforts were often quite effective for mildly retarded persons.

Another possibility was sexuality counseling to teach the girl to not invite and to resist sexual advances. A child development center at the local university offered such a program. It consisted of a counseling group for both the patient and the parents. Such counseling is frequently effective for mildly retarded individuals.

Attempting to place the child in a residential institution was another alternative. Placement would substantially reduce any burdens on the family in caring for the child. In the present case, the one that seemed most appropriate was a state institution for the blind, located almost two hundred miles away. There was a waiting list for admission, and the patient would probably need to improve her skills in personal hygiene before being accepted there. The students resided in that institution nine months per year, living with their families during summers.

Administering Depo-Provera was another possibility. This drug has been used extensively outside the United States as a contraceptive. It is administered by injection, with one shot providing contraceptive protection for about three months. The U.S. Food and Drug Administration has withheld approval of Depo-Provera for contraceptive use because it has been found to cause cancer of the breast and uterus in experiments using beagle dogs and monkeys.[20] It is approved, however, for other uses such as control of menorrhagia (excessive menstrual bleeding) and dysmenorrhea (painful menstruation). After two or three injections of Depo-Provera, the patient usually stops having menstrual periods; the drug suppresses the cyclic changes in hormone levels that cause ovulation and menstruation. The cessation is reversible, but the return of periods after shots are discontinued may take up to eighteen months or longer in some cases. Depo-Provera is sometimes administered to retarded women who cannot manage their menstrual hygiene and whose bleeding is sufficient in amount to cause a problem for their caretakers. Its use for this purpose is considered to be consistent with FDA regulations. A suspected complication of the drug, in addition to its possible carcinogenic effects, is an increased risk of cardiovascular disease with long-term use. Specifically, Depo-Provera belongs to a class of drugs called progestogens, the long-term use of which is associated with an increased incidence of high blood pressure, heart attack, and stroke.[21]

One other option would be to prescribe birth control pills. Not only would conception be prevented, but the menstrual periods would become somewhat more manageable, because the duration of menses would be shortened to about two days. However, birth control pills contain progestogens, and there would be a risk of cardiovascular disease with long-term use. Also, the effectiveness of this approach would be reduced if the patient failed to take the pill regularly. If she missed one day, she could have spotting for about three days. If she went off the pill, she might have heavier menses for a while.

After a discussion of these options, the physician recommended exploring the possibility of in-home training in menstrual hygiene and enrollment of the family in a sexuality counseling group. The parents firmly stated, however, that they were not interested in the programs. They said they did not believe those options were the solution to their problems. A genuine lack of interest in home training would make them, in fact, poor candidates for that program; the training includes teaching the parents to reinforce what the child has been taught, and its effectiveness depends heavily on a commitment by the parents to provide the reinforcement. The parents did state, however, that they were interested in residential placement of the child.

At that point the physician was faced with several alternatives, including the following: (1) carry out the hysterectomy as requested; (2) recommend either Depo-Provera or birth control pills but not perform a hysterectomy; (3) assist in attempted institutional placement; or (4) assist in attempted placement and carry out option 1 or 2.

Various factors were pertinent to the problem of deciding which course to take. One was the autonomy of the parents. The decision in question would have an impact not only on the retarded child but on the other two siblings and the family as a whole. Parental autonomy includes the right to make plans for the family and to take reasonable steps to prevent disruption of those plans. An unwanted pregnancy, in particular, could be a significant interference with family plans. A hysterectomy would eliminate this possibility. Use of Depo-Provera or birth control pills, however, would not completely rule out such a possibility because of the reversible nature of these methods and the fact that their effectiveness is compromised if one fails to take the drugs regularly. Also, making sure she received her pills or shots would simply be one more thing for the parents to worry about. Respect for parental autonomy would suggest performing a hysterectomy.

A closely related factor was the well-being of the family. Because the parents did not want to raise any offspring of the girl, an unwanted pregnancy could place burdens on them—in terms of time, energy, and finances—that would adversely affect their well-being.

Also, the patient's inability to manage her menstrual hygiene would be not only an inconvenience to the family but a potential source of embarrassment as well. It is not unusual in such cases for the retarded child to soil her clothes with menstrual blood at inopportune times, such as in public places or when visiting the homes of family friends.

In opposition to these considerations was the patient's interest in preservation of reproductive capacity. Because her developmental level had improved markedly in the past five years, it was possible she would continue to improve and

Duties to Patient and Family

someday be competent to make her own decisions concerning procreative matters. These considerations suggested that it would be preferable to postpone any procedure that would make her irreversibly sterile. On the other hand, her blindness and deafness might prove to be such serious obstacles to her mental development that she would remain incompetent to make such decisions. It was possible that she would never understand what reproduction is and would never desire to procreate. If she were never capable of raising children, she would be prevented from experiencing the benefits of child rearing. If so, it could be argued that any interest she may have in procreation would be greatly attenuated and that a hysterectomy would not be a violation of any serious right.

With regard to the well-being of the patient, a hysterectomy would have certain advantages. The patient would be permanently free of periods and associated menstrual problems and would avoid the risks associated with long-term use of Depo-Provera and birth control pills. Also, a hysterectomy would eliminate many of the most common types of gynecological pathology, such as uterine bleeding or pain, infections or cancer of the uterus, and benign uterine tumors. It would also eliminate the possibility of anxiety in the event that she became pregnant and did not understand what was happening to her body. On the other hand, if the patient later became capable of raising children and desired to do so, a hysterectomy presumably would adversely affect her well-being.

Another consideration was the well-being of any offspring of the retarded girl. If the patient were to attempt to provide care at some future time for any children she might have, that care could conceivably prove to be deficient in ways that would result in harm. Also, if the patient would be unable to provide care, then being raised without the nurture of a mother (and father, possibly) could be a detriment.

The legal aspects of the situation did not rule out the possibility of a hysterectomy. A similar case had established a legal precedent several years earlier in the state in which the physician practiced. The parents and physician in that case had sought court approval to perform a hysterectomy on a mentally retarded and legally incompetent adolescent who could not manage her menstrual hygiene. The court stated that it did not have the authority to rule on such requests; explicit authority had not been assigned by statute. Therefore, although performance of a hysterectomy would not violate any statute, there was no legal means for the physician to protect himself against the possibility of a civil lawsuit for assault and battery. The risk of a successful lawsuit by the parents did not appear to be great, however, because they would be parties to the putative assault and battery. On the other hand, there had been a case in which a hysterectomy was performed on a mildly retarded woman without her knowledge and in which she subsequently married and desired children.[22] A lawsuit by the retarded woman would be a possibility in that sort of situation.

The physician was aware that a number of other doctors in the community performed hysterectomies on the retarded at the request of parents. If he did not agree to do it, it was possible that the parents would go to another physician.

2.9 Conflict about Maintaining a Brain-Dead Woman for the Sake of Her Fetus

A nineteen-year-old woman had been pregnant approximately twenty-seven weeks when she began having headaches and a stiff neck. The headaches became worse over a week, and her family took her to a hospital in the nearest city, about thirty-five miles away. By the time they arrived, she was comatose, and she was soon diagnosed as having meningitis of unknown cause. The patient's condition steadily worsened in the hospital. Her blood pressure became highly erratic, and it was necessary to give her drugs to elevate her blood pressure above dangerously low levels. She was placed in an intensive care unit under the care of a neurosurgeon. She was put on a respirator, and a Swan-Ganz catheter was inserted into the artery leading to her lungs in order to monitor her blood pressure.[23] In addition, a Foley catheter was inserted into her bladder to collect her urine, and she was fed through a nasogastric tube. A fetal heartbeat was detectable and was normal.

The patient was unmarried and this was her first pregnancy. Her family consisted of her parents, a sister, and two brothers. The family knew the young man who had impregnated her and expressed anger toward him. They had learned about the pregnancy only a couple of months earlier and had been upset by the news. The man was not present at the hospital.

The neurosurgeon told the family that it was possible the patient would not regain consciousness. Understandably, this was very upsetting to them. In spite of their grief, the parents and sister were amicable toward the physician, but the brothers were difficult to deal with. They were angry about the girl's illness and demanded that everything be done to try to save her. The brothers seemed to be making the decisions, with the other family members simply going along. The main concern of the whole family was that the girl get better. The neurosurgeon assured them that he would do everything possible.

Soon the hospital administrators became aware of the case. They raised the question of what medical treatment should be provided to the fetus, in part because they were concerned about the hospital's legal responsibilities. The hospital did not have an obstetrical service, and the administrators asked an obstetrician in the community for a consultation.

After reviewing the case history, the obstetrician met with the family. He explained that although the patient's cognitive functions were impaired, the organ systems that support the fetus were functioning adequately. As long as this condition continued, the fetus could grow and develop normally. Furthermore, this condition could conceivably be maintained until the fetus reached full term. In that event, the patient would eventually go into labor and deliver the infant. He also pointed out that if she went into labor, the method of delivery that would be best for the fetus might be cesarean section. This would be so if, for example, a fetal monitor were being used and it indicated fetal distress or if the uterine contractions did not expel the fetus in an adequate period of time. He explained that a cesarean section would involve risks for the mother, including hemorrhage and postpartum infection. Combined with the difficulty in maintaining her blood pressure, such complications conceivably could result in a fatal deterioration of her condition. She might also have a cardiac arrest during surgery. When informed of these potential risks, the family members said that they did not want anything done for the fetus that would jeopardize their daughter's chances for recovery. This seemed to rule out cesarean section as long as the daughter's condition remained as it was. The family was so overwhelmed by what had happened to the daughter that they could hardly think about the interests of the fetus.

The obstetrician recommended to the neurosurgeon that he try to sustain a satisfactory uterine environment by maintaining the patient's blood pressure, feedings, and adequate levels of oxygen in the blood. In reviewing the chart, the obstetrician had learned that the patient's blood pressure had once dropped to a very low level and that corrective action had not been taken promptly. He urged the neurosurgeon to give close attention to the blood pressure because such periods of low blood pressure in the mother can cause fetal brain damage.

The next day the neurosurgeon told the obstetrician that the patient appeared to be progressing toward brain death, based on the fact that the EEG tracings were showing decreasing electrical activity in her brain.

If the entire brain ceased to function, the patient would be legally dead according to state law. In that event, the physicians might be able to maintain her body functions in an attempt to keep the fetus in utero as long as possible. Although a respirator often cannot prevent the cessation of heartbeat relatively soon after the onset of brain death, in some cases somatic life has been maintained for a number of weeks in pregnant brain-dead patients. The obstetrician recommended that if the patient became brain-dead, an attempt should be made to maintain somatic function for the sake of the fetus. The longer the fetus could be kept in the uterus, the better its chances for survival. One of the major risks associated with premature birth is respiratory distress associated with immature lungs. Premature newborns may suffer chronic lung disease or death even with intensive respiratory treatment. Another major risk is hemorrhages in the infant's brain, which can cause irreversible brain damage or death.

It was also possible that all of the mother's organ systems, including the cardiovascular system, would cease to function. If that happened, one option would be to perform an emergency cesarean section in an attempt to save the fetus's life. With this possibility in mind, the obstetrician recommended that the patient be immediately transferred to the county's public hospital, which had an obstetric service.

The neurosurgeon, however, was opposed to maintaining somatic function if brain death occurred. The very concept of doing so seemed foreign to him. He also opposed transferring the patient to the public hospital, saying that it was difficult to obtain an EEG tracing there. The neurosurgeon later told the obstetrician that the family was also opposed to maintaining the patient if brain death occurred.

A week after admission, the patient became brain-dead. The neurosurgeon informed the parents by phone. He then telephoned the obstetrician to report that the family had agreed to an immediate cesarean section so that they could "put an end to the situation and arrange a funeral." They said, more or less, "If you're going to take the fetus out, do it now." The obstetrician again recommended that the patient's bodily functions be maintained for the fetus's sake, but the neurosurgeon was still opposed.

At this point the obstetrician could either perform the cesarean section as requested or take steps to try to keep the fetus in utero. Although further efforts to persuade the family and the neurosurgeon seemed likely to fail, attempting to obtain a court order was another possibility.

It was uncertain whether a court order could be obtained; there was no clear legal precedent. The applicable legal rules appeared to be those contained in the Uniform Anatomical Gift Act. According to that act, the next of kin may give all or part of a decedent's body to any specified individual for therapy needed by that individual or to any physician for purposes of therapy.[24] There have been no cases in which courts have authorized the use of a decedent's body over the refusal of the next of kin. However, courts have ordered medical procedures against the wishes of pregnant women in order to prevent harm to the fetus. In one case, for example, blood transfusions were ordered for a Jehovah's Witness;[25] in other cases, a cesarean section was ordered against the woman's wishes.[26] These cases recognize the fetus as an individual whom the state has an interest in protecting. However, these cases are disanalogous to the present one because they concern the wishes of competent patients rather than the next of kin of brain-dead patients. A second type of case has involved overruling the next of kin for the sake of incompetent patients. They frequently involve overruling parents in order to treat a child. Such cases could be a precedent for situations in which the incompetent patient is a fetus and the next of kin is a grandparent. Perhaps these two types of cases together would provide grounds for overruling the next of kin's decision concerning use of a brain-dead woman's body for the sake of the fetus. Whether the local court would make such a ruling was an open question.

Although court-ordered treatment might avoid the risks associated with premature birth, it was not clear that such an aggressive approach was best for the fetus. The period of low blood pressure that had occurred might have caused fetal brain damage. If the family did not want to raise the infant, then the presence of brain damage would make it difficult to find adoptive parents. The child might be institutionalized. The physician wondered if survival would be in the infant's best interests in that case. Another consideration was that the meningitis that killed the mother might have been caused by the herpes simplex virus. It is suspected that this virus can cross the placenta and infect the fetus. In a fetus or newborn such infections are extremely serious. The survival rate of newborns with herpes infections is about 50 percent, and among survivors there is a high probability of brain damage.

The well-being of the family was another factor. Perhaps there would be a change of attitude, with the grandparents later deciding that they wanted to raise

Duties to Patient and Family 71

the child. After all, the recent events had been stressful for the family members, and they were now grieving over the daughter's death. Their decision concerning the fetus may not have reflected their considered wishes. If they later provided a home for the infant, promoting the health of the infant now would be in their interests as well as the child's. On the other hand, if the fetus were already handicapped, a court order might have the effect of keeping alive a damaged infant who would otherwise have died. This could prove to be contrary to the grandparents' interests if they later attempted to raise the child.

Another concern was the right of the next of kin to decide the disposition of the decedent's body. It is based on a moral right to conduct the grieving process in the manner most acceptable to the family. This includes a right to privacy and a right to conduct preburial activities in a manner consistent with the family's religious beliefs. Given the deep personal trauma that the death of a family member causes and the need of persons to deal with this crisis in ways that are culturally and religiously familiar, these seem to be important rights. Yet a court order would constitute a direct infringement of them.

There was also a question of who would pay the cost of maintaining the brain-dead patient. Although the patient had been covered by hospitalization insurance, it was uncertain whether the insurance company would pay medical bills incurred after the onset of brain death. Perhaps the patient could be transferred to the county hospital, where the bills would ultimately fall upon the taxpayers. Abandoned infants were cared for at the county hospital, and perhaps an abandoned fetus could be treated there as well.

2.10 Choosing the Method of Delivery for a Fetus with Hydrocephalus

The patient was a twenty-four-year-old woman referred to the university obstetrical service after an ultrasound examination indicated that her fetus had hydrocephalus, an excessive accumulation of cerebrospinal fluid in the brain. At the university another ultrasound showed that the lateral ventricles (spaces within the brain that contain cerebrospinal fluid) were enlarged, confirming the diagnosis of hydrocephaly. The fluid was compressing the brain against the skull. At that time, the diameter of the head was slightly larger than normal for the fetus's gestational age, which was approximately thirty-five weeks. Comparison with the previous ultrasound indicated that the degree of head enlargement was increasing. The second ultrasound exam also showed that the lower portion of the fetus's spine looked abnormal, suggesting that the fetus had spina bifida as well.

Although the prognosis for fetuses with hydrocephalus is generally not good, there is considerable variation in the long-term outcome. Recent developments in treatment have included insertion of a shunt into the brain following birth in order to drain the excess fluid. The survival rate for patients shunted after birth is approximately 86 percent.[27] Among survivors, about 22 to 31 percent have normal cognitive development.[28] Among those with below-normal development, about half are severely or profoundly retarded,[29] and handicaps such as vision defects, paraplegia, and seizures are occasionally present. Among infants who do not receive surgical treatment after birth, the survival rate is reported to be 7 percent or less.[30] Hydrocephalus in utero has a worse prognosis than hydrocephalus that develops after birth because typically there is a longer period before treatment is initiated. The increased pressure of the cerebrospinal fluid destroys brain tissue, and the longer the pressure continues, the greater the degree of damage.

Spina bifida can result in additional handicaps, including partial or total paralysis of the legs, incontinence of bowel or bladder, abnormal curvature of the spine, and difficulty in swallowing. Victims often have associated anomalies such as club feet and dislocated hips. The presence and severity of these conditions vary considerably. Typically, the higher the lesion is located on the spine, the worse the prognosis for physical handicaps. When the fetus is in utero, it is difficult to predict the degree of handicap that will later be present.

The patient and her husband were counseled concerning the ultrasound results and their implications. During the session they both cried. As they walked out, the husband said to his wife, "I'll continue to love you no matter what happens." There was no attempt to make any decisions concerning medical treatment at that time.

A decision, however, would soon have to be made concerning the method of delivery of the fetus. In the obstetrician's view, the options were basically the following: (1) deliver the fetus as soon as its lungs were mature enough for it to breathe on its own—by cesarean section, if necessary—so that a shunt could then be inserted without further delay; (2) carry the fetus to term and perform a vaginal delivery, decompressing the enlarged head if necessary to permit passage through the birth canal; or (3) attempt to insert a shunt into the fetus's head in utero.

The first approach would constitute an attempt to promote the best interests of the fetus. Once outside the uterus, there would be an increased ability to assess the infant's condition and to treat the hydrocephalus safely and effectively. The university's neurosurgeons would be able to insert a shunt consisting of a small plastic tube, one end of which would be placed in a lateral ventricle in the brain. The tube would be passed, just beneath the skin, down the head and neck into the jugular vein, with the other end terminating in the right atrium of the heart. A one-way valve in the tube would permit cerebrospinal fluid to drain from the brain to the bloodstream without backflow, thus reducing the pressure on the brain.

Even at thirty-five weeks gestational age, this approach would involve a trade-off. The risks associated with prematurity, together with those involved in the surgery to place the shunt, would have to be weighed against the risk of further brain damage from the hydrocephalus. The main complications of prematurity include respiratory distress because of immature lungs, which can result in death or chronic lung disease. Hemorrhages in the brain are another major complication, which can cause death or permanent brain damage. The more premature the fetus, the stronger is the argument against delivery. In the judgment of the obstetrician, at thirty-five weeks the trade-off would favor delivery, provided a chemical analysis of the amniotic fluid indicated that the fetal lungs were mature.

The chemical analysis in question is a standard test that measures the ratio of the concentrations of lecithin and sphingomyelin in the amniotic fluid (the L/S ratio). Empirical studies have established that if the L/S ratio is 2 or greater, it is highly probable that the lungs are mature. The test had already been carried out in this case, by means of amniocentesis, and it indicated that the lungs were not yet mature. However, it would be possible to administer steroids to the mother in an attempt to speed up the maturation process. Betamethasone is one steroid used for this purpose, and it normally takes only several days for the effects of this drug to be realized.

The main shortcoming of this approach is that it might require a cesarean section for either of two reasons. First, the fetal head might be too large to pass through the pelvis. Although the fetal head was slightly enlarged now, it might become larger by the time of delivery. Second, attempts to induce labor prematurely are not always successful, and then prompt delivery can be accomplished only by cesarean section.[31]

The second approach would constitute an attempt to minimize the risk of physical harm to the mother by avoiding a cesarean section and its associated risks. The maternal death rate is three to nine per ten thousand cesarean sections, a six- to eleven-fold increased risk compared to vaginal delivery.[32] Additional complications of cesarean section include hemorrhage, infection, and accidental incision of the bladder. Infrequently, a hysterectomy may become necessary to control uterine bleeding. According to a recent study, significant complications other than death occurred in 21 percent of cesarean sections, compared to 4 percent of vaginal deliveries.[33]

If the fetal head were too large to pass through the pelvis, a needle would be inserted into the head or the spinal canal, depending on whether the fetus was emerging head first or feet first. Cerebrospinal fluid would then be extracted in sufficient quantity to reduce the size of the head so that a vaginal delivery would occur. This method of delivery, however, almost universally results in death of the infant within a few days because of the rapid decompression of the head.

The third approach would involve placing a shunt in the fetus's head via a needle inserted through the uterus, using ultrasound to guide the needle. One end of the shunt would be placed in a lateral ventricle, with the other end free within the amniotic sac. A one-way valve would permit excess cerebrospinal fluid to flow into the amniotic fluid. This approach, however, was considered by the obstetrician to be less favorable than the first option because it was still experimental. There was considerable uncertainty surrounding its risks and the likelihood of success. At thirty-five weeks the balance of risks and benefits favored prompt delivery and postnatal shunting (assuming lung maturity could soon be achieved, which seemed likely). Intrauterine shunting would be given greater consideration in earlier stages of gestation, in which fetal lung maturity was weeks away. Therefore, the third option was ruled on out medical grounds.

It would be possible to perform another test to confirm the presence of spina bifida before making a decision about the method of delivery. The test would consist of another amniocentesis followed by measurement of the concentration of alpha-fetoprotein in the amniotic fluid. An elevated concentration would indicate spina bifida. A disadvantage of doing this, however, is that it would take about ten days to obtain the results of the test. There could be progressive brain damage while waiting for the results.

In deciding what he should recommend and/or be willing to do, the obstetrician was faced with two troublesome questions. First, he asked himself if he would be willing to decompress the fetus's head if it came to that. Because this would probably contribute to the death of the fetus, it could be considered an active rather than passive involvement. Second, he asked himself what he would do if the mother refused a cesarean section and the fetus's head was too large for a vaginal delivery. One possibility would be to try to obtain a court order for a cesarean section. In several recent cases courts have authorized cesarean sections against the wishes of the mother in order to protect the interests of the fetus.[34] However, those cases did not involve fetuses with anomalies.

In answering these questions, several considerations were relevant. For one thing, it is widely held that the distinction between killing and allowing to die is a morally relevant one, at least in some cases. It might be argued that even if withholding treatment after the child's birth would be permissible in this case, actively causing death by decompressing the head during delivery is not. On the other hand, it could be claimed that when the prognosis is very poor, head decompression is permissible in order to prevent substantial risks to the mother.

Actively causing the death could also have legal ramifications adversely affecting the physician's own well-being. Although criminal charges have never been brought against an obstetrician for decompressing a fetus's head, even though the procedure has been performed many times, a risk is always present that the local prosecutor might be informed and decide to take action. Also, a civil lawsuit by the parents could not be ruled out. Several cases in which a physician injured a fetus, causing death just after birth, have resulted in wrongful-death lawsuits.[35]

The mother's right to decide what happens to her body was another major concern. It could be argued that the woman's right to self-determination overrides the interests of the fetus in this type of situation. On the other hand, it might be claimed that there is a significant difference between a fetus late in gestation and one early in gestation. It could be argued that while the woman's right to self-determination outweighs the fetus's interests early in gestation, it does not do so near term.

Another consideration was the well-being of the fetus. The presence of handicaps did not necessarily mean that continued life would be contrary to the fetus's interests. On the other hand, if the brain damage and spina bifida were severe, then life might not be a benefit to the fetus. The obstetrician also considered the possibility that the parents might be opposed to inserting a shunt in the event that the infant did not die soon after birth. If the shunting procedure were not going to be performed, then it was highly probable that the infant would die regardless

Duties to Patient and Family 75

of whether the obstetrician decompressed the head. Furthermore, prompt delivery followed by shunt insertion might not be the best choice for promoting the fetus's interests. The shunt procedure would be somewhat painful, and because in about 44 to 48 percent of cases the outcome is death or severe retardation, there might not be significant benefit.

The well-being of the family was another factor. The couple lived in a small rural town about one hundred fifty miles from the university medical center. In that town there were no resources available to help care for handicapped children. The nearest city of moderate size was about sixty miles away. The care of a handicapped child can create serious difficulties for a family, especially when few community resources are available. If the child survived and was cared for at home, the couple would be able to receive governmental financial assistance, amounting to about two hundred fifty dollars per month. Even with this assistance, there might be large debts incurred in caring for the child. The father was a blue-collar worker, and the extended family was not well-to-do.

Commentary

In this chapter we consider a type of conflict between the physician's duties to the patient and the interests of third parties—that in which the third parties are members of the patient's family.[36] Other types of third-party conflicts will be considered in chapters 4 and 5, but conflict between duties to patients and the interests of families deserves separate treatment for several reasons. First, it involves moral considerations that are not present in other third-party conflicts. An example is the professional responsibility to help families cope with emotional distress caused by serious illness of a loved one. Second, this sort of conflict leads us to examine some fundamental questions concerning the role of the physician. To what extent should the physician be concerned about the patient's family in addition to the individual patient? What are the limits, if any, of the physician's duties to the patient when they conflict with family interests? Third, this type of ethical dilemma occurs with sufficient frequency to be a significant issue in clinical medical ethics.

Patient-family dilemmas arise in a variety of situations. One type of case involves conflict between the wishes or well-being of elderly debilitated patients and the interests of their families, as in case 2.1. Another type involves conflicts between the interests of pediatric patients and the wishes or well-being of their parents, illustrated by cases 2.2 through 2.4. There can also be tension between the wishes of parents and the emerging reproductive and sexual autonomy of adolescent patients, as in cases 2.5 and 2.6. Some dilemmas involve reproductive decisions for the mentally retarded, exemplified by cases 2.7 and 2.8. Others involve pregnant women, fetuses, and their families, such as cases 2.9 and 2.10. Thus, the conflicts can take various forms, and the moral interests involved vary accordingly.

Clinical decision making takes place within a legal framework that requires physicians to subordinate the interests of patients to third parties in specified situations. For example, physicians are legally required to report certain ordinarily confidential information to public health authorities, concerning gunshot wounds, abortions, venereal diseases, and other communicable diseases. Family members are sometimes among those protected by such reporting, particularly by the reporting of communicable diseases. Another example is the legal requirement in some states that physicians notify parents before performing abortions on minors, even though minors sometimes prefer strict confidentiality. Although physicians have a strong moral obligation to obey laws, questions occasionally arise concerning whether the duty to obey the law is overridden by other moral concerns. However, the issue of obedience to the law will be considered in chapter 5. The central question of this chapter is the following: Outside of situations in which the law requires physicians to subordinate the interests of patients to family members, how should physicians resolve conflicts between the interests of patients and their families? Our focus on situations unencumbered by such legal requirements is appropriate for two reasons. First, such situations are the more frequently encountered in which genuine dilemmas arise in balancing patient and family interests. Second, the role of the physician vis-à-vis patient and family is brought into sharper focus in such situations.

Many physicians resolve conflicts between the interests of patient and family by applying a traditional principle of medical ethics according to which the physician's primary obligations are owed to the patient. We shall refer to this traditional maxim as the *principle of patient advocacy*. Evidence of the wide acceptance of this principle among physicians includes the frequent assertion of it in their codes and writings. For example, the World Medical Association adopted a physician's pledge known as the Declaration of Geneva, which states, "The health of my patient will be my first consideration."[37] Arnold Relman, editor of the *New England Journal of Medicine,* maintains that "A physician's obligation is primarily to help his patient, and *not* the patient's parents or next of kin or legal guardian."[38] Similarly, neonatologist Mildred Stahlman has said, "I believe, as the Hippocratic oath states, that the physician's first responsibility is to act in the best interests of his patient, then in the interests of the parents, and finally in the interests of society, in that order."[39]

A question naturally arises about why the physician's duty to the patient should take precedence over the interests of the patient's family. Relatively little has been written on this question, despite the important place held by this principle in the ethics of the medical profession. One approach is suggested in a recent essay by Jonsen and Jameton.[40] In discussing the social responsibilities of physicians, they attempt to ground the physician's ethical duties on a conception of the functions and role of the physician. The primary function of the physician, most would agree, has traditionally been to help the sick by exercising skill in diagnosing and treating illness. Although a variety of other activities are carried out by contemporary physicians—cosmetic surgeries, artificial inseminations, elective abortions, sterilization procedures, provision of contraceptives, and promotion of wellness, among others—a central aspect of the physician's role continues to be treatment of the ill. As the "American College of Physicians

Ethics Manual'' puts it, "The primary goals of the physician are to relieve suffering, prevent untimely death, and improve the health of the patient while maintaining the dignity of the person."[41] The main duties associated with the role of the physician, thus described, can be conceived as those that advance the performance of this function. This implies that the physician's primary obligations include, as expressed by Jonsen and Jameton, exercising due care in the process of diagnosing illness and treating patients and having a personal concern for the interests of the patient.[42] Another major duty would be to respect the rights of the patient, with particular attention to those rights whose protection advances the aims of the doctor-patient relationship, such as rights to confidentiality and informed consent. These patient-centered duties, according to this view, should be regarded as uppermost by physicians.

Thus, there are good reasons for the view that physicians should give priority to their patients over family members. However, there is controversy concerning the limits of the physician's duties to the patient when they conflict with family interests; the principle of patient advocacy stated above can be interpreted in either of two ways. On one hand, it is held to imply that the interests of the patient should *always* have priority over the interests of the family. We shall refer to this as the *strict-advocacy* view. On the other hand, it can be interpreted as asserting that the duty to patient is a prima facie one that *normally* takes precedence over family interests but in some circumstances can be overridden by them. We shall call this the *modified-advocacy* view. Although there has been little empirical study of the prevalence of these two views, the strict-advocacy view appears to be the dominant one. One encounters this view frequently in the clinical setting and the medical ethics literature. For example, physician Solomon Papper claims: "As an area of commitment, responsibility to the patient has the highest priority and supersedes, but does not preclude, other obligations. When we assume responsibility for the well-being of another person, all other responsibilities must be placed in the background."[43] In omitting any discussion of possible exceptions to this principle, Papper implies that the responsibilities to the patient always have priority. Hans Jonas, an ethicist, states a similar view in discussing conflicts between the interests of patients and the advancement of medical research:

> In the course of treatment, the physician is obligated to the patient and to no one else. He is not the agent of society, nor of the interests of medical science, *the patient's family*, the patient's co-sufferers, or future sufferers from the same disease. The patient alone counts when he is under the physician's care. . . . [The physician] is bound not to let any other interest interfere with that of the patient in being cured. . . . We may speak of a sacred trust; strictly by its terms, the doctor is, as it were, alone with his patient and God.[44]

To consider another example, many neonatologists strictly adhere to the principle that the interests of the handicapped newborn always take precedence over the wishes and well-being of the infant's family. This view was strongly endorsed by the President's Commission for the Study of Ethical Problems in Medicine and Biomedical and Behavioral Research, which asserted that permanent handicaps "justify a decision not to provide life-sustaining treatment only when they are so severe that continued existence would not be a net benefit to the infant. . . . This is a very strict standard in that it excludes consideration of the negative effects of an impaired child's life on other persons, including parents, siblings, and society."[45] Others have attested that the view that the interests of patient always override those of family is widely held among physicians.[46] These quotations suggest that one conception of what it means to be a physician involves a strict interpretation of the role discussed above. On this view, the physician's service to the patient is of such central importance in defining the role of physicians that allowing family interests to take priority is considered a failure to fulfill that role.

In addition to such statements of attitude, arguments can be put forward in support of the strict-advocacy view. One argument is based on the fact that serious illness typically impairs the ability of the patient to act autonomously. As pointed out in chapter 1, there are several ways in which illness can impair a competent patient's decision-making capacity. First, physical disability may prevent or impede the carrying out of activities that are essential to previously formulated life plans. Such physical impairment may require revision of major life activities and may involve a transition period during which the patient does not have settled long-range plans that can form the basis of personal decision making. Second, illness can interfere with the patient's ability to make considered decisions even when the patient has well-formulated life plans that can provide a framework for decision making. These include a lack of understanding of clinical medicine, which makes it difficult for patients to appreciate the significance of medical information that is provided to them. Affective factors such as fear, anxiety, and pain can also interfere with the ability to assimilate information.

With considerations such as these apparently in mind, Natalie Abrams defends the view that the patient's interests should always come first.[47] She claims that the traditional role of medicine aims to reestablish, in the best possible way, the personal autonomy that is shattered by illness. Giving priority to patients is warranted, she suggests, by the importance of restoring their autonomy. That this is an important goal is revealed, as she points out, by "a desire each one of us has, to be recognized as valuable, responsible, and free moral beings."[48]

Another type of argument, a utilitarian one, is suggested by Robert Veatch. If physicians give priority to third parties in order to pursue what appears to be a greater good at the moment, more total harm than good will be done in the end.[49] To elaborate on this reasoning, it might be claimed that people are more likely to seek health care if they trust doctors, and they are more likely to trust doctors if it is generally perceived that doctors put the interests of patients first. Also, a relationship built on trust has the therapeutic advantages of helping to reduce patient's anxieties and enhancing compliance with the physician's recommendations. Thus, a practice of putting the patient first, if followed by all physicians, would help maximize social utility.

On the other hand, there are reasons that can be put forward in support of the modified-advocacy view. First, giving priority to the patient can involve failure to fulfill professional responsibilities to family members. An example is the responsibility of health professionals to respond to the needs of family members for emotional support when a patient is seriously ill or dying. The basis of such a duty is the principle of beneficence, the family's need in a time of crisis, and the ability of health professionals to provide such emotional support. There are various ways in which physicians can help provide emotional support to family members: carefully explaining the patient's medical condition, prognosis, and treatment; showing concern for the family as well as the patient; reassuring the family that everything reasonable is being done to help the patient; and listening to the concerns of the family. An illustration is provided by case 2.1, involving a seventy-four-year-old woman who suffered a stroke resulting in coma and whose daughter insisted that the previously stated wishes of the patient concerning nontreatment be disregarded. Postponing the withdrawing of treatment would give the physician time to help the daughter understand that the coma was not caused by the delay in taking her mother to see a doctor. On the other hand, immediately withdrawing respirator therapy in accordance with the patient's wishes might cause an exacerbation of the daughter's guilt as a result of the patient's death. Thus, the physician would fail to provide needed counseling to the daughter.

Another professional responsibility is to assist families who assume the task of providing special care for patients. Family needs can be especially great when the patient is debilitated, retarded, or otherwise handicapped. Assistance might involve informing families of available community resources, giving advice about problems, referring the family to paramedical specialists, or offering medical procedures for the patient. An illustration is case 2.8, involving a family caring for a eleven-year-old daughter who was mentally retarded and unable to manage her menstrual hygiene. The least invasive option for the patient was a program to train her to manage her menstrual hygiene, but the parents were not satisfied with the degree of remedy this would provide. Other options included institutionalization, hysterectomy, or giving Depo-Provera, a drug that would eliminate her periods. Each of these options involved potential harms to the patient; therefore, the physician had to weigh these risks against the family's need for assistance in caring for her. If the physician were to reject all these options, his responsibility to help the family would be unfulfilled.

A second reason for the modified-advocacy view is that failure to respect the family's interests can constitute a violation of important rights. An example is case 2.9, involving a brain-dead pregnant woman. One of the physician's options was to seek a court order for the sake of the fetal patient. Doing so, however, would infringe on the family's moral right to decide the disposition of the deceased daughter's body. Such a right is based on important moral concerns such as permitting the family to conduct its grieving in a manner it finds culturally and religiously familiar. Another example is case 2.10, in which spina bifida and hydrocephalus were detected in a fetus at thirty-five weeks gestational age. The obstetrician was faced with the question of what to do if the mother refused consent for a cesarean section. The fetus's condition was treatable, so the approach that would promote the interests of the fetus would be to seek a court order to perform a cesarean section. However, court-ordered surgery would violate important rights of the parents, including the mother's right to decide what happens to her body and the parents' right to participate in decisions concerning treatment of a fetus with serious deformities.

Third, there are circumstances in which usually weighty moral interests of the patient have questionable significance. In case 2.9 involving the brain-dead woman, for example, the moral status of the fetal patient at twenty-eight weeks gestational age was uncertain. Some would maintain—and others would deny— that the fetus has a right to life. Another example is case 2.8 involving the eleven-year-old girl whose parents requested a hysterectomy because of the problem of her menstrual hygiene. An objection to hysterectomies in such cases is that they violate the patient's right to reproduce. However, because of her retardation and other handicaps, it could be questioned whether she had a genuine moral interest in reproducing. Thus, while the physical risks of a hysterectomy procedure were clearly relevant to the decision in this case, it was unclear whether the right to reproduce should be considered.

Fourth, in some cases decisions that favor the patient prevent only minimal damage to the patient's interests while causing substantial harm to the family. Consider case 2.1, involving the daughter who insisted on treatment for her comatose mother. A decision to postpone withholding treatment for a couple of days would constitute only a minor delay in implementing the patient's wishes and was unlikely to cause pain or suffering, given her comatose state. However, failure to postpone seemed likely to result in significant psychological harm to the daughter. In another example, case 2.7, the mother of a mentally retarded twenty-one-year-old pregnant woman requested an abortion for her daughter. The patient's inability to consent to an abortion provided a reason not to perform it. However, the degree to which an abortion would infringe on the patient's interests was diminished by two factors. First, the physical risks of an early abortion would be less than the medical risks to her in carrying the fetus to term. Second, it was doubtful that she had a moral interest in procreating. On the other hand, if an abortion were not done, the mother would have the large burden of caring for the handicapped daughter and raising another child.

Fifth, in some cases, giving priority to the patient is unlikely to promote the patient's interests but is almost certain to harm the family, sometimes in serious ways. For example, in case 2.2 the parents refused treatment on religious grounds for an eighteen-month-old child with neuroblastoma. Although treatment against the family's wishes was an option, the probability that such action would promote the girl's interests was low. On the other hand, court-ordered treatment would put the family through the long ordeal of rigorous treatment for their child, while probably compromising the ability of the staff to provide needed support.

These considerations arising from the clinical and social circumstances of cases enable us to see a number of implications of the strict-advocacy view. One is that the physician's professional responsibilities to the family should be left unfulfilled whenever carrying them out would interfere with the patient's interests. Another is that the patient's interests should be given priority even when doing so violates important rights of the family. A third is that the patient's interests should have primacy even when there are reasonable grounds for questioning the significance of those interests in a particular case. A fourth is that actions on behalf of the patient should be pursued even though they prevent only minimal injury to the patient's interests while causing great harm to the family. Yet another implication is that the patient should be given priority even though the likelihood of advancing the patient's interests is low while harm to the family is nearly certain.

The above considerations call into question the justifiability of the view that the patient always comes first. In addition, there are responses that can be made to the arguments supporting this view. Consider Abrams's arguments that the high value we assign to autonomy justifies such an approach. One objection would point to the other moral values whose promotion can be in conflict with maximizing patient autonomy, such as the well-being and rights of the family, the well-being of the patient, and the physician's responsibilities to the family. Abrams's argument assumes that the good to be achieved in attempting to promote the patient's autonomy always outweighs whatever injury would befall the family. However, it is not clear that this is so, as illustrated by some of the cases in this chapter. Certainly, a defense of that assumption would be needed in order for Abrams's argument to be successful. A second response to her argument is that patients do not always have significantly diminished autonomy. Her argument focuses on situations of serious chronic illness or catastrophic acute illness, in which impaired autonomy is a characteristic feature. However, many encounters between doctor and patient occur in other circumstances, such as the primary care setting. An example in which autonomy is not significantly impaired might involve a competent adult who learns that he is a carrier of a genetic disease and insists on concealing this information from his family. Furthermore, in some cases of chronic illness in which the patient's autonomy is impaired, the chance that a more autonomous state can be achieved is virtually nonexistent. Examples include the comatose patient in case 2.1 and the severely mentally retarded patient in case 2.7. Why, it might be asked, should Abrams's argument apply to cases such as these?

One response to the utilitarian argument is that it applies only to patients who have the capacities to trust their physician, to follow their physician's advice, or to seek medical care in the first place. However, some patients do not have these capacities, one example being very young children. It might be thought that the utilitarian argument can be applied to the parents of child patients, but this approach is not successful either. The utilitarian goals of encouraging parents to seek medical care for their children and to trust pediatricians and follow their medical advice would seem to be promoted as well if not better by alternative principles, such as giving priority to the child's interests unless doing so violates rights of the parents, in which case doing what the parents wish.[50] Thus, the utilitarian argument does not establish that the interests of patients should always come first. At best, it could yield such a conclusion only concerning patients having the capacities in question.

Even with regard to patients having the relevant capacities, however, the argument can be questioned. Such utilitarian considerations seem to provide a good reason for a *prima facie* obligation to the patient but not a convincing reason for an absolute duty. Awareness that physicians *normally* put their patients first would seem to result in greater benefits for society compared to a state of affairs in which, for example, it is generally recognized that physicians are usually not advocates for their patients. The question is whether the added amount of compliance and medical care that would result from an absolute principle of patient advocacy being generally followed, as opposed to a *prima facie* principle, would yield a net benefit to society when the added adverse consequences for families are taken into account. An assumption of the utilitarian argument is that the increment in harm to families would not be greater than the increment in benefit to patients. However, it is not clear that this would be so. An adequate defense of this key empirical assumption would be needed in order for the argument to be successful.

Consideration of the clinical and social factors discussed above suggests a way of formulating the modified-advocacy view. This formulation involves two main elements. First, for each type of situation, it requires identification of the morally relevant factors pertaining to the interests of patient and family. For example, in cases of parental refusal of treatment needed by their child, several factors have a bearing on the child's interests, such as the magnitude of the harm to the child which treatment aims to prevent and the likelihood that action in opposition to the parents' wishes will prevent that harm. Factors pertaining to the family's interests include the magnitude of potential harm to the family resulting from such opposition and the likelihood that such harm would occur. Second, decisions are made by weighing the factors pertaining to the patient against those relating to the family. This approach gives careful consideration to the degree to which the various factors are present in an individual case. Thus, in the example of parental refusal of treatment, the greater the likelihood that treatment will prevent harm to the patient, the stronger the argument for opposing the parents' wishes. On the other hand, the greater the magnitude of the harm to the family, the less compelling is the argument for doing what is best for the patient. If the likelihood that treatment would prevent harm to the patient were relatively low but the expected harm to the family in providing the treatment were relatively large, one might be justified in giving priority to a family's refusal.

Adoption of such an approach is consistent with the view that the physician's primary obligations are owed to the patient. One could continue to hold that there is a *prima facie* obligation to put the patient's interests first. One might even hold that it is a very strong *prima facie* obligation, overridden only when a clear and forceful argument can be made for doing so.

We have identified two opposing views concerning resolution of conflicts between the physician's duty to the patient and the interests of the patient's family—the strict-advocacy view and an alternative that attempts to balance the conflicting values in individual cases. Each of these views has strengths and shortcomings. The main advantage of the strict-advocacy view is its conceptual simplicity, which permits its application in clinical situations to frequently yield a straightforward answer concerning what ought to be done. Thus, this approach is the easier of the two to apply and produces conclusions that are often clear-cut within its own framework.[51] A corollary to its simplicity is the fact that it is psychologically easier on the physician, in that it eliminates many moral conflicts. As Abrams puts it, "If one has a single clear goal or end point, moral conflicts are not as perplexing or agonizing."[52] Although psychological ease does not constitute a moral argument for this approach, it may help account for its attractiveness. The main weakness of the strict-advocacy view is that it fails to give adequate attention to all of the morally relevant considerations, yielding conclusions that sometimes are at odds with our moral intuitions about what ought to be done. For example, as the potential benefit to the patient decreases and the expected harm to the family that would occur in giving priority to the patient increases, it becomes less plausible to assert that the patient's interests should nevertheless take precedence. Such moral intuitions indicate that the strict-advocacy view oversimplifies the moral dimensions of these conflicts.

The major strength of the modified-advocacy view is that it maintains consistency with these moral intuitions by genuinely taking into account the moral considerations pertaining to the family. Its main shortcoming is that it sometimes does not yield clear-cut solutions. Whereas the strict-advocacy approach provides a simple prioritizing rule which easily resolves conflicts between patient and family, the modified-advocacy view requires balancing the morally relevant factors pertaining to the patient and family. It might not provide definitive solutions in gray-area cases where it is unclear whose interests should have priority. Thus, within the framework of this approach there is greater room for disagreement, and the task of giving reasons to support one's decision is more difficult.

As the above considerations suggest, the problem of how to assign priorities to the interests of patient and family in various situations is a difficult one. Yet the way in which a physician weighs these conflicting interests can have significant consequences for patients and families, as illustrated by the cases in this chapter. Further debate on the pros and cons of various approaches appears to be needed, given the potential impact of these decisions on individual patients and their families.

Notes

1. A *stroke* is a rupture or blockage of a blood vessel in the brain which deprives part of the brain of its blood supply and results in loss of consciousness, paralysis, or other symptoms, depending on the location and degree of brain damage.
2. Full-term gestation is thirty-eight to forty weeks; therefore, this infant was about five weeks premature.

3. Placenta previa refers to a placenta located in the lower uterine segment, so that it partially or completely covers the cervical opening. Dilation of the cervix can cause tearing of placental tissue and bleeding. Hemorrhage on the fetal side of the placenta can cause fetal death or brain damage as a result of asphyxia. When placenta previa is diagnosed during labor, cesarean section is necessary to save the fetus's life and minimize maternal bleeding.
4. The normal range of fetal heart rate is 120 to 160 beats per minute. A low heart rate (bradycardia), if severe and prolonged, can cause death or brain damage from poor oxygenation. Epinephrine (adrenaline) stimulates the heart to beat faster.
5. Hyaline membrane disease is a lung disease of premature infants associated with the immaturity of their lungs. It impairs the process of oxygenation of the blood and is life-threatening.
6. The hematocrit is the volume percentage of red blood cells in whole blood. Following hemorrhage, extravascular fluid normally enters the bloodstream, with lowered hematocrit as a result.
7. See, for example, N. N. Finer et al., "Hypoxic Ischemic Encephalopathy in Term Neonates: Perinatal Factors and Outcome," *Journal of Pediatrics* 98 (1981): 112–17; Joseph B. McMenamin, Gary D. Shackelford, and Joseph J. Volpe, "Outcome of Neonatal Intraventricular Hemorrhage with Periventricular Echodense Lesions," *Annals of Neurology* 15 (1984): 285–90.
8. The U.S. Department of Health and Human Services issued regulations in April 1985 implementing the Child Abuse Amendments of 1984. According to these regulations, life-supporting treatment may be withheld only if (1) the infant is irreversibly comatose, (2) attempts to prolong life would be futile, or (3) attempts to prolong life would be virtually futile and inhumane. See Department of Health and Human Services, "Child Abuse and Neglect Prevention and Treatment Program; Final Rule," *Federal Register* 50 (April 15, 1985), pp. 14,877–901.
9. See, for example, Ann Gath, "The Impact of an Abnormal Child upon the Parents," *British Journal of Psychiatry* 130 (1977): 405–10; Jean Holroyd and Donald Guthrie, "Stress in Families of Children with Neuromuscular Disease," *Journal of Clinical Psychology* 35 (1979): 734–39.
10. Studies of parental reactions include Dennis Drotar et al., "The Adaptation of Parents to the Birth of an Infant with a Congenital Malformation: A Hypothetical Model," *Pediatrics* 56 (1975): 710–17; Nan Johns, "Family Reactions to the Birth of a Child with a Congenital Abnormality," *Medical Journal of Australia* 7 (1971): 277–82.
11. M. Zelnick and J. F. Kantner, "Sexual Activity, Contraceptive Use and Pregnancy among Metropolitan-Area Teenagers: 1971–1979," *Family Planning Perspectives* 12 (1980): 230–37.
12. I. D. Rotkin, "A Comparison Survey of Key Epidemiological Studies in Cervical Cancer Related to Current Searches for Transmissible Agents," *Cancer Research* 33 (1973): 1353–67. The causal relationship between early intercourse and cervical cancer is unknown at present. There is evidence that *Herpesvirus Hominus* type 2 and papillomaviruses, which are sexually transmissible, may be carcinogenic agents. An associated factor is that there is an increased amount of cellular replication in the cervix during adolescence, which may make the cervix especially susceptible to the influence of carcinogens. If viral infections are part of the cause, then having multiple sex partners at an early age would also increase the risk for cervical cancer.

13. Hydrocephalus is an excessive accumulation of cerebrospinal fluid in the brain, which can result in head enlargement.
14. *Code of Federal Regulations,* Title 42, Chapter IV, sections 441.203, 441.205.
15. Ibid., section 441.205.
16. In the dilatation and evacuation procedure, the cervix is widened (dilated) by inserting a series of progressively larger metal instruments. The fetus is then removed through the cervical opening by forceps and suction.
17. H. K. Atrash et al., "Legal Abortion Mortality in the United States: 1972 to 1982," *American Journal of Obstetrics and Gynecology* 156 (1987): 610. The figure cited is for the eleven-year period 1972–1982.
18. National Center for Health Statistics, "Advance Report of Final Mortality Statistics, 1981," *Monthly Vital Statistics Report* 33, Supplement, June 22, 1984. The figure cited is for 1981.
19. See, e.g., B. J. Tew, H. Payne, and K. M. Laurence, "Must a Family with a Handicapped Child Be a Handicapped Family?" *Developmental Medicine and Child Neurology* 16, Supplement 32, (1974): 95.
20. *Physician's Desk Reference,* 42d ed. (Oradell, N.J.: Medical Economics, 1988), p. 2123.
21. Richard Lincoln, "The Pill, Breast and Cervical Cancer, and the Role of Progestogens in Arterial Disease," *Family Planning Perspectives* 16 (March–April 1984): 55–63.
22. *Stump et al.* v. *Linda Sparkman and Leo Sparkman,* 435 US 349, 55 L Ed 2d 331, 98 S Ct 1099, 1978.
23. One of the purposes of monitoring blood pressure in the pulmonary artery is to enable the physician to add fluid to the bloodstream to elevate blood pressure without adding so much as to produce fluid congestion in the lungs.
24. A. M. Sadler, Jr., B. L. Sadler, and E. B. Stason, "The Uniform Anatomical Gift Act," *Journal of the American Medical Association* 206 (1968): 2501–6 (see secs. 2 and 3 of the act).
25. *Raleigh Fitkin–Paul Morgan Memorial Hospital* v. *Anderson,* 42 N.J. 421, 201 A. 2d 537 (1964) cert. denied, 337 U.S. 985 (1964).
26. See, e.g., *Jefferson* v. *Griffin Spalding Co. Hospital Authority,* 247 Ga. 86, 274 S.E. 2d 457 (1981).
27. David C. McCullough and Lynn A. Balzer-Martin, "Current Prognosis in Overt Neonatal Hydrocephalus," *Journal of Neurosurgery* 57 (1982): 378–83.
28. John Mealey, Jr., Richard L. Gilmor, and Michael P. Bubb, "The Prognosis of Hydrocephalus Overt at Birth," *Journal of Neurosurgery* 39 (1973): 348–55; John Lorber, "Results of Treatment of Myelomeningocele: An Analysis of 524 Unselected Cases, with Special Reference to Possible Selection for Treatment," *Developmental Medicine and Child Neurology* 13 (1971): 279–303.
29. Ibid.
30. McCullough and Balzer-Martin, "Current Prognosis"; Mealey, Gilmor, and Bubb, "The Prognosis."
31. If the attempt to induce labor failed, there would be an added reason to perform a cesarean section. The process of inducing labor includes rupture of the amniotic membrane, because this is believed to stimulate uterine contractions. However, the amniotic sac is a natural barrier to microorganisms present in the vagina, and a fetus that remains in utero after rupture of the membrane faces a significant risk of

infection. Therefore, a cesarean section would also be indicated to prevent fetal infection.
32. J. A. Pritchard and P. C. MacDonald, *Williams Obstetrics,* 16th ed. (New York: Appleton-Century-Crofts, 1976), pp. 1082–83; J. R. Evrard and E. M. Gold, "Cesarean Section and Maternal Mortality in Rhode Island," *Obstetrics and Gynecology* 50 (1977): 594–97; G. L. Rubin et al., "Maternal Death after Cesarean Section in Georgia," *American Journal of Obstetrics and Gynecology* 139 (1981): 681–85.
33. W. A. Bowes et al., "Breech Delivery: Evaluation of the Method of Delivery on Perinatal Results and Maternal Morbidity," *American Journal of Obstetrics and Gynecology* 135 (1979): 965–73.
34. *Raleigh Fitkin–Paul Morgan Memorial Hospital* v. *Anderson; Jefferson* v. *Griffin Spalding Co. Hospital Authority.*
35. *White* v. *Yup,* 85 Nev. 527, 458 P.2d 617 (1969); *Vaillancourt* v. *Medical Center Hosp.,* 425 A.2d 92 (Vt. 1980).
36. We use the term *interests* to refer not only to a person's well-being but to all of a person's moral interests, including interests in having one's autonomy and rights respected.
37. World Medical Association, "Declaration of Geneva," *World Medical Journal* 3 (1956): 10–12. Similarly, the International Code of Medical Ethics requires that "Any act, or advice which could weaken physical or mental resistance of a human being may be used only in his interest." See *World Medical Association Bulletin* 1 (October 1949): 109, 111.
38. Arnold Relman, "Treating Children without Parental Consent," in M. Basson, ed., *Troubling Problems in Medical Ethics* (New York: Allen Liss, 1981), p. 109.
39. Mildred Stahlman, "Ethical Dilemmas in Perinatal Medicine," *Journal of Pediatrics* 94 (1979): 519. Contrary to Stahlman's assertion, the Hippocratic oath does not state explicitly that the physician's first responsibility is to act in the best interests of the patient, nor does it address the interests of parents and society. As Veatch points out, the historical roots of the view that only the interests of the patient are to be considered are obscure at present. See Robert Veatch, *A Theory of Medical Ethics* (New York: Basic Books, 1981), p. 155.
40. Albert Jonsen and Andrew Jameton, "Social and Political Responsibilities of Physicians," *Journal of Medicine and Philosophy* 2 (1977): 376–400.
41. American College of Physicians, Ad Hoc Committee on Medical Ethics, "American College of Physicians Ethics Manual," *Annals of Internal Medicine* 101 (1984): 131.
42. Jonsen and Jameton, "Social and Political Responsibilities," pp. 382, 383.
43. Solomon Papper, *Doing Right: Everyday Medical Ethics* (Boston: Little, Brown, 1983), p. 6.
44. Hans Jonas, "Philosophical Reflections on Experimenting with Human Subjects," *Daedalus* (1969): 238 (emphasis added).
45. President's Commission for the Study of Ethical Problems in Medicine and Biomedical and Behavioral Research, *Deciding to Forego Life-Sustaining Treatment* (Washington, D.C.: U.S. Government Printing Office, 1983), pp. 218, 219. A similar position was recently taken by the American Academy of Pediatrics Committee on Bioethics. See its report, "Treatment of Critically Ill Newborns," *Pediatrics* 72 (1983): 565–66.
46. See, e.g., Tom Beauchamp and Laurence McCullough, *Medical Ethics: The Moral*

Responsibilities of Physicians (Englewood Cliffs, N.J.: Prentice-Hall, 1984), p. 133; Veatch, *A Theory of Medical Ethics,* pp. 155, 156.
47. Natalie Abrams, "Scope of Beneficence in Health Care," in Earl Shelp, ed., Beneficence and Health Care (Boston: D. Reidel, 1982), pp. 183–98.
48. Ibid., p. 197.
49. Veatch states and opposes this argument in *A Theory of Medical Ethics,* pp. 155, 156.
50. We are not advocating this principle, but we cite it in order to point out the shortcomings of the utilitarian argument.
51. This is not meant to imply that there is always a clear answer to the question of what action would best promote the interests of the patient. Some of the problems involved in making such a determination are explored in chapter 3.
52. Abrams, "Scope of Beneficence," p. 196.

3
Deciding for Others

3.1 A Bedridden and Cognitively Impaired Elderly Patient

James A., an eighty-year-old man, was brought to the emergency room because he was having difficulty breathing. A medical workup revealed that he was dehydrated, malnourished, and anemic and had a urinary tract infection. The breathing problem was a result of pneumonia of his left lung. He was accompanied by one of his daughters, Olivia, who reported that he had "slowed down" considerably during the past two years. She said that his appetite had decreased markedly, that he had lost weight, and that his sight had worsened so much that she considered him blind. Before a previous hospital admission two months earlier, he had been ambulatory and was living with his seventy-eight-year-old wife. Following that hospitalization he had been taken to Olivia's home. She said that since then he "hadn't done anything"—he had not eaten, walked, or talked. He stayed in bed all the time, hardly moving, and was fed by a nasogastric tube that had been placed when he was in the hospital. His immobility had caused contractures of both legs and several decubitus ulcers.[1] His legs were bent at the knees and were in an immobile position with the heels near the buttocks.

In the hospital his treatment included antibiotics for the infections, three units of packed red blood cells for the anemia, and a Foley catheter to collect his urine. Fluids, electrolytes, and multivitamins were provided by an IV line, and feedings were given via a nasogastric tube. Nursing care for the ulcers included washing them with hydrogen peroxide and turning the patient every three hours.

Although James was conscious, his interaction with others was minimal. When staff members talked to him or asked him questions, he would not respond in any way. When awake, he would simply lie in bed and stare at the wall. Another of his daughters, Amelia, said that he had spoken briefly when she was present, but she could not understand what he said. During two of her subsequent visits he had not spoken at all. The physician found that the patient would react only to stimuli that ordinarily would be deeply painful. After several days of nutrition and hydration therapy, there was no improvement in mental status or physical activity. His internist believed that the patient had a type of chronic brain syndrome known as senile dementia, in which there is a decline in mental functioning caused by atrophy of brain cells. It was very unlikely that there would be a significant recovery of his cognitive functions. Senile dementia involves progressive degeneration and is eventually fatal. The average survival time after onset is about five years.

Although James had twelve children, only his wife and daughters Olivia and Amelia lived in the same city as the patient. In addition to taking care of James, Olivia was raising three children. She worked as a maid for a motel chain, and her husband was deceased.

The physician discussed the patient's condition with the wife and two daughters. He explained that the patient would probably survive with continued treatment, but it was highly unlikely that he would regain a capacity for independent living. In fact, significant improvement in mental status and ability to interact with others was doubtful. The physician then asked if the patient had ever expressed any wishes concerning life-prolonging treatment if he were to become seriously debilitated, but family members could not recall any such discussion.

Because the patient's prognosis seemed poor in terms of quality of life, the physician was faced with two difficult and closely related questions. First, would continued treatment be in his best interests? In particular, the physician wondered if the antibiotic treatment of the pneumonia was truly in his interests. Before the introduction of modern antibiotics, pneumonia had been referred to as "the old man's friend." Perhaps the most humane thing would be to allow the pneumonia to take its course. Second, should he raise the question of withdrawing the antibiotics with the family, and, if so, should he make a recommendation or give the family an opportunity to make the decision with minimal influence from him?

The physician's options included the following: (1) continue to treat the pneumonia and provide all measures necessary to maintain life; (2) recommend withdrawing the antibiotics and, if the family agrees, then withdraw them; (3) continue to treat the pneumonia but recommend to the family that resuscitative efforts not be carried out if a respiratory arrest occurs, and, if the family concurs, write a "Do not resuscitate" order; or (4) explain the various options and tell the family he will do whatever they want.

The question of whether treatment would promote the well-being of the patient was central to the physician's quandary. One aspect of this question concerned what weight, if any, should be given to various factors indicative of the patient's quality of life, such as the patient's ability to have affective relationships with other persons; the degree to which the patient's cognitive abilities are impaired; the ability to formulate and carry out plans and daily activities; and the extent to which the patient experiences pleasures and pains. Admittedly, it was difficult at that time to determine what James was experiencing. There was little indication that he was having any pleasurable experiences. It was also unclear how painful the contractures and decubitus ulcers were to him. Responsive only to deep pain stimuli, he might be experiencing very little discomfort.

If treatment would be in the patient's best interests, that would constitute strong support for option 1. If, however, the interests of the patient were unclear, then other considerations might gain in importance. One of these was the well-being of the family. James would need considerable care if he survived, and the attempt to provide care at home could be a large burden for the family. Although relief could be provided by sending the patient to a nursing home, a continuation of the patient's condition in a nursing home could itself exact an emotional toll on the family.

The autonomy of the family was another important consideration. Although option 4 seemed the one that most fully respected family autonomy, options 2 and 3 also gave substantial weight to this concern.

Another factor was the physician's own well-being, which could be affected by legal ramifications. The lack of clear legal rules about withholding treatment made it uncertain what was legally permitted. If the patient were allowed to die by the withdrawal of antibiotics and that was reported by someone to the local prosecutor, there would be a risk of criminal prosecution. On the other hand, several recent court decisions could be interpreted as supporting the withdrawal of antibiotics in at least some cases.[2] Even so, whether such interpretations would actually provide a successful legal defense was unclear. Although the likelihood of criminal prosecution seemed low, the magnitude of the potential adverse impact on the physician was great enough to make this a real consideration.

If the possibility of withholding treatment were discussed with the family, another issue concerned the manner in which the topic should be presented. The physician wanted to avoid placing the entire burden of the decision on the family, because he believed it could later produce feelings of guilt if they decided to let their loved one die. He was inclined, therefore, to avoid laying out the options and asking the family to decide. He believed he could provide emotional support to the family by assuming part of the burden of the decision. These considerations supported making a recommendation concerning treatment and giving the family an opportunity to accept or reject it.

3.2 Who Should Decide for a Patient in Persistent Vegetative State?

A thirty-nine-year-old woman had been having pain in her abdomen during the previous month. An ultrasound examination revealed stones in her gallbladder, and she was admitted to the hospital for surgical removal of the gallbladder. She had a history of diabetes mellitus and suffered one of its complications, autonomic neuropathy (damage to the autonomic nervous system, which controls involuntary bodily functions). In her case the nerve damage symptoms included orthostatic hypotension (lowering of blood pressure upon standing) and gastroparesis (decreased stomach motility) resulting in delayed gastric emptying.

During administration of anesthesia in the operating room, her heart rate dropped far below normal, and she suffered a cardiac arrest. Efforts to resuscitate were immediately begun. Atropine and epinephrine were given to stimulate the heart, while artificial breathing was provided using oxygen and a hand-held squeeze bag. Cardiopulmonary resuscitation eventually restored the patient's heartbeat and blood pressure, and a continuous infusion of isoproterenol was begun to continue stimulating the heart. The surgery was aborted, and the patient was taken to the intensive care unit, where respirator treatment was begun.

In the ICU the patient was only partially responsive. She would grip hard upon command, responded to noxious stimuli, and could flex and extend her arms, but otherwise she seemed unconscious. An electroencephalogram was abnormal, indicating moderate to severe cerebral injury caused by the reduced oxygenation that occurred when her heart stopped beating.

The cardiac arrest had been quite unexpected in this relatively young woman who, except for gallstones and diabetes, appeared to be in fairly good health. The arrest was not caused by error in the administration of anesthesia but was a rare and unpredictable reaction to the anesthetic drug. A consultant suggested that although the cause was unknown, her autonomic neuropathy might have played a role.

After two weeks she no longer responded to commands or performed purposive behavior. In response to stimuli that ordinarily would be painful, she grimaced and exhibited decerebrate posturing of her arms.[3] She would withdraw her legs somewhat to such stimuli. Although her pupils were not reactive to light, she blinked when loud noises occurred. She also had roving eye movements, which can occur when there is severe brain damage. Such eye movement is not purposive behavior, and there was no evidence of visual perception. The consulting neurologist stated that these signs and the lack of improvement during two weeks strongly suggested that the patient was in a persistent vegetative state, in which there is brain-stem function but absence of activity of the higher brain. In this condition there are sleep-wake cycles and occasional bodily movements and moaning. However, such patients irreversibly lack awareness.

Although it was possible that the patient was not in a persistent vegetative state, the few patients who have regained consciousness after a prolonged period of unconsciousness have been severely disabled. Although the degree of permanent injury has varied, it has typically included inability to speak or see, distortion of the limbs, and paralysis.[4] Because there was brain-stem function, this patient was legally alive.

Although she no longer required respiratory support and had been moved to a ward, her care involved antibiotics for pneumonia, and she was being fed by means of a nasogastric tube. Blood levels of glucose (sugar), albumin (protein), and electrolytes such as potassium were being monitored in order to prevent harmful levels. The patient was being turned in her bed periodically to prevent pressure sores. A jejunostomy[5] was also being considered because the nasogastric tube feedings were not effectively providing nutrition as a result of the patient's gastroparesis.

The patient's husband and eleven-year-old son had been at her bedside frequently since the cardiac arrest. The physician discussed the poor prognosis with the husband and explained that a decision would have to be made concerning continuation of treatment. After it was determined that the patient's wishes were not known, the physician recommended that no aggressive efforts be continued. The husband, however, was unwilling to accept this approach, claiming that there was still a chance she would recover. He said that if God wanted her to get well, she would. Although he was willing to forgo cardiopulmonary resuscitation if she had another cardiac arrest, he wanted everything else provided, including respirator treatment if needed, antibiotics for the pneumonia, and monitoring of blood levels. This expression of denial concerning the poor prognosis was not his first. Unlike everyone else, he had repeatedly insisted that his wife responded to commands. For example, he would claim that his wife moved her fingers, even though nurses who were also observing saw no movement.

Treatment was continued while an effort was made to counsel the husband. If he could be brought to accept the poor prognosis, then he might agree to withholding aggressive treatment. A second neurological consultation confirmed the diagnosis of persistent vegetative state. After this corroborating report, the patient's son no longer visited frequently, but the husband continued to be at the hospital most of the time. Continuing efforts to help the husband overcome his denial were unsuccessful. It became apparent that his attitude reflected more than a simple psychological defense mechanism. Rather, his firm conviction that his wife might recover was based on strong religious beliefs. He belonged to a church whose tenets give prominence to belief in divine providence and do not accept medical prognosis at face value. He believed that God might heal her, and his faith required him to maintain this hope.

The medical and nursing staff were very concerned because of the apparent futility of continued treatment and the potential financial burden to the family. Although the patient's insurance would pay for hospital costs, home care or a nursing home would be more appropriate if her acute medical problems were resolved. The husband had decided against home care. He was concerned about the impact on the eleven-year-old son of the wife being in the home in her condition. He also thought that the amount of care she required would be more than he could handle. If the patient were transferred to a nursing home, the insurance would pay for only the first one hundred days.

The physician and nurses responded to several complications in the patient's condition. The patient's blood level of protein had dropped markedly, because of poor nutrition caused by her gastroparesis. The low protein caused pronounced edema, so treatment with an intravenous infusion of albumin (protein) was necessary.[6] Because the patient's nutritional status was deteriorating, the jejunostomy operation was performed. As a complication of her diabetes, there were wide swings in her blood sugar, including hypoglycemic episodes (low blood sugar), which required administration of glucose and close monitoring.[7] In addition, the patient began to develop pressure sores which required daily cleansing.

Because the husband and physician had different views concerning continuation of treatment, a central question concerned whose wishes should be followed. Transferral to a nursing home was not a viable option at that time because the patient's acute problems required hospital care. Alternatives available to the physician included the following: (1) Inform the husband that he will provide supportive measures such as nursing care for bed sores. However, life-sustaining procedures such as correcting blood levels and respirator treatment would not be employed. (2) Do what the husband wants, providing all lifesaving measures except cardiopulmonary resuscitation. (3) Follow the course previously recommended without telling the husband this is being done. (4) Attempt to negotiate a compromise approach with the husband.

In decision making for incompetent patients, the self-determination and well-being of the patient normally have priority. Given the goal of promoting these values, several considerations support the customary approach of permitting the patient's family to be the surrogate decision maker. First, the family is usually most knowledgeable about the wishes and values of the patient. Second, the family is usually most concerned about the patient's welfare. There are two widely recognized exceptions to this customary approach, but neither was applicable in this case. First, if the patient were unavoidably dying, the physician would not need the consent of next of kin to withdraw aggressive therapy; but in this case it could not be concluded that the patient was dying. Second, it is sometimes proper to override a next of kin's decision that is clearly contrary to the patient's interests; but this patient's lack of consciousness made it doubtful that continued treatment would cause pain or other harm to her.

However, when patients are irreversibly unconscious and their wishes are unknown, there are considerations opposing the approach of letting the family decide. It can be argued that life can benefit or harm someone only if the individual is conscious or has a potential for consciousness. Because irreversibly unconscious patients are beyond our capacity to affect their well-being, patient-centered values that the customary approach aims to promote cannot be affected. Moreover, allowing family decisions for continued treatment of irreversibly unconscious patients has two drawbacks. First, long-term treatment can negatively affect the family's well-being by prolonging emotional distress and causing financial hardship. Second, treatment can constitute a suboptimal allocation of the scarce time and resources of health professionals. There might be other patients with greater potential for recovery; therefore, spending a large amount of time with an irreversibly unconscious patient can diminish overall patient welfare. These considerations support option 1.

On the other hand, there are reasons for following the customary approach when patients are irreversibly unconscious. First, families are significant social units responsible for decisions intimately affecting their members. Encroachments of family autonomy should be very restricted concerning personal matters on which there is wide diversity of opinion in society. Some families might find significant meaning in the continued care of an unconscious loved one. To override such choices in order to prevent harm to families, it might be argued,

Deciding for Others 95

is unjustifiable paternalism. Second, if treatment is terminated before family members have worked out their acceptance of the loss of the patient, their adjustment might be more difficult after the patient's death. Respecting the family's wishes helps ensure that treatment is withdrawn only when the family is psychologically prepared. Thus, these considerations concerning family autonomy and well-being favor the family as final decision maker, thereby supporting option 2.

From the physician's point of view, legal considerations also favored the second option. The risk of a wrongful-death lawsuit later being initiated by the husband seemed much lower with this approach, compared to option 1. Admittedly, such a suit would be successful only if the physician had a legal duty to provide life-prolonging care, and the law is unclear concerning whether there is a duty to treat in such cases. Even if not successful, a suit would probably harm the physician, nurses, and hospital because of the time, expense, and stress involved in a legal defense.

Pros and cons could also be advanced concerning the third option. Like option 1, it might protect the family from harms involved in long-term care. Furthermore, if the husband were not aware that needed treatment was being withheld, then the risk of a lawsuit would be lessened. On the other hand, because the husband was present most of the time, he might realize that necessary treatment was not being given. An important consideration against this option is that it would be deceptive, because the intent would be to mislead the husband concerning treatment plans.

The fourth option would seek a compromise, such as continuing monitoring and correction of blood levels but withholding antibiotics if pneumonia occurred again. However, the husband's insistence on continued treatment suggested that he had compromised as much as he was willing in agreeing to no cardiopulmonary resuscitation. Moreover, a compromise might result in prolonged survival if the only complications that developed were ones it had been agreed would be treated.

3.3 Nasogastric Tube Feedings for an Elderly Stroke Patient

B.P., an eighty-six-year-old woman, was admitted to the hospital after a probable stroke. Her son, with whom she lived, reported that for two days she had been unable to speak or communicate and appeared to have decreased use of her left arm and leg, could not swallow food, and would choke when given water. Because she appeared to be dehydrated, an intravenous line was started to provide glucose and water.

The patient's health had steadily declined over the last three years. She had had several mild strokes impairing use of the limbs on both sides of her body. She had also suffered from retinal hemorrhages which were unsuccessfully treated with laser surgery. She was completely blind in one eye and could see only broken patterns or shapes with the other eye. In the last year, she had been diagnosed as having congestive heart disease and postural hypotension, a condition in which blood is not pumped in adequate quantities to the brain when the patient is upright, causing loss of consciousness. As a result, she had had several bad falls and was generally confined to bed.

The son told the attending physician that she had rapidly declined during the last six months. On some days, her orientation to person, place, and time was very poor. She had also had rather uncharacteristic mood swings, being frequently depressed and frustrated by her physical disabilities. A former teacher of French literature, she had avidly pursued her educational interests during retirement. But with the loss of her eyesight, she could no longer read or watch television. Her son said that on two separate occasions they had emotionally intense discussion in which his mother stated that the quality of her life was no longer acceptable. She said, "I cannot get around, I cannot watch television, I cannot read—what is life without such things?" She said that she had had "a beautiful life" but that she "couldn't live forever" and was "ready to die." However, she continued to conscientiously take her heart medications.

The assessment of a consulting neurologist was that B.P. suffered a serious blockage of the middle cerebral artery, resulting in the death of some brain tissue. The stroke had impaired various reflexes and muscular control on her left side, as well as her ability to swallow and speak. He estimated that there was only a one-in-four chance that B.P. would recover her ability to swallow. He was also pessimistic that she would recover her ability to speak or that her mental confusion would resolve.

The neurologist recommended that a nasogastric tube be placed to provide B.P. with adequate nutrition. Such a tube is inserted through the patient's nose, down the throat, and into the stomach and can be left in place indefinitely. The external end can be unclamped to insert essential nutrients in liquid form. Flexible tubes approximately 2.5 mm in diameter are normally used. Patients often find these tubes to be uncomfortable but rarely painful. Side effects of tube feedings include diarrhea, distension, vomiting, and imbalances of essential nutrients, but these problems can be resolved with appropriate changes in the content of the feedings or the procedures used to administer them. For patients who fail to recover the ability to swallow, a permanent tube is often surgically inserted through the stomach wall.

The attending physician discussed the neurologist's recommendation with B.P.'s son. He explained that the tube feedings might only be necessary temporarily, although they were not optimistic about his mother's chances for returning to her level of functioning before the latest stroke. The son quietly but firmly indicated that he did not believe that his mother would want the feeding tube. He said that it did not matter whether she might return to her previous level of functioning. In their private discussions, she had said that that level of functioning was no longer acceptable. Thus, even if only necessary on a temporary basis, the feeding tube could not make the quality of her life satisfactory. The physician decided to wait to see whether the patient's ability to swallow and speak might return spontaneously. In the meantime, the intravenous hydration and feeding of the patient (with sugar water) was continued.

Deciding for Others 97

After six days there was no sign that B.P. would recover her ability to speak or to swallow or that her mental confusion would resolve. The physician faced a difficult decision. The patient's son had insisted that his mother would not want the feeding tube. However, the patient had not made an informed decision to reject the feeding tube. Her wishes could only be inferred from statements about her desire to continue living. They might have only been expressions of her depression and frustration, as well as implicit requests for continuing support and assistance from her son. It was another step to the conclusion that she intended to refuse life-prolonging treatments. After all, she had continued to take her heart medication. Given doubt about her precise wishes, it might be appropriate to err on the side of sustaining life.

A second concern was that B.P.'s death did not appear imminent. This fact clearly distinguished her situation from that of the terminally ill patient whose death is inevitable within a few hours or days. In the latter case, the use of life-prolonging treatments is literally a useless, unjustifiable burden to the patient. But in B.P.'s present case, use of the feeding tube might sustain the patient's life for an indefinite period.

Indeed, this feature of the case generated considerable conflict. One resident said bluntly that the physician was discriminating against the patient based on her age. He said that the attending physician was assuming that nontreatment is acceptable for a person who is eighty-six years old, although he would probably sustain the life of a nondying patient with a similar condition who was thirty years younger. In effect, a decision not to insert the feeding tube reflected an unarticulated theory that an elderly person's life may be brought to an "appropriate" close.

A final concern related to the impact of nontreatment on the hospital staff. The attending physician thought that it would take about a week for the patient to die if the intravenous hydration were also discontinued. If the latter therapy were not also withdrawn, the patient might live for three weeks or longer. Consequently, the staff would be required to care for the patient for quite some time, watching her slowly deteriorate, without being able to provide further assistance. This situation might create considerable stress among the personnel responsible for the patient's care.

3.4 A Prolonged Stay in the Neonatal ICU

A male infant weighing two pounds two ounces was born at his mother's home in a rural area. The child was premature at twenty-nine weeks gestational age and suffered a cardiopulmonary arrest at birth. He was taken to the county emergency room and was put on a respirator. He survived, but his blood pH was below 7.0, indicating severe asphyxia. The child was transferred the same day to a regional neonatal intensive care unit.

The child did poorly in the unit. Soon after admittance his hematocrit[8] fell sharply, and there was marked decrease in physical movement. These signs suggested an intracranial hemorrhage, a development correlated with brain damage. At two weeks of age he still could not breathe on his own, a problem the attending physician believed reflected brain injury caused by asphyxia and hemorrhage. Standard drug treatment (theophylline) was begun to stimulate breathing. There was still relatively little physical movement. Subsequently, the infant developed bronchopulmonary dysplasia, a type of persisting lung damage caused by the prolonged respirator therapy. Also, a CT scan of the brain revealed a porencephalic cyst—a region in which there is an absence of brain tissue—in the left frontal area.

By two months of age the infant was off the respirator but continued to have numerous medical problems. He had apnea and bradycardia[9] two to eight times per nursing shift, and resuscitation by means of a hand-held squeeze bag was required about once every three to five days. A sample of spinal fluid contained blood, indicating another intracranial hemorrhage. There were occasional seizures, so the patient was put on phenobarbital. When oral feedings were attempted, it was found that the baby did not have a suck reflex, so feedings had to be continued by nasogastric tube. The infant could not swallow, resulting in the accumulation of secretions in his throat, so frequent tracheal suctioning was necessary to prevent suffocation. An endotracheal tube was inserted for suctioning and to facilitate use of the resuscitation bag. Two weeks of physical therapy directed at stimulating a sucking response had no success. Also, the infant developed contractures of the legs as a result of his inactivity. To help with this, the physical therapist carried out range-of-motion exercises regularly on the baby's legs.

The child's mother was twenty years old and lived with her own mother in a small house with electricity but no running water or telephone. Water was carried to the house from a nearby well, and the nearest telephone was at a neighbor's house approximately one mile away. The mother and grandmother had a car, but it was old and not very reliable. This infant was her second child. The father of the patient did not live with the mother, nor were they married. However, he described their relationship as very close. He worked in a nearby town, and they saw each other frequently.

From the outset, the family had shown considerable concern for the baby. A week after the infant was admitted, the father and grandmother visited the NICU while the mother was recovering from the recent childbirth at home. The grandmother was concerned about the infant's small size and asked whether he would survive. The resident said that the baby was still in critical condition but that there was hope for survival. Quality of life was not discussed. The grandmother said that the mother was depressed and anxious about the infant. After she recovered, the mother joined the grandmother in visits to the nursery on weekends. The father also visited when possible.

The mother had recently taken a job at a bread factory near her home. Unfortunately, this employment made her ineligible for Medicaid. The social worker applied for assistance from her state, but if the request were denied the charges would become the mother's responsibility and would probably have to be absorbed by the hospital.

Deciding for Others

A new resident took over the case and met with the parents to discuss discharge plans. He explained that although the infant was finally off the respirator, he was still having episodes of apnea and bradycardia, so someone at home would have to be able to resuscitate the infant with a bag resuscitator. Because he had heavy secretions in his throat, he would have to be suctioned regularly. Also, his feedings would have to be given by nasogastric tube. It was also explained that the infant had brain damage, but the possible ramifications of this were not discussed. The mother seemed to be somewhat overwhelmed by all of this but wanted the infant to return home. She was especially concerned about nasogastric tube feedings and preferred that he be taking feedings normally before discharge. The grandmother was concerned about their ability to care for the baby without running water or a phone. It was decided that they would try to learn how to carry out the necessary nursing care. This might take some time; they could come to the hospital only on weekends because of the distance involved.

The mother and grandmother continued to come in regularly on weekends to learn how to care for the infant, but they became increasingly doubtful that they would be able to provide adequate care. The social worker maintained contact with the father by phone. He seemed to be very interested in the baby and tried to visit on weekends. He told her that he had discussed the infant's problems with the mother and that they both wanted him to leave the hospital. However, neither parent believed they could provide the kind of care he would need.

At this point the attending physician began to have doubts about whether continued resuscitative efforts would be in the infant's best interests. His clinical experience with similar handicapped infants suggested that even if the infant remained alive until discharged from the NICU, he would probably not survive outside the unit. The degree of close, around-the-clock nursing care needed to maintain the child's breathing is typically found only in an intensive care unit. The neurologist who was consulted said that the prolonged lack of physical movement and absence of suck and swallow reflexes indicated severe brain damage. Although it was not possible to reliably predict the degree of impairment, it was highly probable that there would be serious retardation if the infant survived. He might never be able to walk.

The alternative courses of action for the attending physician included the following: (1) enter a do-not-resuscitate order into the chart; (2) enter an order permitting resuscitation by "bagging" but not by means of a respirator; (3) discharge the infant to home and provide an apnea monitor to alert the mother whenever the infant stopped breathing; (4) attempt to place the infant in an institution; or (5) allow the infant to remain in the NICU indefinitely, maintaining the present level of aggressive therapy.

The physician discussed the question of resuscitation with the parents and grandmother. They hoped the infant would live, but they did not know what to say about the use of "heroic" efforts. The father said that such decisions were up to the doctors because of their medical expertise.

The social worker tried to identify a facility in the infant's home state that could provide long-term care. One institution accepted such children, but only for thirty days. Another did not admit children below the age of five. Yet another could take the child for only twenty days. In short, no institution could be found to provide long-term care.

The social workers were in favor of telling the mother that the child was going to die and giving her the option of letting him die at home. The mother, however, rejected this option. She was unwilling to accept the child's death as inevitable and said that if he died at home she might feel responsible.

A conference of the NICU staff was held to decide what to do. Several persons were concerned about the infant staying in the NICU indefinitely. The cost of a bed alone was $275 per day. Additional costs arose for special treatments, drugs, and tests, of which there were many in this case. The question was raised of whether the hospital was obligated to continue providing such costly treatment.

But other staff members felt differently. One resident thought that too much emphasis was being placed on the intellectual potential of the child. He noted that a significant percentage of the unit's patients had handicaps but that treatment decisions were not made on that basis. He suggested that from the child's perspective, continued life might be beneficial in spite of retardation. Because the medical staff is supposed to protect the child's welfare, he also did not think that financial costs were relevant to the decision. Although he agreed that the child was likely to die, he favored the continuation of aggressive therapy.

A nurse participant was quite uncomfortable with the idea of withholding all resuscitative measures. She agreed that if the child could be kept alive only by frequent use of the artificial respirator, then it was not in his interest to have aggressive resuscitative efforts continued, because this meant he had no hope for life outside the NICU. On the other hand, she pointed out that it is everyday nursing practice in the unit to use the squeeze bag to restore spontaneous breathing. She felt that disallowing resuscitation by this means was, from a nursing standpoint, much like failure to feed the child—a denial of ordinary care. If ordinary care were all that the infant needed to be maintained alive, then it was surely in his interest to provide it.

But another resident said that if the case was genuinely hopeless, he did not see how any resuscitative measures could serve the child's interests.

As the hour for the conference drew to a close, the assembled staff failed to reach a consensus on the issue of resuscitation.

3.5 Deciding Treatment When the Preliminary Diagnosis Is Trisomy 18

A female infant was born four weeks prematurely, weighing three pounds fourteen ounces. She was having difficulty breathing, so she was taken to the intensive care nursery and given oxygen therapy. A physical examination revealed numerous congenital abnormalities, and a diagnosis of trisomy 18 syndrome[10] was suggested by the following: clenched hands, overlapping of the index fingers over the third fingers and the fifth fingers over the fourth, simian crease on one hand, "rocker-bottom" shaped feet with protruding heels, low-set malformed ears, organomegaly (enlarged internal organs), and a heart murmur. X-ray examination revealed an enlarged heart, confirming the presence of a heart defect, most likely a ventricular septal defect[11] or a coarctation (narrowing) of the aorta. In addition, the infant had an esophageal atresia, a condition in which the esophagus does not extend to the stomach. A geneticist was consulted, and he considered it highly likely that the tentative diagnosis was correct. However, confirmation required a karyotype, a photomicrographic representation of the chromosomes that would reveal the extra number 18 chromosome. Blood was drawn for the karyotyping, which would take approximately two weeks.

Newborns with trisomy 18 syndrome have a poor prognosis. Thirty percent die within the first month and 50 percent by two months. Approximately 10 percent survive the first year but are severely mentally impaired.[12] Death is usually sudden and caused by factors that are unknown, even after autopsy. In rare cases the extra chromosome is a partial one, a condition that can result in longer survival, sometimes to adulthood. In such cases there is less profound but nevertheless severe mental retardation.

Several life-support measures were being provided to the infant. Water containing dextrose and essential electrolytes (such as sodium and potassium) was being provided via an intravenous line. The levels of oxygen and carbon dioxide in the blood were being monitored frequently in order to provide appropriate oxygen therapy. The concentrations of various electrolytes in the blood were being monitored to prevent harmfully abnormal levels. Also, treatment was being provided for a rising level of bilirubin in the blood.

Bilirubin is a waste product normally broken down by the liver. Premature infants often have immature livers that do not adequately process the bilirubin, resulting in an accumulation in the blood. Excessive levels can result in brain damage or death. The infant was currently being treated using "bili lights," which decompose the bilirubin in capillaries near the surface of the skin. If this did not work, an exchange transfusion could be performed. In this procedure blood is removed from the infant and replaced with blood having a relatively low concentration of bilirubin.

Other life-support measures were being considered. First, because feeding by mouth was ruled out, intravenous nutrition would be required. Second, it was possible to surgically correct the esophageal atresia, thereby enabling the infant to take fluids and nutrition by mouth. Third, the heart defect would probably be amenable to surgical correction when the infant was somewhat older, if she survived.

The parents were informed of the infant's condition and poor prognosis. They and the physician wanted to do whatever would best promote the well-being of the infant, but it was not clear what action would do this. There were various options, including the following: (1) Provide all treatments, including surgical correction of the esophageal atresia, regardless of the karyotype results. (2) Until the results of the karyotype are obtained, provide all life-sustaining treatment except surgery. If trisomy 18 is confirmed, withhold all life-support measures except hydration and nutrition. (3) Until the karyotype results are obtained, withhold all lifesaving measures except hydration, nutrition, and oxygen. If trisomy 18 is confirmed, withhold all life-sustaining support. (4) Immediately withhold all life-sustaining support and keep the infant warm, dry, and as comfortable as possible.

The issue of what would be best for the infant involved a number of considerations. First, there were questions concerning which procedures were necessary to provide comfort. Would withholding fluids or nutrition cause discomfort? Would excessive bilirubin levels produce suffering? Unfortunately, the answers are unclear because it is difficult to ascertain what the intensive care nursery patient is experiencing. Some would claim that sensation is attenuated because a neonate's nervous system is not fully developed. Others have reported giving morphine when treatment is withheld to prevent discomfort.

Second, there was the question of whether quality-of-life considerations other than pain should enter into the decision. On one hand, it could be asserted that there are certain cognitive abilities that make life particularly beneficial to humans, such as self-reflection, the ability to formulate and carry out personal plans, and the ability to have interpersonal relationships. If the patient did not survive infancy, she would never develop these important benefit-conferring abilities. Thus, briefly prolonging her life would not yield significant benefits to her.

On the other hand, it might be argued that there is an obligation to provide life-support measures because of uncertainty concerning the infant's prognosis. The child might not have trisomy 18 or any other fatal syndrome. Given this uncertainty, it might be best for the infant to receive all life-support treatments, at least until the prognosis concerning survival and quality of life is more clearly known.

Others would argue that quality-of-life considerations should not influence the decision—that life should be preserved because it has inherent value. This sanctity-of-life viewpoint supports option 1. However, when this case occurred there were no government regulations requiring that quality-of-life considerations be excluded.[13]

In addition to the well-being of the infant, several other considerations were relevant to the decision. First, prolonged treatment could have a significant emotional impact on the family. During such treatment the family's experience might include frequent trips to the hospital, participation in difficult medical decisions affecting the well-being of their infant, constant worry about the infant's condition, and grief about her plight.[14]

Also, the financial expense of care might be significant. Because the infant was a Medicaid patient, a large portion of the costs would be paid by the government. If the infant were to remain in the intensive care nursery for a considerable time, the total costs could be high. A one-month stay, for example, might cost thirty-five thousand dollars or more.[15] Furthermore, it was uncertain how long the patient would require intensive care. If complications developed, the infant might remain in the hospital several months or longer.

Another consideration was the allocation of the nurses' and physicians' time.

If a large amount of time were devoted to this patient, the time available to care for others might be reduced. Assuming others have a greater chance for recovery, this could result in a failure to optimize overall patient benefit. For example, in exchange transfusions the blood is withdrawn and replaced in small increments. The procedure requires two persons, usually a nurse and physician, and takes approximately an hour and a half. The level of bilirubin in the blood may soon rise again, necessitating additional exchange transfusions. Thus, this procedure can require a significant investment of time. The view that such allocations are inappropriate supports options 3 and 4.

Even if certain procedures could ethically be withheld, some would argue that fluids and nutrition must be provided.[16] It might be claimed that the physician's action would be the cause of death by dehydration. As such, it would be indistinguishable from actively killing, such as by lethal injection. This would differ from situations in which the disease could be said to cause death, such as withholding cardiopulmonary resuscitation from a terminal patient. Because the rule of avoiding killing should always be followed,[17] withholding fluids and nutrition is impermissible. In reply, it could be argued that if it were not for the esophageal atresia, the infant would be given food and water by mouth. Thus, if death from dehydration occurs, the disease (esophageal atresia) would be a causal factor.

Another argument against withholding nutrition is that our sentiments and emotions cause us to be repelled by the thought of starving someone to death, even when it might be for the patient's own good. Thus, it might be claimed that there is a rule against allowing people to starve to death. In opposition to this view, it could be argued that fluids and nutrition would only extend the dying process, thereby prolonging the suffering of the infant and the parents. Because this would produce more harm than benefit, such treatment should not be provided.

3.6 Risk/Benefit Assessment of Surgery for a Child Suffering from Strokes

The patient was an eleven-year-old girl first seen at the pediatric medical center three years earlier. Her parents had noticed that A.C. had weakness on her left side and that her speech was unusually slow. This prompted them to take the child to a local pediatrician, in whose presence she suffered a focal seizure involving her left arm. He quickly made arrangements for her admission to the hospital. By the time the family arrived at the hospital, A.C. was having approximately one seizure per half-hour. The weakness of her arm and leg on the left side had progressed to partial paralysis, which also affected the left side of her face. Although her consciousness was not impaired, her speech was slow and labored. It was suspected that she had suffered a stroke.

Subsequent diagnostic assessment included cerebral angiography, a procedure allowing X-ray visualization of the arteries in the head. This test revealed a 60 percent narrowing (stenosis) of her right internal carotid artery, a major vessel supplying blood to the brain. There was also a mild stenosis of her middle cerebral artery, a major vessel supplying a portion of the brain controlling many sensory, motor, and cognitive functions. Although these obstructions accounted for her stroke, the cause of the arterial disease could not be determined. Other diagnostic results suggested that A.C. suffered from some underlying congenital abnormality. For example, she had an unusually short stature, a horseshoe-shaped left kidney, a small obstruction of the ureter from this kidney to her bladder, and she was slightly retarded. However, no recognized syndrome could be identified.

A.C. was one of four children. The family lived in a small, isolated farming community comprised primarily of two large extended families. There were numerous consanguinous marriages, including that of her parents. Although the family's farmhouse had inside plumbing, all water was provided by a well. The family had no radio or television and did not receive a newspaper. The father worked as a farm laborer, and neither he nor his wife had attended high school. A.C. had required special education during her first years in school but was later placed in regular classes. Her parents seemed to be very loving and concerned.

During the initial hospitalization, the child's seizures were controlled with high doses of Dilantin. Within three weeks, her left-sided paralysis resolved, and she was able to walk with a limp. Her recovery was progressing well, and it was therefore assumed that blood was now being adequately supplied by other vessels in her head. She was placed on a maintenance dose of Dilantin and discharged.

The child's condition remained unchanged for three years until she suffered another stroke. That morning, her parents observed weakness on her right side, inappropriately childish behavior, and much-decreased spontaneous communication. After they arrived at the hospital, she developed partial paralysis of her right leg and arm.

The new diagnostic assessment revealed complete closure (occlusion) of her left internal carotid artery (the other main vessel supplying the front of the head), with the former partial obstruction of the right internal carotid artery remaining stable. Although a specific cause for the child's disease had not been isolated, her neurologist thought that it was progressive and would ultimately cause her death. No effective medical therapy was available, so he requested an evaluation by the neurosurgery service.

After his review, the neurosurgeon met with the neurologist and attending pediatrician. He indicated that it was technically feasible to perform a surgical procedure (called a carotid endarterectomy) to remove the blockage from the unclosed carotid artery. This procedure involves opening the carotid artery and cutting the plaque and other foreign material away from the wall. He pointed out that endarterectomy for the completely occluded vessel was not recommended, because it has been found possible to remove the obstruction from an occluded vessel in only 10 percent of operative cases, while incurring the usual risk of operative mortality or morbidity. Nevertheless, opening the other carotid artery might improve the volume of blood reaching the key areas of the brain impaired by the child's strokes.

But the neurosurgeon expressed uncertainty about whether the risk/benefit ratio justified surgical intervention. On one hand, the child might not survive for long without surgical intervention. This concern was supported by available information about the "natural history" of vascular disease of this sort. In a fourteen-year study of carotid artery disease, patients with stenosis of one carotid artery and complete occlusion of the other were followed for an average of fifty-one months while receiving only medical therapy.[18] Of 103 patients, 5 died within the first two months, 3 as a result of severe strokes. Of the remaining 98 patients, 33 percent later suffered new strokes, and half were fatal. (At the termination of follow-up, 51 percent were dead from all causes.) The three physicians agreed that A.C.'s risk of soon having another stroke might even be higher, given the steady progression of her disease.

On the other hand, surgery posed clear risks for the patient. In the above-mentioned study, 108 patients with stenosis of one internal carotid artery and occlusion of the other were treated surgically. Twenty-eight percent died within two months after surgery, and 15 percent suffered grave complications. (By contrast, only 5 percent of the medically treated group succumbed during the first two months after admission to the study.) Although the actual degree of risk for these patients is now much lower, the fact that this patient had advanced carotid artery disease and had suffered two moderately disabling strokes suggested that her risk of surgical mortality or morbidity was significantly higher than the current risk (less than 2 percent) for patients who have no symptoms of stroke at the time of surgery. The neurosurgeon's opinion was that the operative risk of surgical mortality or morbidity was above 10 percent. The most serious danger was that the child might suffer another stroke as a result of surgery. This risk derived from the fact that normal blood flow is always somewhat interrupted during surgery, and this child's other carotid artery could not compensate for this reduction in blood flow to the brain, because it was completely occluded.

The second problem with surgery concerned its potential efficacy in altering the natural progression of the child's arterial disease. In the study already described, patients in both the surgical and nonsurgical treatment groups were followed for an average of fifty-one months. Leaving aside the 28 percent of the surgical patients who died within two months after surgery, long-term follow-up showed that 51 percent of the medically treated patients were dead at the end of the observation period, compared to 35 percent in the surgically treated group. Thus, patients incurred the risks of surgical mortality and morbidity in exchange for only a 16 percent improvement in overall survival for the four-year period after surgery. One interpretation of these findings is that surgical intervention often fails to alter the progress of the underlying vascular disease. As a result, blockage of arteries develops in other locations and produces fatal injuries. The aggressive nature of A.C.'s arterial disease suggested that she might fit into this category.

Subsequent to this meeting, the attending pediatrician had several conversations with the parents. He was very open in explaining the uncertainties about the child's care. The limited knowledge and education of the parents made it very difficult to convey the subtleties of the clinical assessment or to discuss the relevance of the statistical data. But the pediatrician was able to explain that serious dangers attended either course of action (surgery or nonsurgery) and that, even if successful, it was possible that the surgery might not significantly prolong their daughter's life.

On each occasion, the parents expressed deep concern and exhibited much emotional distress. But they did not offer any determinate opinion about what should be done. Rather, they were highly deferential to the physician's authority and conveyed a deep trust in his ability to handle their daughter's care in the most beneficial way. Quite clearly, they did not feel emotionally able or sufficiently knowledgeable to make a choice.

Thus, the decision fell squarely on the shoulders of the pediatrician, and there was much to consider. Successful surgical repair of the child's artery might lengthen her life somewhat, providing more time to share with her family. His professional inclination was to not stand idly by while the vascular disease caused progressive disability and eventual death. Nevertheless, he recognized that the surgery might actually have little impact on the rate at which the disease process compromised the child's quality of life. Moreover, if the most serious risks of the surgery materialized, they would be cutting short what precious time the child and her family might have together. There was much to be said for leaving the child and the family alone, allowing their lives together to go on normally as long as possible. How long this would be was hard to say; a catastrophic stroke might occur in five months or five years.

3.7 Responding to a Family's Decision for Laetrile

The patient was a fourteen-year-old girl who began having pain in her extremities several months before hospitalization. At first her parents thought these problems were "growing pains." Within four months, however, her pain was so severe that she began to limp. Her feet grew swollen, and she developed a low-grade fever. Two weeks later, the symptoms worsened with severe bruising, nosebleeds, and fatigue. She was finally brought to a local hospital and found to have acute lymphocytic leukemia. She was referred to a university hospital and entered a research treatment program.

Her treatment involved three stages: an initial period of intensive therapy with prednisone, vincristine, and daunomycin, designed to induce remission within four weeks; a two-week segment of radiation to protect the central nervous system from leukemic cells; and a thirty-month regimen of methotrexate and mercaptopurine to maintain the remission. She achieved complete remission of her disease within three weeks. After the radiation therapy, maintenance therapy proceeded uneventfully for eight months, until leukemic cells were found in her cerebrospinal fluid, indicating a relapse. Leukemic cells soon reappeared in her bone marrow.

It was clearly explained to her parents that because bone marrow relapse had occurred during therapy, it was no longer realistic to expect a cure for their daughter's cancer. (This judgment was based on the failure of almost all previous patients to achieve long-term, disease-free survival after bone marrow relapse during therapy.) Nevertheless, the girl's life might be extended for an additional two or three years if relapse therapies were effective. The family consented to the child's entry into a research study for relapsed patients, and she quickly achieved a complete second remission.

About four months later, during the maintenance phase of her relapse therapy, the patient and her mother came to the outpatient clinic for a regular checkup. The mother revealed that after the initial relapse, she had decided to take her daughter to Mexico for laetrile treatments. The mother said she had a vision in which God told her she must take her child to Mexico to save her life. She had also been encouraged by friends and relatives to seek these treatments. The patient had received two months of therapy in Mexico while also taking her regular chemotherapy.

The new treatment program consisted of laetrile, "metabolic" therapy, rectal enzymes, and a special diet. She was currently taking a 0.5 gram tablet of laetrile four times each day. The "metabolic" therapy involved megadoses of vitamins A, B, C, and E, as well as pancreatic enzymes. The diet involved restrictions of dairy products, meats, refined-flour products, salt, and caffeine-containing substances. It encouraged fresh fruits and vegetables, whole-grain breads and cereals, and nuts such as almonds.

The decision to try laetrile was accompanied by a noticeable change in the mother's attitude. After her daughter's relapse, she seemed to expect the worst outcome in every respect. She often expressed fears that she had done something to cause her daughter's problems. She constantly sought advice from all staff members about her daughter's condition and care and required constant reassurance about the usefulness of what was being done. By contrast, the mother now seemed confident that her daughter would be cured. She was praying constantly, and her faith in the present course of action was being fully sustained. She tried to explain the benefits of laetrile therapy to each staff member and even asked them to assist in providing this therapy.

The attending physician was not sure how to respond. He knew that parents are rightly permitted considerable discretion in decisions relating to their children's medical care. Although the courts have often overridden the decisions of parents to seek unconventional forms of care, the clearest situation is when the child's life is endangered without proper therapy, the conventional treatment has a high probability of success and is not life-endangering, and the unconventional approach has no scientific basis or merit. In this case it was probably no longer possible to save the child's life with available therapy, nor was the mother preventing her daughter from receiving it. Besides, the regular chemotherapies involved calculated dangers of their own, such as toxic effects on organ systems and increased susceptibility to life-threatening infections and hemorrhages. Thus, the mother's actions appeared within the scope of legitimate parental discretion.

When the patient was asked how she felt about the laetrile treatments, she said, "They're all right . . . it's not too bad." She did express a willingness to continue with laetrile if it was what her mother thought best. The impression was that she was ambivalent about the laetrile but wished to please her mother.

Concern for the patient's well-being made the physician reluctant to ignore the matter. There is little evidence that laetrile is effective. One research study involved 178 patients with various kinds of solid tumors, for whom standard therapy offered no hope of cure or prolongation of life. Patients received laetrile therapy, including the "metabolic" component, but there was only one partial response in the entire group.[19] (However, no leukemia patients were involved in this study.) Moreover, amygdalin, the active substance in laetrile, breaks down into benzaldehyde and free cyanide, the latter being highly toxic. Blood cyanide levels can rise to potentially lethal levels, and some deaths from laetrile-induced cyanide poisoning have been reported. This danger is most serious when patients take more than three daily doses or more than one tablet at a time or when they consume large amounts of almonds. The almonds contain a significant level of beta-glucosidase, which maximizes the breakdown of laetrile into cyanide.[20] In addition, manufactured laetrile tablets have often been found to contain microorganisms, which might cause serious infection in a patient whose defenses against microorganisms are already compromised by standard therapy. Finally, a majority of laetrile patients experience "minor" toxic reactions, including nausea, vomiting, headaches, and dizziness. The patient had suffered these symptoms periodically in recent weeks. (Similar symptoms are also very common with standard chemotherapy.) Thus, the laetrile therapy would probably increase the child's discomfort and could needlessly shorten her life.

On the other hand, the physician recognized the dangers of addressing the issue in an aggressive way. Intense initial discussions with the mother about the dangers of laetrile therapy left her completely unshaken in her belief that the child should continue to go to Mexico. Stern insistence on stopping the laetrile treatments might cause her to remove the child from regular treatment, resulting in the absence of useful therapy and the inability to follow the child's status. Similarly, any attempt to draw out the patient's feelings might cause friction to develop between mother and child. The mother appeared to need the laetrile option to support her overt denial of the ultimate outcome. Nevertheless, the mother's emotional needs were being satisfied at the expense of the child. Beside the concern about the effects of the laetrile regimen on the child's quality of life, the physician was worried about the chance of life-threatening cyanide poisoning or infection from the laetrile tablets. Possibly the mother needed a firm challenge to break the hold of her current approach to her child's treatment.

Options available to the physician included the following: (1) insist that the laetrile treatments be stopped if the mother wished her daughter to continue to receive regular therapy; (2) bring the daughter into the discussions, trying to break down the mother's inability to consider the feelings of the child and the dangers to her; (3) drop the whole subject, and proceed as if nothing had happened; or (4) go along with the mother's desire to receive assistance in providing the laetrile (maybe surreptitiously substituting sugar pills when possible).

3.8 Selecting Therapy for a Mentally Retarded Teenager

An ethics committee associated with a clinic for mentally retarded patients met at the request of a gynecologist. His patient was an eighteen-year-old woman with mild mental retardation caused by Noonan's syndrome, a genetic disease. Characteristic features of Noonan's syndrome include short stature, a webbed neck, low-set or malformed ears, a shield-shaped chest, and mental retardation. There is evidence that Noonan's syndrome is an autosomal-dominant genetic disease, implying that offspring of afflicted persons have a 50 percent chance of inheriting the disease. Also, the disease is believed to have variable expressivity, meaning that its severity varies in different people. Thus, the mental retardation can vary from mild to severe, although usually it is mild.

Recent psychological testing revealed that the patient's mental development was approximately that of an eleven-year-old. She had been raised at home by her parents, who had no other children, and she was attending a special school that provided vocational training. Upon reaching the age of majority (eighteen), she had been declared legally incompetent, and her mother had been appointed guardian. However, the patient was capable of self-care to some degree, including managing her own menstrual hygiene.

The patient's mother had brought her to the clinic because she had seizures and severe cramping pain during her periods. Standard anticonvulsant medications had not eliminated the seizures, which typically occurred several times during menstruation. The gynecologist was very concerned about the seizures because they can be fatal. The treatment he selected was Depo-Provera, a drug sometimes used to prevent dysmenorrhea (painful menstruation). Depo-Provera suppresses the cyclic changes in hormone levels that cause ovulation and menstruation. After several injections, patients stop having periods. This cessation is reversible, with periods resuming after injections are stopped. An injection every three months will continue the suppression of periods.

The patient had been receiving Depo-Provera for several months, and it had effectively stopped her periods, thereby eliminating the seizures and cramping. However, the patient had begun to have a mild amount of breakthrough bleeding, a menstruallike bleeding that is a common side effect of Depo-Provera. The issue the physician presented to the ethics committee concerned the action to be taken if the breakthrough bleeding became worse. In a heavy case there can be bleeding every day. The amount of bleeding is usually not enough to cause anemia or other serious medical problems but is a nuisance to patients and a significant interference with their comfort.

If the bleeding became serious, one option was the use of birth control pills. The pill might not cause breakthrough bleeding. Moreover, birth control pills would produce relatively light periods, lasting only a couple of days, and might eliminate the patient's seizure problem. However, at the age of fourteen she had been on birth control pills and developed deep-vein thrombosis, requiring hospitalization. Such thrombosis is a complication believed to be caused by the estrogen hormone in birth control pills, and it involves formation of blood clots within the vessels. This is a serious condition; the clots can break off, travel in the bloodstream, and become lodged in arteries causing fatal pulmonary embolus, heart attack, or stroke. Because of these risks, the physician was opposed to giving this patient the pill and had initially selected Depo-Provera.

Another therapeutic approach would be to use an alternative drug that eliminates periods. The only commercially available drug was danazol, which would eliminate periods without the risks of thrombosis. The main disadvantage is that it costs about one hundred dollars per month, considerably more than Depo-Provera. The patient's mother had rejected this option, stating that she could not afford it.

A third option was to continue use of Depo-Provera. However, this approach would not only fail to eliminate the discomfort and annoyance of breakthrough bleeding, but it would involve an increased risk of cardiovascular disease associated with long-term use of the drug. Depo-Provera is a progestogen, a type of drug whose long-term use is associated with an increased incidence of high blood pressure, stroke, and heart attack.[21]

Fourth, the physician could perform a hysterectomy. Although this would eliminate periods and the discomforts associated with them, it was uncertain whether it would prevent seizures. The seizures might be directly associated with the cyclic changes in levels of hormones produced by the ovaries, which would not be eliminated by a hysterectomy. If a hysterectomy did not eliminate the seizures, however, additional measures could be taken. One approach would be to surgically remove the ovaries, but without the estrogen produced by the ovaries, the patient would develop osteoporosis (brittle bones), perhaps by middle age. Although estrogen pills can help prevent osteoporosis, the previous thrombosis caused by estrogen in birth control pills provided a strong reason against using estrogen. A medically preferable course would be to resume Depo-Provera injections if a hysterectomy did not eliminate seizures. Without a uterus, there would be no breakthrough bleeding. Thus, the seizure problem could be managed in a way that avoided the nuisance of constant vaginal bleeding.

A fifth approach would be to seek court authorization of a hysterectomy and perform the procedure only if a court order is obtained. Because the patient was mentally incompetent, court review would give added protection to her interests. Moreover, court authorization would reduce the physician's risk of legal liability.

Because of the risks of birth control pills and the mother's rejection of danazol, the third, fourth, and fifth options appeared to be the only viable ones. The gynecologist was seeking the committee's view concerning which of these options would be ethically preferable if the bleeding became heavy.

In the ensuing committee discussion, various considerations were mentioned. A clergyman on the committee suggested that a hysterectomy should not be performed. He said that patient autonomy would be promoted by postponing the procedure. Although the patient was currently incompetent, she might later develop the capacity to make her own decisions concerning procreative matters. Second, it could be argued that she had an interest in preserving her reproductive capacity. Although she had stated that she did not wish to have children, she might later change her mind. Furthermore, although there was doubt about whether she would be able to provide adequate care to children, this possibility could not be ruled out. Third, the well-being of the patient could be adversely affected by performing a hysterectomy. If she later had the capacity and desire to raise children, she would be prevented from experiencing the benefits of having her own children and might suffer psychological harm. Also, there are physical risks associated with hysterectomy, including excessive bleeding, infection, and risks of general anesthesia.

However, a physician on the committee argued that other factors related to the patient's well-being supported performing a hysterectomy, provided the patient would assent. He pointed out that surgery might avoid the long-term risks of Depo-Provera and would eliminate the discomforts associated with ongoing breakthrough bleeding. Also, if a hysterectomy were not performed and the patient later attempted to become pregnant, there would be an interval before pregnancy during which she would again have periods and be subjected to the risks of seizures. He also suggested, in opposition to the clergyman, that the patient's autonomy might be enhanced by a hysterectomy, through the elimination of the disruptive effects on her daily life of constant bleeding. Not only would she be free of the hygienic tasks involved, but she might also be more free to go places and do things if such bleeding were eliminated.

An administrator then spoke up. She believed that the interests of potential offspring were relevant to the decision. Any child of the patient would apparently have a 50 percent chance of acquiring Noonan's syndrome. Moreover, there is currently no prenatal test for this condition. It might be argued that when parents intentionally conceive a child with knowledge of such risks and an afflicted child is born, that child is wronged. A hysterectomy would preclude the wronging of offspring in this way.

A lawyer who was present added that the well-being of the physician could be affected. If a hysterectomy were performed and the patient later wanted children, she might sue the physician. Although a court order authorizing a hysterectomy would help protect the physician from such a suit, courts in this state do not authorize hysterectomy unless it is necessary to protect the welfare of the incompetent person. Because it was not clear that a court would consider a hysterectomy necessary to protect this patient's interests, seeking court approval might involve considerable time and expense, to no avail.

3.9 Birth Control for a Retarded Woman

Julie was twenty-one years old and mild to moderately retarded. At a visit to her gynecologist five months after giving birth to her first child, she and her doctor discussed contraception. She was taking birth control pills, but she had been using them when she became pregnant and admitted that she had difficulty remembering to take them. The gynecologist was concerned that the pill might again fail to be an effective method of birth control. The patient expressed a strong desire for effective contraception or sterilization. She had a boyfriend with whom she was living who was not mentally retarded and who had fathered her child. She said that he was nice to her and that they loved each other. They had maintained a steady relationship and would have married except that she would have stopped receiving her welfare checks. He was thirty years old, divorced, and had three children from a previous marriage. Neither of them wanted more children.

The physician had asked a social worker to provide information about the patient's home situation. The social worker reported that the patient's family gave her little support. They were alienated from each other for reasons that were not clear. The patient was learning to cook and keep house. She was able to read and write at a very elementary level and could take care of herself and the baby. However, a recent checkup had revealed that the child, although normal, was developing slowly, perhaps because of inadequate adult-child stimulation.

A guardian had previously been appointed by the local court to make medical decisions for the patient. Within the past year she had been evaluated by a psychologist for competency to consent to sterilization. She seemed to have a rudimentary understanding that it was an operation to prevent her from having babies. However, she had difficulty understanding other aspects of the procedure such as its irreversible nature and the pros and cons of the various methods of sterilization and contraception. The psychologist's opinion was that she was not competent to give informed consent for sterilization.

The physician considered the various methods of contraception. The patient said she preferred not to use a diaphragm because she and her boyfriend found it inconvenient. An intrauterine device (IUD) was another possibility, but its use would increase her risk of pelvic infection, especially since she had a history of pelvic and urinary tract infections.[22] The physician was concerned that an IUD would cause an infection and that the patient would delay seeking medical help, as retarded persons sometimes do. If she waited too long, she could develop a pelvic abscess, which can be life-threatening. For this reason he was firmly against an IUD.

Another method is to give Depo-Provera, a drug widely used as a contraceptive in other countries. As discussed elsewhere in this book, it works by suppressing the woman's normal cyclic changes in hormone levels, thus preventing ovulation and menstruation. It is administered by injection, with a shot providing contraceptive protection for about three months. The effects are reversible, and periods resume after the shots are stopped. Depo-Provera is not approved as a contraceptive by the U.S. Food and Drug Administration (FDA) because it has caused cancer of the breast and uterus in experiments using beagle dogs and monkeys. It is approved, however, for other uses and is therefore available.

The approaches that could be recommended by the physician included the

Deciding for Others 113

following: (1) switch to Depo-Provera; (2) continue using birth control pills and enroll in a training program to help her remember to take her pills; (3) seek court authorization for sterilization by tubal ligation; or (4) ask the boyfriend to consider having a vasectomy.

The various options had advantages and disadvantages. Depo-Provera would involve some risk to the patient's health. It is a progestogen, and there is an association between long-term use of progestogens and an increased incidence of cardiovascular disease, including high blood pressure, heart attack, and stroke.[23] Another problem was that although lack of approval as a contraceptive by the FDA did not make it illegal to prescribe Depo-Provera for this purpose, the physician's potential liability would be great if there were an adverse reaction. In a court of law it would be difficult to defend using it rather than approved contraceptive methods. The gynecologist was concerned about potential liability.

The local public health department offered sexual counseling classes for retarded women which included training to remember to take their birth control pills. But the patient might forget to take the pill for a day or two while being trained and could become pregnant. Therefore, birth control pills were less likely than Depo-Provera to fulfill her desire to prevent pregnancy. Another problem was a risk of producing birth defects in the fetus if she continued taking the pills, not knowing she was pregnant. The progestogens in birth control pills are believed to sometimes cause heart and limb defects.[24] In addition, long-term use of birth control pills would have the risk of cardiovascular disease associated with progestogens.

A troubling aspect of tubal ligation was the high probability that it would be irreversible.[25] Women sometimes regret tubal sterilization for various reasons, a common one being divorce followed by a desire to have a child with a new mate.[26] Although the possibility of a later change of heart does not affect the right of a fully competent woman to consent to sterilization, a retarded woman's lack of sophistication regarding personal relationships raises concerns about allowing her to exercise this option. She might have an unrealistic view concerning the permanence of her current relationship. Because preservation of reproductive capacity is of value, it can be argued that less restrictive means of birth control should be tried when patients are incompetent. Another factor is the risk of the tubal ligation procedure, which includes anesthesia risk, infection, and injury to bladder, intestines, or ovaries. However, these are probably no greater than the risks of long-term use of birth control pills or Depo-Provera.

On the other hand, sterilization has advantages. It is highly effective and avoids the inconvenience of taking pills or shots. Moreover, it would avoid the prospect of the patient having other children to whom she might be unable to give adequate financial support or maternal care. It can be claimed that this popular method of birth control should be available to retarded women who want it and that the patient deserved a full hearing in court to explore the possibility of sterilization. The competency of mild to moderately retarded individuals is often not clear-cut, and there might be opposing testimony on this point. Perhaps the court would declare her competent to consent to sterilization. If the court considered her incompetent, on the other hand, it was bound by common-law principles to approve sterilization only if that were in the patient's best interests. Whether the court would find it to be in her interests was an open question.

Perhaps the fourth option would best promote the well-being of the patient; it avoids any risks or invasive procedures for her. It might be argued, however, that one should not ask the boyfriend to undergo an irreversible procedure when reversible methods for the patient are available.

3.10 A Family's Lack of Commitment

The patient was a fifteen-year-old boy who was moderately mentally retarded and had a long history of renal problems. He was born with a blockage in his lower urinary tract, a bladder neck obstruction, which caused bilateral hydronephrosis,[27] and an infection in his left kidney. When he was one year old the left kidney was surgically removed after an abscess formed in it. The obstruction was treated by a ureterostomy, in which the right ureter was disconnected from the bladder and brought to the surface of the abdomen. This required that he wear a plastic bag in order to collect the urine from the right kidney. Because the ureter went directly to an opening in the abdomen, there was a risk of infection of the ureter, and the patient developed a urinary tract infection seven times between the ages of seven and fifteen as a result of poor personal hygiene. These repeated infections contributed to a progressive deterioration of the right kidney. Hydronephrosis, caused by the many infections, became a recurring problem and contributed to the kidney damage. He had also developed hypertension, caused by the renal disease.

His full-scale Wisconsin IQ score was 40. His verbal skills were approximately at the level of an early-grade-school child. He could, for example, play simple card games such as "War" but would sometimes be unsure which card was higher.

He was being followed at an outpatient clinic, with an attempt being made to control his high blood pressure with drugs and to prevent urinary tract infections by means of antibiotics. However, the patient's mother frequently failed to make him take his medications or to bring him to the clinic for his appointments, apparently for several reasons. First, the boy had behavioral problems that included misbehavior in class and truancy from school. His mother claimed that she was unable to control him or to make him take his medicine. Second, the patient's family seemed unwilling to make the extra effort needed to bring about compliance with the treatment plan. After each failure to keep an appointment, the mother would say she had been ill, an excuse the clinic staff seriously doubted. Third, the family's socioeconomic condition may have been an obstacle to compliance. The patient lived with his mother and eight of his eleven siblings in a four-room apartment in a housing project. The patient was the youngest of the children. The parents were separated, and the father provided only thirty dollars per week. A substantial percentage of the family's income consisted of monthly government payments, available to families with handicapped children living in the home. The patient's medical bills were paid by Medicaid.

The patient was admitted to the hospital because various clinical signs, including uremia, lowered creatinine clearance, increased diastolic blood pressure, and anemia, indicated end-stage renal disease.[28] The purposes of the admission were to reevaluate the patient's renal function and to assess the ability of the patient and the family to manage his chronic illness. They were told that he needed dialysis and possibly a kidney transplant. It was explained that successful dialysis required that the patient follow a special diet, take his medications, and show up regularly for dialysis. However, the parents did not appear to be interested in making that commitment. Furthermore, no one in the family was willing to donate a kidney. According to one of the patient's sisters, no one would donate because the patient was "different" from everyone else in the family.

The patient was discharged with medications to take at home. He was to take Apresoline for his high blood pressure and Amphojel to correct an elevated phosphorus level. In addition, he was put on a low-protein, low-salt, low-potassium diet restricted to twenty-five hundred calories a day. If he would follow that diet, then the need for dialysis might be prevented or postponed. A dietitian began meeting with the mother to explain the diet and help her maintain it.

However, the patient continued to neglect both his medications and the dietary restrictions. He ate high-sodium snacks such as potato chips at every opportunity, a habit that, as was explained to him and his parents, could prove lethal. The dietitian suggested that the mother keep a food diary to monitor what the patient ate, but she didn't think she could do it because the patient ate things when she was away from home and other family members would not help.

Further deterioration of his condition resulted in the need for another hospitalization in order to bring down his blood pressure. Even in the hospital, he would sneak out of his room and go to the vending machines, where he would get potato chips and other snacks. He seemed unable to comprehend his medical condition or the effects of his behavior on his health. His mother also seemed to have only a limited understanding of his medical problems.

A pediatric nephrologist was consulted to explore the possibility of dialysis and transplantation. After reviewing the situation, the nephrologist stated that the patient should not be considered for dialysis or transplantation, because the patient and the family could not be expected to follow the rigid regimen required for those treatments. The previous failures by his family to make him take his medicines, follow his diet, and keep appointments would make dialysis futile. With regard to transplantation, the necessary regimen would include taking immunosuppressive drugs daily. Failure to do so would result in rejection of the kidney. Thus, transplantation was bound to fail for similar reasons.

An additional obstacle to transplantation was posed by the patient's ureterostomy. Because he would need to take immunosuppressive drugs, the risk of infection originating at the urine collection bag and spreading to the new kidney would be significant, especially considering the patient's history of many infections. An infection could result in the loss of the new kidney. It might be possible to circumvent this problem by eliminating the ureterostomy and reconnecting the ureter to the bladder. One difficulty with this approach is that the bladder, after years of nonuse, might not function properly. However, the potential of the bladder to function properly could be assessed before surgery by inserting a catheter into the bladder through a needle puncture, filling the bladder with saline, and observing whether the patient could void. If the patient did not void at first, it would be possible that repeated filling of the bladder in this manner would eventually result in proper functioning. On the other hand, proper functioning might never occur.

Because the patient was retarded, the physician considered institutionalizing him so that he could be dialyzed regularly with good supervision. However, the social workers reported that there were no facilities for the retarded that could supervise long-term inpatient dialysis. He then asked the social workers whether the state could take custody of the patient for the purpose of either ordering the parents to comply with the treatment regimen or placing the boy in a foster home where there might be better supervision. They replied that the court would probably not consider this a clear enough case of child abuse or neglect to warrant removing the child from the home. Another reason why the court would probably not intervene was that it was not clear that a court order could remedy the situation. For one thing, the treatment in question was not a one-time course of therapy after which the boy could be returned to his family. Second, it was not clear that the patient's family was capable of supervising him adequately, even if motivated by a court order. Third, it was unlikely that foster parents could be found who would be willing to assume the large task of supervising the boy's treatment. Developmentally disabled children are difficult to place, and the potential burdens on a foster family involved in long-term dialysis would make placement even more difficult.

An attempt was made to persuade the patient's adult siblings to supervise his dialysis, but none was willing and able to assume that responsibility. The options therefore were limited but included the following: (1) Attempt medical management without dialysis or transplantation. This would involve further efforts to maintain the patient on a diet, to control his blood pressure with drugs, and to prevent urinary tract infections. (2) Continue trying to arrange for dialysis or transplantation without involving the courts. This would include a new attempt to increase the family's vigilance in caring for the patient and to find another nephrologist to supervise dialysis or a surgical team willing to perform the transplant. (3) Petition the local court to take custody of the patient so that an attempt could be made to place him in foster care. If adequate supervision of the child could be arranged, plans for dialysis or transplantation could be made.

Various considerations were pertinent to the patient's well-being. The first approach would not save the patient's life. His blood urea nitrogen was steadily rising, and he would soon die without regular dialysis or a kidney transplant. However, this approach would allow the child to remain in familiar surroundings until he died and would spare him the pain and suffering connected with the more aggressive interventions, which were not likely to succeed.

There were also trade-offs associated with the second option. Arranging for further therapy without removing the patient from his present environment would avoid some emotional stress and give the child a chance for a longer life. But the difficulties with compliance meant that the child's suffering might be exacerbated and the chance of treatment success undermined. For example, in the case of dialysis there would be a need to implant an access catheter, which would be a potential source of painful infection that was more likely without proper hygienic care. Moreover, if the patient ate or drank excessively, as seemed likely, he would feel very sick until the next dialysis. Thus, the dialysis might not extend his life for long and could result in substantial suffering.

The third course of action held out the best prospect for prolonging the child's life, especially if carefully supervised foster care could be arranged. This might relieve the compliance problem, although it was unclear whether anyone could ensure adequate compliance of this young man. But this course of action would remove the child from a home where, for all his problems, he seemed quite happy. There was also the basic fact that both dialysis and transplantation carried the prospect of additional suffering without great hope of success. For example, the transplantation surgery and the urinary tract surgery would cause considerable pain. The urinary tract surgery itself could result in hydronephrosis, which might further damage the right kidney and hasten the child's death. Similarly, the unwillingness of family members to donate a kidney meant that a cadaver organ would have to be used. This increased the probability that the patient's body would reject a transplanted kidney.

Commentary

Some of the most controversial cases in medical ethics involve choosing what is best for persons unable to speak for themselves. Much attention has been given to decisions about use of life-sustaining technologies for incompetent patients with compromised quality of life. However, other important matters can be at stake, such as avoidance of disfigurement or amputation, preservation of reproductive capacity, or continuation of home care rather than institutionalization. Patients for whom substitute decision making is most commonly needed fall into several categories. First, adults who were previously competent are sometimes unable to speak for themselves because of debilitation or terminal illness. Although a fundamental principle in such circumstances is to pursue the course of action the patient would choose if able, it is often unclear what the patient would want. Most people do not prepare living wills or other advance directives. In many cases patients have never discussed preferences concerning medical treatment with family or friends. Sometimes family and friends are not available to advise physicians about the patient's preferences. Cases 3.1 through 3.3 illustrate the ethical problems in making treatment decisions under such conditions. Second, decisions must be made on behalf of children who have serious illnesses. Sometimes the problem concerns whether to withhold treatment from newborns with serious birth defects, exemplified by cases 3.4 and 3.5. Other situations involve choosing among alternative therapies when the selection is value-laden, as in cases 3.6 and 3.7. Third, persons who are mentally retarded are sometimes incompetent to make their own decisions. Cases 3.8 and 3.9 illustrate decisions concerning hysterectomies and birth control for retarded women, and in case 3.10 the physician must decide how to treat a chronically ill retarded boy whose family appears to have diminished concern for him.

Two main questions can be distinguished. First, what principles should be followed in trying to choose what is best for an incompetent person? This is usually referred to as the *substantive* issue. The second is the *procedural* question: Who should make these decisions? We begin with the substantive question.

The Patient's Best Interests

A central issue in many of these cases arises because the patients suffer from handicaps, pain, or other effects of disease that adversely affect the quality of their lives. For example, seriously debilitated adults often suffer a diminished capacity to interact with others. Similarly, impaired newborns often have reduced potential for cognitive development, and the mentally retarded sometimes have a significantly limited capacity for rational decision making. In choosing what is best for these patients, two main views can be identified. According to one view, regarding these impairments as morally pertinent in deciding what is best for the patient denies the full status of personhood to the patient. Decisions about what would best promote the patient's interests should consider what would be appropriate for any person, regardless of degree of handicap. According to the second view, handicaps and suffering can in some cases be morally relevant to judgments about the patient's best interests. On this view, what is best for persons with these incapacities can vary from one person to the next, depending on the specific situation.

The differences between these two views can be explored by examining their implications for the three types of patients considered in this chapter. Case 3.1 illustrates situations involving debilitated adults. James A. was an eighty-year-old man believed to have senile dementia. Although conscious, he did not respond in any way when addressed. His immobility had caused several bed sores as well as severe contractures of both legs. A diagnosis of pneumonia was made after the patient developed difficulty breathing. With effective antibiotic therapy, the patient would survive, perhaps living a number of years. Without treatment, the pneumonia would probably be fatal.

According to the first view, the patient's cognitive impairments and lack of capacity for affective relationships are not relevant to the questions of whether treatment would promote his interests. The pneumonia should be treated because the patient's life has inherent value. In the context of such life-or-death decisions, this view is usually referred to as the sanctity-of-life approach. As Daniel Callahan explains, "the *meaning* of the 'sanctity of life' is that of signifying the ultimate respect we are willing to accord human life. It expresses a willingness to treat human life with consideration, to give it dignity, to commit ourselves to its furtherance."[29]

Endorsements of this view are not difficult to find, particularly among physicians, whose training emphasizes the saving of lives. The following comment is representative: "[Even] when a case seems hopeless, the physician is morally obligated to fight for this human life with all the weapons at his command. No physician has the right to give up, no matter what the pressures to 'let the patient die in peace and dignity.' "[30]

The second view, on the other hand, holds that the diminished abilities are relevant because they affect the patient's quality of life. Life has value insofar as it enables one to pursue activities cherished by human beings. Treatment decisions must consider whether patients will be able to engage sufficiently in valued activities to make continued life in their interests. One who holds a quality-of-life view might conclude that James A.'s prospects are so dismal that continued life is not in his interests. If so, comfort-providing care, but not lifesaving treatment, should be administered.

A similar issue arises with respect to cases involving young children. An example is case 3.4, in which a premature infant suffered a cardiopulmonary arrest and severe asphyxia at birth. Subsequent intracranial hemorrhages caused additional brain damage. In the intensive care nursery the infant would frequently stop breathing and have a very low heart rate. These emergencies required resuscitation and administration of oxygen. Whether the infant would survive was unclear, but it was likely that there would be serious retardation. The child might remain bedridden and never talk. The physician had doubts about whether continued resuscitation would promote the interests of the child.

The first view holds that a serious diminution of cognitive potential is not relevant to treatment decisions. It is illustrated by an early version of the Department of Health and Human Services (HHS) "Baby Doe" regulations, which held that withholding life-sustaining treatment from impaired newborns constitutes discrimination against the handicapped. According to HHS, "It is only when non-medical considerations, such as subjective judgments that an unrelated handicap makes a person's life not worth living, are interjected in the decisionmaking process" that discrimination occurs.[31] Similarly, Paul Ramsey states that "the standard for letting die must be the same for the normal child as for the defective child. If an operation to remove a bowel obstruction is indicated to save the life of a normal infant, it is also the indicated treatment of a mongoloid infant."[32] According to this view, continued use of life-preserving measures would be required to promote the best interests of the infant in case 3.4. The second view, however, considers quality-of-life factors important in choosing what is best for impaired newborns. It might conclude that expected quality of life falls below a minimal level necessary for life to be beneficial to the infant, so that there is no obligation to resuscitate.

A similar conflict of views arises concerning withholding medical hydration and nutrition. Because the infant in case 3.4 was unable to suck or swallow, continued survival required artificial feeding. Those who hold that the child's lack of potential for normal development is not ethically relevant would conclude that nutrition and hydration should not be stopped. Because provision of food and water is a symbolic expression of care and concern, as well as life-sustaining, withholding it would fail to respect his status as a person. For example, HHS regulations assert that "the basic provision of nourishment, fluids, and routine nursing care is a fundamental matter of human dignity, not an option for medical judgment. Even if a handicapped infant faces imminent and unavoidable death, no health care provider should take it upon itself to cause death by starvation or dehydration."[33] On the other hand, those who claim that the infant's handicaps are relevant might conclude that all life-sustaining medical procedures, including provision of fluids and nourishment, should be withheld if doing so would not increase suffering.

The third type of situation is illustrated by case 3.8, involving an eighteen-year-old woman with mild mental retardation caused by Noonan's syndrome. The patient's cognitive functioning was approximately that of an eleven-year-old, and she had been declared legally incompetent. Although capable of managing her menstrual hygiene, she had been having seizures and severe pain during her periods. She was treated with Depo-Provera and experienced a mild amount of breakthrough bleeding as a side effect. If it became heavier, the only viable alternatives would be to continue Depo-Provera in spite of bleeding or to perform a hysterectomy. The issue was whether a hysterectomy to eliminate such bleeding would be in the patient's best interests.

The first view again would maintain that the patient's cognitive impairments are not relevant to the decision. An illustration is found in a recent court decision concerning an eighteen-year-old profoundly retarded woman.[34] She had heavy menstrual bleeding as well as bleeding between periods and was unable to manage her hygiene. Efforts to control the bleeding with drugs had failed, and the woman's guardian sought court authorization for a hysterectomy. The judge inquired whether the procedure would be medically indicated for a woman of normal intelligence with similar problems. The woman's physician testified that if she were mentally normal he would not recommend a hysterectomy. Based on this information, the judge ruled that it could not be concluded that a hysterectomy would promote the interests of the patient, and the authorization was denied. Thus, the first view would emphasize that the patient has the same rights as persons with normal cognitive ability, including a right of noninterference with the capacity to reproduce. With regard to the patient with Noonan's syndrome, this view suggests that a hysterectomy would not be warranted. Rather, a trial period might be recommended to see if the patient could cope with the bleeding. If possible, a decision about hysterectomy should be postponed to see if the patient might become competent to make the decision for herself. According to the second view, this case should be decided by weighing the various factors pertaining to the patient's interests. The patient's moral interest in procreating, potential for competency, wishes, and personal comfort would be carefully assessed. The mental retardation would be relevant to deciding what is best for the patient. If the patient would never be capable of raising children, then she would be prevented from experiencing the rewards of child rearing. This would presumably diminish her moral interest in procreating. Assuming the patient were to assent to hysterectomy, giving up the ability to bear children to avoid years of constant uterine bleeding might be a reasonable way to secure her interests.

We have seen that two approaches to the problem of choosing what is best for another can be identified. The first view emphasizes respecting the patient's status as a person. The second view asserts that decisions should take into account the well-being of patients in addition to their rights and status as persons. The terms *sanctity of life* and *quality of life* are widely used in the context of life-or-death decisions, but there is no standard terminology to depict these views as they apply to a wider range of situations. Therefore, we shall refer to the first view as the *inviolateness-of-persons* view. According to this view, respect for persons requires that the lives and bodies of persons be considered inviolable. Our behavior toward others should be firmly guided by concerns such as respect for life, preservation of the physical integrity of the body, and respect for the reproductive capacities and decisions of persons. Thus, it is a central feature of this view that respect for patients is to be secured by adherence to certain rules designed to protect the inviolateness of persons, such as the lives of persons should be preserved; adequate food and water should not be withheld from persons; persons should not be sterilized without their informed consent.[35] We shall call the second approach a *beneficence-centered* view. This view considers all the interests of patients, but beneficence is emphasized because when the patient's wishes are unknown, an important guiding principle in surrogate decision making should be concern for the patient's well-being. According to the beneficence-centered view, decisions should be individualized based on the specific patient's needs, rather than based on firm rules designed to preserve the inviolateness of the lives and bodies of persons.

The Inviolateness-of-Persons View
Various arguments can be put forward in support of the inviolateness-of-persons view. One is that the human capacities or states protected by the rules have inherent value, rather than a value that is dependent on the person's ability to pursue cherished activities. Because these states are inherently valuable, their protection is always required. The specific form of the argument depends on which rule one is considering. Perhaps greatest attention has been given to the rule that the lives of persons should be preserved. Arguments that human life has inherent value have been based on both religious and philosophical considerations. Within the framework of Christian thought, the fundamental idea is that human life's inherent value derives from God. Paul Ramsey explains:

> ... one grasps the religious outlook upon the sanctity of life only if he sees that this life is asserted to be *surrounded* by sanctity that need not be in a man; that the most dignity a man ever possesses is a dignity that is alien to him.... A man's dignity is an overflow from God's dealing with him, and not primarily an anticipation of

anything he will ever be by himself alone. . . . The value of a human life is ultimately grounded in the value God is placing on it.[36]

Furthermore, human life is viewed as a gift from God of which we are stewards. As Norman St. John-Stevas puts it, "Man is not absolutely master of his own life and body. He has no *dominion* over it, but holds it in trust for God's purposes."[37] On this view, our stewardship requires the preservation of life. Others have argued that human life's inherent value does not derive from its being created by a God who finds it valuable. Edward Shils, for example, suggests that its value can be ascertained by direct human experience. In Shils's words, "The idea of sacredness is generated by the primordial experience of being alive, of experiencing the elemental sensation of vitality and the elemental fear of its extinction. . . . The question still remains: is human life sacred? I answer that it is, self-evidently. Its sacredness is the most primordial of experiences.[38] According to Shils, this direct perception of the sanctity of life can be appreciated by the religious believer and nonbeliever alike.

Another approach to defending the inviolateness-of-persons view focuses on the consequences of not following the rules in question. This type of argument has two principal forms. The empirical-wedge argument is concerned to show that if policies were adopted permitting violation of the rules in some cases, they would result in a widening of the range of cases in which exceptions are made. Judgments about quality of life can be misinterpreted as judgments about the *worth* of a life. Thus, some might perceive that they have free rein to withhold treatment from those they disvalue, such as the aged, the insane, or the socially unproductive. Furthermore, withholding treatment in cases such as those of the elderly debilitated man (case 3.1) and the brain-damaged newborn (case 3.4) might open the door to *positive* killing of defective infants and the elderly.[39] Another adverse consequence is suggested by Ramsey: "If the defective infants are not to be treated, they can be used in medical research, enabling their lack of actual potential to benefit others by experimentation."[40] Thus, patients might be subjected to experimental hazards or discomforts inconsistent with the respect that is owed to them.

The other form of argument is the logical wedge, which is concerned with the logical consequences of not following the rules. It relies on the principle of universalizability, which requires that cases not different in any morally relevant way be handled similarly. The argument seeks to undermine rival positions by showing that their conclusions about specific types of cases must be logically carried over to other cases in which the same conclusions are clearly unacceptable. To illustrate this argument, consider the recent case of Sharon Siebert, a forty-one-year-old severely brain-damaged nursing home patient.[41] She required artificial feeding since she could not swallow and was confined to bed or wheelchair. Her cognitive functioning was approximately that of a two-year-old. She could speak only a few intelligible words and expressed herself by movements of her hands, eyes, and facial muscles. She was able to participate in simple activities such as tic-tac-toe and could express some likes and dislikes. Her level of awareness was described by a friend who said, "I have seen terror come into [her] eyes a few times when during illnesses she has felt gagged by vomit."[42] Upon learning that a do-not-resuscitate order had been written by Siebert's physician, the friend obtained a restraining order to prevent its implementation.[43] A proponent of the logical-wedge argument might ask what morally relevant difference there is between Siebert's situation and that of the patient in case 3.1. If a position that supports withholding treatment in case 3.1 based on quality-of-life factors cannot identify the relevant difference, then it is logically committed to the same conclusion in the Siebert case. Assuming that it is morally obligatory to provide treatment to Siebert, the quality-of-life position is thereby shown to produce unacceptable consequences. Similar arguments could be leveled at those who advocate withholding treatment from impaired newborns or performing hysterectomies for the mentally retarded on quality-of-life grounds.

On the other hand, replies can be made to these various arguments. Consider the view that life has inherent value apart from its quality. A major problem with the religious argument is that it relies on its religious presuppositions. Nonbelievers will consider this approach unacceptable, because it rests ultimately on tenets of religious faith. As Daniel Callahan points out, because "a considerable portion of humanity is not Christian and does not accept this foundation for the sanctity of human life, . . . it does not readily provide a consensual norm to which all men can have recourse."[44] Philosophical attempts to defend the sanctity of life also involve serious problems. Perhaps the main difficulty with Shils's argument is that an individual's claim to experience something as inherently valuable does not demonstrate that it actually has inherent value. At best, it reveals a subjective evaluation—that the individual in question regards the thing as valuable. Furthermore, it seems that many persons do not share this experience with Shils. In the absence of a wide agreement concerning such experience, there is no basis to move beyond a mere subjective judgment to the more objective claim that life has inherent value. As Callahan puts it, "People frequently experience something as valuable which later reflection shows to be lacking in value, and it is common for different groups of people to experience different things as valuable."[45]

In reply to the empirical-wedge argument, the mere possibility of adverse consequences is not grounds for rejecting a policy concerning withholding treatment. To be persuasive, the argument would have to provide evidence that such consequences are likely. As Bok has pointed out, evidence might include the following: a large rise in the number of cases placing a burden on society, ignorance of the effects on the victims, the inability of victims to resist, or conscious efforts by persons who desire or would profit from such consequences.[46] The main weakness of the argument is that there is little evidence to suggest that such factors will result in the feared consequences. Moreover, recent history has seen an increasing consciousness in our society concerning the rights of persons who are defenseless in varying degrees, such as the mentally retarded and infants with birth defects. These rights have been bolstered by government regulations, statutes, court cases, and institutional policies. This increased concern and its embodiment in the law provide a counterforce to social factors of the sort identified by Bok.

A response to the logical-wedge argument would focus on the identification of morally relevant differences between cases. It can be argued that it is possible to distinguish *some* cases in which life-prolonging treatment should be withheld from cases, such as that of Sharon Siebert, in which it should not. For example, one can distinguish Siebert from individuals who are irreversibly unconscious, on the grounds that permanent absence of awareness is a morally relevant difference. Moreover, unlike James A., the elderly patient in case 3.1, Siebert is capable of participating in pleasurable activities involving social interaction, and some might consider this an important difference. Thus, proponents of the beneficence-centered approach can satisfactorily respond to the logical-wedge argument by pointing out differences between cases that from the perspective of the beneficence-centered view are morally relevant.

Not only can these replies be made to the arguments supporting the inviolateness-of-persons view, but there is an important argument that can be made directly against it, namely that it leads to conclusions in some cases that are at odds with our intuitions. We might consider case 3.2, involving a thirty-nine-year-old woman who entered a persistent vegetative state following cardiac arrest during surgery. Various life-support measures were being provided, including nasogastric tube feedings and antibiotics for pneumonia. The question arose whether such aggressive measures should be continued. The patient had not previously expressed wishes concerning treatment under such circumstances. According to the sanctity-of-life approach, efforts to maintain the patient's life should be continued. It seems doubtful, however, that the interests of the patient require life-prolonging treatment in such cases. Another example involves the eighty-year-old man discussed in case 3.1. The question arose whether resuscitation, including use of a respirator if needed, should be carried out if cardiopulmonary arrest occurred. Although the sanctity-of-life approach would seem to require such measures, withholding respirator treatment with the approval of the patient's family appears to be morally permissible in such a situation.

The Beneficence-Centered View

A strong consideration in support of the beneficence-centered view is that it yields conclusions that conform more closely to our intuitions. On the other hand, there are a number of serious difficulties in developing a beneficence-centered approach. One involves identifying criteria for determining that a patient's quality of life is so impoverished that life-prolonging treatment should not be provided. Advocates of this approach would generally agree that there is no obligation to prolong life when death is imminent or when coma is irreversible, but these are not the problematic cases. The greatest difficulty involves patients who have a potential for continued life in a conscious but seriously compromised state. With regard to such individuals, two general views concerning quality of life can be distinguished. According to one view, efforts to maintain life should be carried out only if it is reasonable to believe that the patient would have a *meaningful life.* Different views concerning what constitutes a meaningful life have been suggested, ranging from possession of the "potential for human relationships"[47] to the ability to be self-supporting and to live independently.[48] The second view maintains that life-preserving treatment promotes the patient's interests only if continued life would be of *benefit* to the patient.[49] The major difference between these views is that two different comparisons are involved. The first view implicitly compares the patient's expected quality of life with a norm of human capacity. When that quality of life is sufficiently below the norm, the life is considered not to be meaningful. The second view compares the patient's expected life with the absence of life. It asks whether continued life would be better for the patient than death itself. If the positive experiences would outweigh the negative ones (e.g., pain and suffering), then continued life is regarded as benefiting the patient. It is the second view that provides the appropriate framework for our discussion, for two reasons. First, the meaningful-life view overlooks the possibility that a life might provide net benefit to the individual who lives it, in comparison to nonexistence, even though it is substantially below some norm of human ability. Second, judgments about whether life is meaningful come close to, and perhaps are indistinguishable from, judgments about the worth of a life as seen by another, as opposed to its value to the person who lives it.

The difficulty lies in choosing criteria for judgments concerning whether continued life would benefit the patient. According to one view, occurrence of pleasurable experiences with enough frequency and duration to outweigh the patient's painful experiences is sufficient to make continued life a benefit.[50] In case 3.1, for example, if James A. is capable of experiencing simple pleasures and is generally free of pain, then the pneumonia should be treated. However, other criteria take into account the ways in which cognitive abilities confer benefit to a person's life. For example, one might consider the patient's ability to formulate and carry out personal plans and to experience the cognitive features of interpersonal relationships. Because these abilities were greatly diminished or absent for James A., it might be concluded that continued life does not promote his interests. The resolution of this issue is an important problem facing the beneficence-centered approach, and it is unclear how it should be resolved.

Even if the problem of selecting quality-of-life criteria can be resolved, deciding what will benefit a patient involves other difficulties arising from the clinical and social dimensions of situations. One problem is the occasional need to balance disparate goods without a generally agreed-upon framework for assigning priorities. An illustration is case 3.9, involving a twenty-one-year-old mild to moderately retarded woman who desired contraception or sterilization after giving birth to her first child. She was opposed to using a diaphragm because she and her boyfriend found it inconvenient. An IUD had been ruled out because the patient had a history of pelvic infections and would be at significant risk of infection associated with its use. Her difficulties in remembering to take birth control pills created a risk that she would become pregnant again if she used them. Another option was to seek court authorization for sterilization by tubal ligation. However, the patient had been interviewed by a psychologist who raised questions about her competency to consent to sterilization. Moreover, the sterilization would probably be irreversible. Thus, it was not clear how to balance preservation of reproductive capacity, obtainable with birth control pills, against the increased likelihood of preventing pregnancy that would accompany the tubal ligation.

A second problem in clinical decision making is that there is often considerable uncertainty about the patient's prognosis. The case of the infant who suffered severe birth asphyxia (3.4) is an example. It was not known whether continued aggressive treatment would result in long-term survival. Also, it was not possible to reliably predict the degree of handicap that would be present if the infant survived. Another illustration is case 3.6, involving an eleven-year-old girl who had suffered two strokes from an arterial disease of unknown cause. One approach to treatment involved surgery to remove the plaque that was occluding main arteries supplying blood to her brain. Alternatively, a medical approach not involving surgery could be attempted. The available data suggested a greater mortality rate during the two-month period following surgery, compared to medical treatment. However, the data also indicated that surgery increases the probability that the patient would be alive four years after diagnosis, compared to the medical approach. Given these differences between the medical and surgical therapies, it was uncertain which one would better promote the interests of the patient.

A third problem is that there often is uncertainty about what the patient is experiencing. In case 3.1, for example, the extent to which James A. was experiencing pain from bed sores and leg contractures was unclear. There was also uncertainty about his degree of awareness of his surroundings. Similar questions arise in case 3.5, involving a premature infant with trisomy 18 syndrome and esophageal atresia. Because of immature liver function, the level of bilirubin (a waste product) in the blood was rising, threatening to cause brain damage or death. Various treatments might be provided, including surgical correction of the esophageal atresia, intravenous fluids and nutrition, and blood transfusions to lower the bilirubin level. In deciding whether withholding treatment would be best for the patient, one question concerned what procedures would provide comfort or prevent suffering. Would withholding intravenous fluids and nutrition cause the infant discomfort? Would high bilirubin levels cause suffering? The answers to these questions were unclear, because it is often difficult to ascertain what the intensive care nursery patient is experiencing.

To summarize this discussion, each of the two main views identified has strengths and weaknesses. A major strength of the inviolateness-of-persons approach is its relative ease of application in clinical practice. To the extent that its rules are clear, their application is rather straightforward, avoiding the task of balancing various ethical consideration in the context of each case. Another strength is that it safeguards against treating patients, whether inadvertently or otherwise, as though they do not have the full status of personhood. Such protection is important, given recent incidents in which the moral status of patients has been inadequately acknowledged.[51] A main weakness of the inviolateness-of-persons approach, however, is that it is at odds with our moral intuitions in some cases. In its exclusive focus on protection of moral status, it results in some patients not being treated in ways most conducive to their well-being.

A major strength of the beneficence-centered view is that it avoids some implausible conclusions of the inviolateness-of-persons approach. By taking account of the various factors bearing on the patient's well-being, as well as the facts of specific situations, it yields conclusions tailored to the needs of individual patients. A main weakness is that this approach is relatively difficult to apply in clinical practice. Not only are there disagreements over suitable criteria of well-being, but there are often uncertainties concerning prognosis as well as the patient's subjective states. Furthermore, because judgments about quality of life might be confused with judgments about the worth of a life, the beneficence-centered approach lends itself to potential misapplication.

Who Should Decide?

There are several reasons why the question of who should make the decisions is important. First, interests other than those of the patient are often affected. For example, patient and family interests can conflict, as illustrated in chapter 2. Similarly, physicians treating incompetent persons can face legal risks in withholding treatment or performing sterilization procedures.[52] Also, society's concern to control health-care expenditures can sometimes conflict with the patient's interests. These various interests might be given differing weight, depending on who makes the decision. Second, there are often obstacles to determining what action would best promote the patient's interests, as discussed above. This suggests that even when decisions aim at the patient's welfare, the quality of the decision might be affected by the choice of decision maker.

Policies concerning who decides can take various forms, but the ones seriously being considered fall into three categories. First, regulatory bodies external to the institution caring for the patient can stipulate the decisions. This approach involves enforcement of substantive principles selected by the regulatory body. An example is the federal "Baby Doe" regulations which state principles for withholding treatment.[53] Second, the decisions can be made by ethics committees at the institution providing care. Committees could formulate principles to be followed, and selected cases could be presented to the committee for resolution. Third, the decisions can be made by the patient's family with advice and counsel of the physician. For purposes of this discussion, we shall conceive this approach as encompassing varying degrees of influence by the physician on the decision. Combined forms are also possible, in which some decisions are made by one party and some by another. However, focusing on these three basic options will facilitate discussion.[54]

A major way in which these options differ is in the extent to which the decision maker is directly involved in the clinical situation. Thus, physician and family have immediate involvement in the circumstances requiring a decision, while ethics committees and regulatory bodies are furthered removed from individual clinical cases. With this feature in mind, let us consider the strengths and weaknesses of these approaches.

Regulatory Bodies

Decision making by regulatory bodies involves enforcing substantive principles. Upon reflection, it is apparent that the only way a regulatory body could specify decisions in individual cases is by adopting a rule-oriented approach. Because the beneficence-centered approach involves balancing the factors present in a specific case, adoption of it by a regulatory body would require relinquishing decision making to others who are more directly involved in the situation. It is no surprise, therefore, that when regulatory decision making has been implemented—notably the "Baby Doe" regulations—the enforced principles have embodied the inviolateness-of-persons approach.

In evaluating the regulatory option, we need to consider the pros and cons of enforcing the inviolateness-of-persons approach. One major advantage is that to the extent its enforced rules are clear and straightforward, there will be comparative ease in applying them in the clinical setting. Another strength derives from the fact that the rules would apply to all. This would tend to promote a principle of justice according to which similar cases should be handled similarly. A further advantage is that this option would prevent serious abuses resulting from undue influence of the interests of family, physician, or hospital. The weaknesses of this option also include those of the inviolateness-of-persons approach. Specifically, the regulatory option prevents individualized judgments based on the facts of specific cases. As pointed out earlier, this can result in failure to address the needs of individual patients and yield conclusions at odds with our intuitions. Another major drawback is intrusion into an area of decision making that has traditionally been a family responsibility.

There are degrees to which regulatory bodies might influence decisions. Short of dictating decisions, regulations might establish a framework of general principles to guide decisions. Alternatively, regulatory bodies could specify procedures to be followed. Such forms of influence, however, do not involve decision making by the regulating agency and are versions of the other two options.

Ethics Committees

Ethics committees constitute an option with several potential strengths. Like regulatory bodies, they can counteract undue influence of family and physician interests. Moreover, they could accommodate the need for individualized decisions better than regulatory agencies. They can promote the goal of considering all relevant information and, depending on their composition, can offer expertise in pertinent areas, such as the availability of community resources. Also, they might resolve disputes between family and physician, avoiding more expensive and cumbersome legal proceedings. In spite of these potential advantages, however, committees may lack firsthand knowledge of the case and might not be as capable as families and physicians in basing decisions on the specific patient's needs. Another concern is that, like the regulatory option, committee decision making would intrude on family responsibility. One practical consideration is that clinical decisions must occasionally be made without great delay, which may preclude prospective committee deliberation. Another is whether an institution's officials would consider the committee worth the expenditure of time and effort by its personnel. If a committee is not felt to be worth the effort, there might be institutional pressures to minimize its activities.

Ethics committees might function in useful ways other than making decisions. For example, they can function in an advisory capacity, making nonbinding recommendations to physicians and families. In this role, they might enhance the decision-making process by presenting alternative ethical viewpoints, identifying options, addressing legal concerns, and helping to ensure that all relevant facts are considered. Given the problems in decision making posed by clinical and social circumstances discussed above, the quality of decisions could perhaps be enhanced by committees acting in an advisory capacity. Because committees would not be making treatment decisions, these activities would be part of an approach in which choices are made by families and physicians.

Families and Physicians

The third option, in which decisions are made by families and physicians, has several points in its favor. It involves decision making by those closest to the actual clinical situation. This permits decision makers to have a firm grasp of the unique features of the particular case. This seems essential in trying to identify what is best for the patient. Also, this option preserves an important area of family responsibility. Another consideration is that it permits the interests of the family to influence decisions. Those who believe such interests should have influence in at least some cases will consider this a strength. However, those who believe that decisions should be based strictly on the best interests of the patient will perceive this as a weakness. Although this option appears to have greater potential for undue influence of family interests, it is doubtful that abuses occur often.[55] Concern that only the patient's interests should count does not, however, rule out this option. Regulatory bodies could establish a framework for decision making according to which the patient's interests are the only consideration, while allowing families and physicians to interpret this requirement in each case. This would counteract tendencies to let other interests take priority. Another weakness is that families and physicians sometimes lack knowledge necessary for well-considered decisions. This shortcoming might be remedied by use of committees in an advisory capacity. An additional problem is that similar situations might be decided differently by different families. Thus, this option might not satisfy the justice-based concern that similar cases should be handled similarly.

Taking into account the pros and cons of each option, decision making by families and physicians appears to be the preferable approach. First, not only does regulatory decision making imply a rule-oriented approach, but regulatory bodies and ethics committees are farther removed than families and physicians from the actual clinical circumstances. Thus, they are less likely to tailor decisions to the needs of individual patients. Second, decision making by government agencies or institutional committees constitutes a serious intrusion into an area of family responsibility. Although such intrusion might be justifiable if it were necessary to prevent serious harm to patients, the abuse of patients' interests appears to be a rare occurrence. Third, although decision making by families and physicians has shortcomings, these can perhaps be diminished by the enactment of regulations or the use of ethics committees in an advisory role. Appropriate federal guidelines might foster the similar treatment of similar cases. In addition, guidelines or committee review can help prevent undue influence of the interests of families and physicians. Committees serving in an advisory role can also help families and physicians deal with difficulties in deciding what would best promote the patient's well-being.

In conclusion, substantive and procedural issues are interrelated in significant ways. Regulatory bodies assuming the role of decision maker would have difficulty utilizing the beneficence-centered view because of its emphasis on individualizing decisions. In addition, the shortcomings of the inviolateness-of-persons view weigh against decision making by regulatory bodies. Acceptance of the beneficence-centered view favors assignment of the decision-making role to families and physicians. However, problems in choosing what would promote the patient's well-being and potential conflicts of interest suggest that decision making by families and physicians might be improved by the assistance of ethics committees or regulatory frameworks.

Notes

1. A contracture is a deformity of a joint that results from its being held immobile. The associated muscles become weak and shorten, so that the patient is unable to straighten the affected limb. At first contractures are usually correctable by physical therapy, but they become more difficult to correct with passage of time. Contractures are a common problem among bedridden elderly patients. Decubitus ulcers, also called pressure sores, result from prolonged pressure between any bony prominence and an external object such as a mattress, so that the tissues between them are deprived of their blood supply and disintegrate. The sores begin as abscesses beneath the skin and later burst through the skin to form large ulcers. Decubitus ulcers are another common problem among bedridden patients.
2. *Barber v. Superior Court,* 147 Cal. App. 3d 1006, 195 Cal. Rptr. 484 (1983); *In the Matter of Claire Conroy,* 486 A. 2d 1209 (N.J. 1985).
3. Decerebrate posturing of the arms refers to a state in which the arms are stiffly extended at the elbows, the forearms are pronated (palms turned outward), and the wrists and fingers are flexed. This rigidity of the arms indicates damage of the upper brain stem.
4. The President's Commission for the Study of Ethical Problems in Medicine and Biomedical and Behavioral Research, *Deciding to Forego Life-Sustaining Treatment* (Washington, D.C.: U.S. Government Printing Office, 1982), p. 182.
5. In a jejunostomy operation, an opening is created between the jejunum (upper part of the small intestine) and the surface of the abdomen. This permits the patient to be fed by pouring a special formula through the opening directly into the jejunum.

6. Edema is an excess accumulation of fluid in the intercellular spaces of the body. Edema was undesirable in this case partly because it would promote the formation of pressure sores. Also, pulmonary edema can promote respiratory distress in a patient with pneumonia.
7. Because the brain utilizes glucose as its energy source, brain function would deteriorate as hypoglycemia progressed, and additional permanent brain damage could result.
8. The hematocrit, as defined earlier, is the volume percent of red blood cells in whole blood.
9. Apnea is cessation of breathing; bradycardia is slowness of the heartbeat.
10. Trisomy 18 syndrome is a genetic disease caused by the presence of an extra number 18 chromosome in each cell.
11. A ventricular septal defect is an opening in the wall separating the two ventricles of the heart. The opening permits blood to flow directly from one ventricle to the other, bypassing the lungs.
12. David W. Smith, *Recognizable Patterns of Human Malformation*, 3d ed. (Philadelphia: W. B. Saunders, 1982), p. 15.
13. Such regulations became law in 1985. See U.S. Department of Health and Human Services, "Child Abuse and Neglect Prevention and Treatment Program; Final Rule," *Federal Register* 50 (1985), pp. 14,877–901, esp. p. 14,888.
14. For an account of parental experience during prolonged treatment, see Robert Stinson and Peggy Stinson, "On the Death of a Baby," *Atlantic Monthly* 244 (July 1979): 64–72.
15. Ciaran S. Phibbs, Ronald L. Williams, and Roderic H. Phibbs, "Newborn Risk Factors and Costs of Neonatal Intensive Care," *Pediatrics* 68 (1981): 313–21. According to this report, sixty-five neonates with major congenital anomalies requiring surgery (excluding cardiac surgery) were hospitalized an average of thirty-three days, at an average total cost of $18,569, in 1977 dollars. Taking into account health-care price inflation, this is equivalent to $34,891 in 1985 dollars. Annual health-care inflation rates are reported in U.S. Bureau of the Census, *Statistical Abstract of the United States: 1985*, 105th ed. (Washington, D.C.: U.S. Government Printing Office, 1984).
16. The 1985 "Baby Doe" regulations also prohibited withholding nutrition and hydration. U.S. Department of Health and Human Services, "Child Abuse and Neglect Prevention," p. 14,888.
17. Active killing would not only violate a moral rule but would be illegal.
18. William Fields and Noreen Lemak, "Joint Study of Extracranial Arterial Occlusion: X. Internal Carotid Artery Occlusion," *Journal of the American Medical Association* 235 (1976): 2734–38.
19. Charles Moertel et al., "A Clinical Trial of Amygdalin (Laetrile) in the Treatment of Human Cancer," *New England Journal of Medicine* 306 (1982): 201–6.
20. Charles Moertel et al., "A Pharmacologic and Toxicological Study of Amygdalin," *Journal of the American Medical Association* 245 (1981): 591–94.
21. Richard Lincoln, "The Pill, Breast and Cervical Cancer, and the Role of Progestogens in Arterial Disease," *Family Planning Perspectives* 16 (March–April 1984): 55–63.
22. IUD use is associated with a three- to ninefold increased incidence of pelvic infection. H. W. Ory, "A Review of the Association between Intrauterine Devices and Acute Pelvic Inflammatory Disease," *Journal of Reproductive Medicine* 20

(1978): 200–204. The risk of infection among IUD users is increased if there is a history of pelvic infections. David N. Danforth, ed., *Obstetrics and Gynecology*, 4th ed. (Philadelphia: Harper and Row, 1982), p. 276.
23. Lincoln, "The Pill, Breast and Cervical Cancer."
24. Ronald A. Chez, "Proceedings of the Symposium 'Progesterone, Progestins, and Fetal Development,'" *Fertility and Sterility* 30 (July 1978): 16–26.
25. It is possible to reconnect the fallopian tubes of women who have been sterilized. The success rate varies with the method of tubal ligation used and the type of surgical reconnection. Results are best when microsurgery techniques are used to rejoin the tubes. Reported rates for pregnancy after microsurgery average about 56 percent. A. Henry, W. Rinehart, and P. T. Piotrow, "Reversing Female Sterilization," *Population Reports*, Series C, No. 8 (September 1980) Baltimore, Johns Hopkins University.
26. R. M. L. Winston, "Why 103 Women Asked for Reversal of Sterilization," *British Medical Journal* 2 (1977): 305–7.
27. Hydronephrosis is the accumulation of urine within the kidney caused by obstructed outflow. It causes distension and damage to the organ.
28. Uremia is a toxic condition caused by an excessive accumulation in the blood of substances ordinarily eliminated in the urine. The condition occurs when the kidneys lose most of their ability to remove waste products from the blood. Creatinine is one of the substances that the kidneys remove from the blood. Creatinine clearance is a measure of the rate at which the kidneys remove creatinine. A decreased clearance is a reliable indicator of impaired kidney function.
29. Daniel Callahan, "The Sanctity of Life," in D. R. Cutler, ed., *Updating Life and Death* (Boston: Beacon Press, 1969), p. 200.
30. Louis P. Pertschuk and Albert S. Heyman, "The Physician's Responsibility in 'Hopeless Cases,'" *Journal of the American Osteopathic Association* 64 (1965), p. 618. Similar views are expressed by the following: David A. Karnofsky (letter), *CA: Bulletin of Cancer Progress* 10 (January–February 1960): 22–23; Franklin H. Epstein, "Responsibility of the Physician in the Preservation of Life," *Archives of Internal Medicine* 139 (1979): 919–20.
31. U.S. Department of Health and Human Services, "Nondiscrimination on the Basis of Handicap Relating to Health Care for Handicapped Infants," *Federal Register* 48 (1983): 30,847.
32. Paul Ramsey, *Ethics at the Edges of Life* (New Haven: Yale University Press, 1978), p. 192.
33. Department of Health and Human Services, "Nondiscrimination," p. 30,852.
34. In re *Guardianship of Gloria Sue Lambert*, No. 61-156 (Tenn. Ct. App. Oct. 29, 1976).
35. Different versions of the inviolateness-of-persons view formulate the rules in different ways. Some incorporate certain exceptions into the rules. For example, one might hold that the lives of persons should be preserved except when imminent death is unavoidable. Writings that propound versions of the inviolateness-of-persons view include the following: Callahan, "The Sanctity of Life," pp. 202–11; Thomas J. O'Donnell, *Medicine and Christian Morality* (New York: Alba House, 1976), pp. 41–134; John Marshall, *Medicine and Morals* (New York: Hawthorn Books, 1960), pp. 65–76, 97–110; and Gerald Kelly, *Medico-Moral Problems* (St. Louis: Catholic Hospital Association, 1959), pp. 5–11, 149–67.
36. Paul Ramsey, "The Morality of Abortion," in D. H. Labby, ed., *Life or Death:*

Ethics and Options (Seattle: University of Washington Press, 1968), p. 71.
37. Norman St. John-Stevas, *The Right to Life* (New York: Holt, Rinehart and Winston, 1964), p. 12.
38. Edward Shils, "The Sanctity of Life," in Labby, ed., *Life or Death*, pp. 12, 18–19.
39. This type of argument is stated, e.g., by Kevin D. O'Rourke, "Christian Affirmation of Life," in D. H. Horan and D. Mall, eds., *Death, Dying, and Euthanasia* (Frederick, Md.: University Publications of America, 1980), p. 365.
40. Ramsey, *Ethics at the Edges of Life*, p. 209.
41. Jane D. Hoyt, "No Dr. Blue/Do Not Resuscitate," *Bioethics Quarterly* 3 (1981): 128–32.
42. Ibid., pp. 128–29.
43. Ibid., p. 132.
44. Callahan, "The Sanctity of Life," p. 190.
45. Ibid., p. 191.
46. Sissela Bok, "The Leading Edge of the Wedge," *Hastings Center Report* 1 (December 1971): 10.
47. Richard McCormick, "To Save or Let Die: The Dilemma of Modern Medicine," *Journal of the American Medical Association* 229 (1974): 175.
48. John Lorber, "Spina Bifida Cystica: Results of Treatment of 270 Consecutive Cases with Criteria for Selection for the Future," *Archives of Disease in Childhood* 47 (1972): 854.
49. Carson Strong, "The Tiniest Newborns," *Hastings Center Report* 13 (February 1983): 17.
50. A view along these lines is stated in Richard Brandt, "Defective Newborns and the Morality of Termination," in M. Kohl, ed., *Infanticide and the Value of Life* (Buffalo: Prometheus Books, 1978), p. 49.
51. See, e.g., James H. Jones, *Bad Blood: The Tuskegee Syphilis Experiment* (New York: Free Press, 1981); Robert M. Veatch, "Experimental Pregnancy," *Hastings Center Report* 1 (June 1971): 2–3.
52. See, e.g., Dennis L. Breo, Doug Lefton, and Mark E. Rust, "MDs Face Unprecedented Murder Charge," *American Medical News*, September 16, 1983, p. 1. For a case in which medical practitioners were sued after sterilizing a mentally retarded woman, see *Sparkman* v. *McFarlin*, 552 F. 2d 172 (CA 7 1977).
53. U.S. Dept. of Health and Human Services, "Child Abuse and Neglect Prevention and Treatment Program."
54. Other decision makers might be physicians acting alone and courts. These approaches do not appear feasible, however. Elimination of the next of kin's consent, in favor of the physician's decision, would be considered unacceptable by most because it infringes on family authority. Courts generally are insufficiently familiar with the clinical setting to unilaterally formulate comprehensive and satisfactory policies. Moreover, oversight of all decisions would be too cumbersome. Court involvement is more feasible when it is limited to the occasional case requiring clarification of law or involving disagreement between families, physicians, and hospitals.
55. In its regulatory impact analysis, the U.S. Department of Health and Human Services acknowledged that the number of cases of unjustifiable withholding of treatment is not large. See "Child Abuse Prevention Program," p. 14,887. A similar view is expressed by John C. Moskop and Rita L. Saldanha, "The Baby Doe Rule: Still a Threat," *Hastings Center Report* 16 (1986): 9.

4
Medical Research Involving Human Subjects

4.1 Limited Consent in Alcoholism Research

Alcoholism is a disease with devastating social consequences. It is estimated that 8 to 10 percent of American men and 3 to 5 percent of American women are alcoholics. Each year there are almost two million alcohol-related deaths in the United States. Some are the direct result of profound alcohol intoxication. Other deaths result from medical conditions that are induced or exacerbated by chronic alcohol dependence. Alcohol abuse also figures in more than two hundred thousand accidental deaths, including 50 percent of auto fatalities. It is estimated that alcoholism is a fifteen-billion-dollar drain on the economy each year, resulting from lost work time, property damage, and health and welfare services for alcoholics and their families.

Despite our growing knowledge about the behavioral and physiological changes associated with alcohol addiction, it is estimated that more than half of the alcoholic patients seen by physicians are not diagnosed. This phenomenon may be the result of wide variations in overt symptoms, the preconceived notions of physicians about the "typical" presentation of alcoholics, and the cultural taboos that encourage persons to hide or deny their symptoms. A partial solution would be the development of a convenient test that physicians could use to screen patients for alcohol dependence. This tool would not replace in-depth diagnostic assessment but could be used to select patients for more intensive evaluation.

The institutional review board (IRB) at the medical college was reviewing a research protocol designed to evaluate potential screening mechanisms. One was a list of four questions that can be asked of patients during routine history taking. The questions asked whether the patient (1) feels he or she should drink less, (2) is annoyed by others criticizing his or her drinking habits, (3) feels guilty about drinking, and (4) takes a drink some mornings to relieve nervousness or overcome a hangover. The other mechanism involved assessment of the blood levels of various chemical substances, using a mathematical formula that correlates certain levels of these chemicals with alcohol dependence. The chemical indicators include urea nitrogen, uric acid, total bilirubin, lactate dehydrogenase, and other substances found in the blood. The capacity of these tests either individually or in combination to pick out all and only alcoholic patients was to be evaluated by using the more extensive Interview Schedule for Alcohol Use as the baseline test to confirm the presence or absence of alcoholism.

The methodology of the study required one thousand subjects, including medical, surgical, and psychiatric inpatients as well as medical outpatients. A research nurse would meet with each subject during an outpatient visit or soon after admission to the hospital. After securing consent, the nurse would ask the four questions and perform a venipuncture, drawing five tablespoons of blood for the laboratory data analysis. The subject would also be administered the Interview Schedule for Alcohol Use.

However, in order to receive accurate answers to interview questions, the investigators could not fully explain the purpose of the study. If it were explained that they were evaluating tests for detecting alcohol addiction, patients who abused alcohol and sought to avoid detection might give deliberately false answers or decline to participate in the study. Consequently, the usefulness of the four questions in routine clinical history taking (where their specific purpose would not typically be explained to the patient) could not be accurately determined. Similarly, utilization of the Interview Schedule for Alcohol Use as the baseline instrument for confirming alcohol addiction might be severely compromised. To circumvent these problems, the investigators proposed telling prospective subjects only that they were "studying the relationship between alcohol use and the results of routine blood tests." Moreover, the potential benefits of the study were to be vaguely described as helping physicians "to understand how to take care of patients in the future." Rather than naming the test interviews, the investigators would indicate only that they would ask "some questions." However, the research procedures, their minimal risks, and the provisions for maintaining confidentiality of the data were to be fully described in the consent interview.

The protocol sparked a sharp debate among committee members. A lawyer asserted that the IRB should not approve the protocol. He maintained that it was neither morally nor legally proper to perform invasive procedures (the venipuncture) without adequately informed consent. Under the law, nonconsensual touching of one's person is equivalent to assault and battery. Moreover, he noted that the questions to be asked, although not physically invasive, dealt with highly personal matters. Failure to secure adequately informed consent for discussion of these matters constituted an invasion of privacy.

However, a colleague of the principal investigator defended the study based on its social importance. She pointed out that an easily usable screening mechanism for covert alcoholism could pay rich dividends in bringing many patients into treatment before occurrence of its most devastating consequences. But this required testing of potential screening mechanisms—without fully adequate consent by subjects. She argued that society often chooses to abridge the rights of persons when matters of considerable social importance are at stake. This situation seemed analogous, and therefore some abridgment of the right to informed consent seemed justified.

The chairperson of the committee noted that federal regulations permit some aspects of informed consent to be deleted when (1) the research involves no more than minimal risk, (2) the waiver or alteration will not adversely affect the rights and welfare of subjects, and (3) the research could not be practically carried out without the waiver or alteration. He believed that the protocol met these requirements. Clearly, the research presented no more than minimal risk, because only venipunctures were involved. The minimal degree of risk also meant that the welfare of the subjects would not be adversely affected. Moreover, the token invasiveness of the venipuncture suggested that the subjects' rights would not be materially compromised.

Another committee member pointed out that the consent document did not involve lying to subjects. That is, the investigators were not making statements about their purpose deliberately intended to lead subjects to believe things to be true that the investigators knew to be false. Rather, the researchers were merely limiting the information being provided. Thus, the moral duty of truth telling would not be violated by this consent document.

But the lawyer rejected these claims. He agreed that society sometimes abridges personal rights to promote compelling social interests. But he argued that these decisions are usually made by elected representatives of the public. This was a much more defensible procedure than the decisions of a university IRB, most of whose members were medical investigators.

He also took issue with the assertion that the rights of the subjects would not be adversely affected. Even though the risks were negligible, the investigators intended to perform an invasive procedure without adequate consent. Any nonconsensual touching, he insisted, is a clear violation of an important personal right. Moreover, he maintained that there were special violations of privacy involved. Prospective subjects least inclined to participate would be persons with drinking problems they wanted to conceal. Failing to inform them of the purpose of the study would trick them into revealing a serious personal problem.

Finally, he dismissed any moral standing that might be gained from the claim that the consent process did not involve lying. The consent procedure would clearly deceive subjects regarding the purpose of the study. This stretched the principle of truth telling just as much as lying. At the very least, he thought the investigators should be required to inform potential subjects that the research design necessitated that not all information relevant to informed consent was being revealed.

However, the primary reviewer moved that the protocol be approved as presented, and his motion was seconded by another panel member.

4.2 Disclosure of Preliminary Results in a Randomized Clinical Trial

Osteosarcoma is a cancer that usually begins in a long bone of the arm or leg and later spreads to the lungs. It primarily affects adolescents. Before 1970, patients were treated with surgery alone. If there was no evidence at diagnosis that the cancer had spread beyond the affected limb, the arm or leg was amputated. If the disease had already spread (metastasized) to the lungs, no treatment was given, because all patients with metastases died. Unfortunately, even among patients who were apparently free of metastases at diagnosis, fewer than 20 percent survived disease-free for longer than two years following amputation.

Early in the 1970s two new drugs, adriamycin and methotrexate, were found to cause regression of the tumor. Recognizing that many patients may have undetected micrometastases at diagnosis, some investigators began to examine the usefulness of giving chemotherapy after amputation but before spread of the disease became apparent (adjuvant chemotherapy). The results were striking. In 1974 two investigative groups reported that about 50 percent of patients having no evidence of metastases at diagnosis survived disease-free for more than two years when treated with adjuvant chemotherapy for one year after amputation. Throughout the remainder of the 1970s various regimens were investigated and similar results achieved.

During this same period, diagnostic techniques were also changing. In the 1960s physicians used chest X rays to look for lung metastases. But in the 1970s they began to use CT scans, which provide cross-sectional views of the chest. Comparison studies showed that this method could detect lung metastases that remained hidden on standard X rays. This raised serious questions about using the treatment results with pre-1970 patients, who received amputation alone, as the baseline for measuring the comparative efficacy of amputation followed by adjuvant chemotherapy. Specifically, cancer specialists were concerned that the dismal results with amputation alone might reflect the inability of pre-1970 X-ray techniques to detect lung metastases already present in many patients. Using the new diagnostic techniques to identify patients without lung disease, amputation alone might achieve much better results in the more accurately diagnosed group. The issue was important because most adjuvant chemotherapies have serious, sometimes life-threatening side effects. If amputation alone is just as effective in curing the disease, chemotherapy should not be used.

After a small preliminary study suggested that amputation alone might also achieve 50 percent two-year disease-free survival, a large national study was initiated. Patients without evidence of lung disease at diagnosis were randomized to receive either amputation alone or amputation followed by one year of adjuvant chemotherapy. The statistical design of the study required that ninety-nine patients be randomly assigned to each arm of the study before the more effective treatment could be determined at a 95 percent confidence level.[1] Patients who refused to be randomized would be allowed to choose between the two treatments.

It quickly became apparent that patients receiving amputation alone were doing more poorly than the group receiving chemotherapy. Of the first thirty-four patients receiving chemotherapy, only three had experienced spread of their disease. By contrast, twenty-two out of thirty-one patients receiving amputation alone had developed metastatic cancer. Because spread beyond its place of origin in the affected limb usually signifies irreversible disease, projected survival rates were much poorer for the latter group.

The question arose regarding whether prospective subjects and their families should be apprised of the preliminary results. Some investigators believed that they were morally obligated to disclose this information. According to the theory of informed consent, prospective subjects should receive whatever information a "reasonable person" would need to make the choice most consistent with his or her values and interests. This includes information concerning the relative benefits and risks of alternative treatments. In this case, survival might depend on which treatment a patient received. Moreover, whether the patient would be exposed to a year of highly toxic chemotherapy depended on the choice made. Given these high stakes, any "reasonable person" would want to know how other patients were faring as one item of information relevant to the decision.

Some biostatisticians rejected this reasoning. They argued that a "reasonable person" would want to interpret relevant data using appropriate statistical methods. These methods indicated that the preliminary results did not yet permit the conclusion that one treatment option was significantly better than the other. There were two reasons. First, the preliminary outcomes might be the result of early chance entry of more "poor prognosis" patients into the amputation-only arm of the study than into the chemotherapy arm. Second, some biostatisticians considered the patients who had chosen their therapy to be not evaluable in determining the better treatment. They feared subtle differences between subjects choosing the respective options, with regard to general health status or psychological profile, which might affect results for the different treatments. Thus, differences in outcome for the two groups might not represent differences in the efficacy of the treatments themselves. Because only thirty of the first sixty-five patients had accepted randomization, the data were even more preliminary, from a statistical perspective, than suggested by the total number of patients.

In light of these concerns, it could be argued that a "reasonable person" would not need the preliminary data; he or she would not be able to draw any statistically defensible inference about the most efficacious treatment. From a more practical standpoint, the average person could only be misled by the preliminary data. Typical subjects, not understanding the relevance of biostatistical theory, would conclude from raw preliminary data that chemotherapy was more effective when, in fact, there was no statistical basis for this conclusion.

However, critics noted that the statisticians were assuming that a person could make a reasonable inference regarding the most effective treatment only by using the criterion of a statistically significant difference between treatments as defined in the study protocol. (A statistically significant difference required enough subjects to determine at a 95 percent confidence level that there was more than a 20 percent difference in two-year disease-free survival rates for the two treatments.) But there are other reasonable ways to choose a treatment. When a patient faces a potentially fatal disease and cannot wait for the study to be completed before choosing a treatment, then the current raw percentage of disease-free patients in both treatment groups seems a reasonable basis for making a choice. In short, a "reasonable person" would want the information.

Those who defend nondisclosure of preliminary data appealed to other considerations. Thus far, even subjects who refused randomization were distributing themselves equally between the two treatments. However, investigators feared that if preliminary data were disclosed, most prospective subjects would choose chemotherapy. For lack of adequate numbers of patients in the amputation arm, the study would not be completed and no scientifically valid conclusions would be possible.

This outcome would have two serious moral consequences. First, treatment for osteosarcoma patients without lung metastases at diagnosis would continue without any firm knowledge about the optimal therapy. A goal of cancer therapy research is to find treatments that achieve acceptable percentages of disease-free survival while keeping serious side effects at a minimum. Failure to complete this study would result in the indefinite use of highly toxic chemotherapies, because the use of adjuvant chemotherapy had become standard treatment.

Second, many investigators believed that they had an obligation to subjects recruited at the outset of the study to complete it. In entering the study, they had agreed to undergo the additional diagnostic tests (X rays, venipunctures, bone marrow aspirations, etc.) that are utilized to carefully monitor the progress of research subjects. They were also willing to accept unforeseeable risks that might result from the therapies. In exchange, the investigators were making a tacit promise to design and execute the study in a way that made their commitments and sacrifices worthwhile. If disclosure of preliminary information was likely to result in the study not being completed (for lack of subjects entering one arm), then adoption of a policy of routine disclosure was tantamount to breaking faith with the subjects recruited early in the study.

4.3 Constraints on Consent in a Phase I Clinical Trial

J.P. was a thirteen-year-old girl whose family resided in a small city. Her father was a factory worker; her mother had devoted her married life to raising their three children, of whom J.P. was the youngest. The family was close-knit and religious. J.P. had always been a sickly child, and she had been cared for by her mother. They had an unusually close relationship. For example, they frequently talked at length about how their relationship was progressing. J.P. was also a popular girl, and had friends both at school and in the youth group at church.

J.P. began having pain her right flank about five months earlier. When a mass appeared on her lower back, she was admitted to the hospital for a diagnostic workup. An exploratory biopsy revealed a soft tissue mass astride a segment of the lower spine (the third lumbar vertebra). It was also determined that a portion of the vertebra (the transverse process) had been completely destroyed. Pathological examination of a biopsy specimen indicated that the mass was a malignant tumor arising from the vertebra (flat bone osteosarcoma). Its precise location made complete surgical excision impossible. Because the location of the tumor also precluded the use of radiation, J.P. was entered into a research protocol for treatment with high-dose methotrexate, a chemotherapeutic agent. The plan was to attempt shrinkage of the tumor until the mass became completely resectable.

At the time of diagnosis, the oncologist had several lengthy discussions with the girl's parents. He explained that flat bone osteosarcoma was very rare and that there was little experience in treating it with drugs. However, past results suggested that the probability of their daughter surviving was less than 5 percent. He believed that the only chance for survival was to surgically remove the tumor after shrinkage by chemotherapy. Although the probability figure was not shared with J.P., she was told that her condition was very serious.

Unfortunately, the mass continued to grow, and two further changes in chemotherapy failed to halt its progression. Within four months, ultrasound revealed a right abdominal mass which filled the abdomen and extended out the back. The right kidney was displaced laterally, and the aorta and inferior vena cava were displaced anteriorly. Physical examination revealed a large mass extending from the ribs to the pelvis and measuring 12 by 12 cm. On the back, the mass measured 16 by 17 cm.

As the child's tumor became progressively larger, the parents were told that there was no longer any hope of survival. However, they continued to express hope that other drugs might cause regression of the tumor. Moreover, both the parents and the patient exhibited considerable denial about the eventual outcome. For example, they continued to actively discuss J.P.'s education, social activities, and career plans.

During the course of her third chemotherapeutic regimen, J.P. was brought back to the hospital in considerable pain and no longer able to sit up. The oncologist told J.P.'s parents that she would begin to deteriorate rapidly. He believed that there was spinal cord involvement and that bladder and bowel incontinence, as well as paralysis of the lower limbs, could occur. But the parents pressed the physician about the availability of further drugs. In fact, they were adamant about their willingness to try any possibility. They still firmly believed that God would help their child.

While the parents were visiting with the physician, the nurse-practitioner had a long discussion with J.P. Because she was highly narcotized with dilaudid for relief of her pain, she alternated between periods of euphoria and hopefulness and a more somber outlook. She also appeared to have mixed feelings about further drug therapy. On one hand, she said that she did not want another drug because she was tired of being sick to her stomach and because her abdominal pain made vomiting so difficult. She also wanted to go home. (Though she had asked her parents to take her home several times, her mother hoped she could stay because management at home had become so difficult.) On the other hand, J.P. said she did not want her mother upset. She also wished to do something for her parents, who she felt needed to be repaid for all they had given her before and during her illness. She knew her mother was still hopeful, and J.P. herself still believed that God would help her. So it would be all right with her if she received another drug.

One remaining alternative was to enter J.P. in a phase I clinical trial of the chemotherapy AMSA. A phase I study is the initial stage of drug testing in humans. With cancer chemotherapies, eligible subjects are persons who have terminal cancer and have been unsuccessfully treated with conventional or "front-line" experimental therapies. The primary purpose of a phase I trial is to identify the toxic effect of the drug at various dosage levels and to determine the maximum tolerable dose at which it can be given. Secondarily, the investigation also involves noting any antitumor effects of the drug. The information gained from a phase I trial is used to establish the appropriate dosage of the drug for later trials of its antitumor effectiveness singly and in combination with other drugs.

In designing a phase I trial, an initial dosage is determined on the basis of previous clinical trials in other human populations and in animals. A series of escalating dosages is then designated. Three patients are entered at each dosage level, and each patient receives only that dosage for the duration of his or her involvement. If prohibitive toxicity does not occur at a given level, the following three patients are entered at the next dosage level. The study is discontinued when a prohibitive toxicity is reached. An individual patient's participation is discontinued when there is either unequivocal progression of the disease or prohibitive toxicity from the drug. The early dosage levels are usually such that no toxic effects and no anticancer results occur; at higher dosages toxicity becomes common and some regression of tumor possible.

The staff met to discuss J.P.'s participation in the phase I trial. The oncologist indicated that she met the technical criteria for eligibility and would be the first patient entered at a dosage of 110 mg per square meter.[2] At this dosage, some toxicity was expected, primarily nausea and decrease in blood cell production. Two previous patients in the study had achieved slight tumor regression, and antitumor activity at this new dosage level was possible.

However, the nurse-practitioner raised serious concern about the family's continuing denial of the girl's impending death. She felt that they would accept any new drug without fully considering its implications for the child's welfare. She reported that although the patient had indicated a willingness to continue treatment, it was based primarily on a concern for her mother's needs. The nurse felt that allowing her to participate in the study for this reason was inappropriate; her physical suffering might be exacerbated. She proposed that the family be strongly urged to make arrangements for J.P. to receive terminal care in an extended-care, skilled-nursing facility near her home (which was seventy miles away), where the whole family could be with her regularly and provide their fullest support to her and one another.

A resident physician who was caring for J.P. took a somewhat different view. He felt that the needs of the parents were quite important. They would need assurance in the coming years that "everything possible" had been done. Failing to allow their child to enter the trial might seriously compromise their psychological adjustment after her death. Moreover, he thought that if the purpose of the study, the expected toxicity, and the low probability of benefit were carefully explained, then the parents would be able to make a sensitive decision. Although he agreed that they showed considerable denial, he said that this is not uncommon and is one way of easing the emotional suffering caused by the impending death of one's child. He also suggested that because most parents exhibit some denial, it is difficult to determine when it becomes so serious as to make consent insufficiently informed or voluntary. If the presence of denial were taken as an indication against the possibility of informed consent, phase I trials in children might never be completed. Because these trials are very important in developing new treatments for children with cancer, the only recourse is to handle the consent situation as conscientiously as possible.

A psychologist pointed out that children and parents sometimes gain satisfaction from participating in clinical cancer trials. Some dying adolescents experience considerable anguish and guilt about "failing" their parents. Although J.P. might not wish further therapy on her own account, it might ease her psychological burden to undergo the treatment her parents wished. Moreover, parents and children sometimes find that helping future patients by participating in a clinical trial is one way of giving meaning to their tragic circumstances. On the other hand, the psychologist thought that it would be best if the staff could break through the denial of both parents and child and prepare them for the child's impending death. But he did not know whether this "ideal" course of action would succeed.

4.4 Proxy Consent for Incompetent Trauma Patients

The IRB chairperson asked Dr. G. to present the first protocol to the committee. She began by noting that valid informed consent of subjects or their proxies should be obtained before the initiation of research. She pointed out that this can be difficult when prospective subjects are incompetent and authorized proxies suffer from decision-making impairments. An example would be research in the intensive care unit involving trauma victims, illustrated by the first protocol. Family members typically are distraught over the injury to their loved one. Emotional shock and stress can interfere with their ability to assimilate information and appreciate the implications of the patient's participation in a research study. This makes it difficult to obtain valid proxy consent and raises questions about such research, she said, particularly when there are risks to the subject not present in standard therapy.

The purpose of the proposed research was to ascertain the effects of blunt trauma on the body's ability to utilize and excrete lidocaine.[3] This information would enable physicians to better determine proper dosages for trauma victims. Lidocaine is a drug often used for trauma patients to correct irregularities of heartbeat rhythm. Although dosages for nontrauma patients are well established, the proper dosage for trauma patients was unclear because the body's natural response to trauma might alter the effects of lidocaine in two ways. First, trauma might slow its elimination from the body, resulting in higher blood levels in comparison to nontraumatized patients. Slower elimination was suspected because lidocaine is broken down by the liver, and trauma causes reduced blood flow to the liver, possibly reducing liver activity.[4] Second, trauma might inactivate some of the lidocaine circulating in the blood by increasing the attachment of protein molecules to lidocaine.[5] This was postulated because trauma causes an increase in the amount of a certain protein circulating in the blood, alpha-1 acid glycoprotein (AAG), which binds to lidocaine. If the net effect of these two bodily responses to trauma were to increase the level of free (not bound to proteins) lidocaine, then adverse reactions to excessive doses could occur. If, on the other hand, the net effect were to decrease the amount of free lidocaine, then its therapeutic effects might not be achieved. Thus, it was important to learn the effects of trauma on lidocaine levels.

The subjects would be adult blunt trauma victims with an Injury Severity Score (ISS) of 10 to 40 and a Trauma Score (TS) greater than or equal to 10.[6] Patients with scores in the ranges indicated would have significant injury but would be likely to survive. Some, if not all, would be incapable of giving consent. Shortly after admission, consent would be sought from the patient or next of kin, as appropriate. All subjects would receive standard care for their injuries. In addition, various procedures would be performed for research purposes. First, a single dose of lidocaine would be administered during the first and seventh days following the injury. After each dose, ten blood samples would be collected over a six-hour period, using an indwelling catheter in the subject's forearm. Blood levels of free and bound lidocaine would be measured in each sample. Second, a single dose of indocyanine green would also be given on days one and seven. Because its rate of elimination provides a known measure of liver blood flow, the blood levels of indocyanine green would be measured by taking eight blood samples over a twenty-minute period following its administration. Thus, the effects of liver blood flow on lidocaine levels would be assessed by comparing the degree of blood flow with levels of lidocaine in the blood. Third, on days one through seven, a blood sample would be drawn daily to measure serum concentrations of AAG and albumin (another major protein that binds with lidocaine). The effects of AAG would be ascertained by comparing these protein levels with the levels of free and bound lidocaine.

The potential risks and benefits to subjects were carefully outlined in the research protocol. The doses of lidocaine and the blood tests would be administered solely to collect research data and would not benefit the subjects. At therapeutic levels lidocaine can produce various adverse reactions. Relatively minor and reversible ones include drowsiness, dizziness, tinnitus (ringing in the ears), double vision, and vomiting. Possible severe reactions include convulsions, hypotension (low blood pressure), respiratory arrest, and cardiac arrest. The researchers were proposing to minimize the risk of an adverse reaction by using a dose of lidocaine (1 mg/kg)[7] below the recommended therapeutic level, and only one dose would be given on each test day. Also, patients whose medical condition (such as hypotension or congestive heart failure) would exacerbate the effects of an adverse reaction would also not be entered into the study. The dose of indocyanine green to be administered (0.5 mg/kg) was the standard dose for this type of test. This dye solution contains a small amount of sodium iodide, and its main risk is an allergic reaction by patients sensitive to iodine. Such reactions can involve headache, profuse perspiration, pruritis (itching), hives, hypotension, and difficulty breathing. Although rare, cases of severe reactions, including at least one death, have been reported.[8] For this reason, patients with a known allergy to iodine would be excluded from the study. In the event of an allergic reaction, medical assistance would be readily available in the trauma unit. Although administration of indocyanine green and associated blood samples were primarily for research, the data obtained might benefit a subject by aiding in the diagnosis of liver damage if present. The risks associated with the drawing of blood would include infection at the venipuncture site, bruising, pain, and fainting. The amount of blood drawn for research purposes would be about six ounces (approximately twelve tablespoonsful), a quantity whose loss would not be medically harmful.

Following Dr. G.'s review of the protocol, discussion by committee members ensued, during which several options were advocated, including (1) approval of the protocol as written; (2) approval with the proviso that the investigators obtain "deferred consent" from next of kin; (3) approval with the proviso that the research be restricted to competent trauma patients; or (4) disapproval of the protocol.

A pharmacologist argued for approval as written; he believed that knowledge about the proper dosage of lidocaine would be useful in treating a large number of future trauma patients. Moreover, this knowledge could only be obtained by studying trauma victims. He pointed out that the statistical risk of injury to subjects was very low, and subjects whose liver function progressively worsens because of their traumatic injury might benefit from detection of this problem.

Dr. G., however, opposed this approach. She believed that the stresses experienced by family members would seriously impede their ability to make considered decisions. She pointed out that federal regulations concerning research require valid informed consent of subjects or their legally authorized representatives whenever forgoing fully adequate consent would adversely affect the subject's rights or welfare.[9] Because proxy consent by a family member who might be familiar with the patient's wishes helps protect the patient's right to self-determination, research on previously competent adults without valid proxy consent would infringe that right. Moreover, because proxy consent is an instrument for protecting the welfare of patients, invalid proxy consent would weaken this protection.

She suggested that deferred consent might provide a way of balancing the social benefits of the research and the concern for patients' interests. According to this approach, the investigators would delay seeking informed consent from next of kin, perhaps until two days after the traumatic injury. At that time family members usually would be under less stress and better able to make an informed decision. Families would nevertheless be informed at the time of admission that the patient would be entered in a research project. They would thus have an opportunity at that time to inquire further and even refuse consent. Furthermore, she thought it would protect the family's emotional well-being to delay consent, because it might add to the family's stress at the time of admission to engage in a consent interview. The physician's duty to provide emotional support to families could be better carried out by deferring a full discussion of the research.[10]

However, another physician on the committee argued that because deferred consent occurs after the entry of the subject into research, it cannot justify the initiation of research procedures. Such justification must be based on other considerations. For example, it might be argued that the importance of the knowledge to be gained from the research outweighs the minor infringement of patients' interests that would occur in delaying proxy consent. He claimed that such an argument would be acceptable only if risks to the subject are low in the interim between initiation of the research procedures and the obtaining of proxy consent. However, he did not believe the risks during this interval would be low, because patients allergic to iodine could have a serious reaction to indocyanine green. Based on these risks, he believed that incompetent patients should not be used in the study. He recommended approval of the protocol only if the investigators were willing to restrict the research to competent trauma patients.

Another committee member suggested that family members usually know when adults are allergic to iodine. He suggested that incompetent patients would be adequately protected by asking the next of kin whether the patient had such an allergy.

Yet another member was doubtful that the surrogate would necessarily know about an allergy. She pointed out that there have been cases of allergic reactions in patients with no previous reactions to iodine. In addition, she argued that even when trauma victims appear competent, the validity of their consent to nontherapeutic research can be questioned. First, affective factors such as emotional shock and fear may interfere with the patient's ability to make a considered decision. Second, because trauma patients are highly vulnerable and dependent on the trauma unit staff for immediate medical care, consent might not be adequately voluntary. She urged the committee to disapprove the protocol based on concern for the interests of subjects.

4.5 Undue Inducement in the Recruitment of Research Subjects

Federal regulations specify that investigators shall seek consent "only under circumstances that provide the prospective subject . . . sufficient opportunity to consider whether or not to participate and that minimize the possibility of coercion or undue influence" (*Code of Federal Regulations* 45, sec. 46.116). Moreover, institutional review boards must ensure that "appropriate additional safeguards" are created to protect the rights and welfare of prospective subjects, especially "Where some or all of the subjects are likely to be vulnerable to coercion or undue influence, such as persons with acute or severe physical or mental illness, or persons who are economically or educationally disadvantaged" (*Code of Federal Regulations* 45, sec. 46.111).

In this case, a biochemist on the research committee raised serious doubts about whether a proposed study satisfied the prohibition against "undue influence." The protocol involved treatment for polycystic ovarian disease (PCOD). Patients with this syndrome usually undergo normal growth and pubertal development but before age twenty-five experience the onset of irregular menses, with eventual prolonged periods in which they do not ovulate and fail to have regular menstrual bleeding. Besides serious infertility problems, many patients have hirsutism, a condition involving the presence of excessive bodily and facial hair. Approximately 40 percent are also obese. When biopsied, their ovaries are found to be enlarged and to contain multiple clear cysts. Causative factors in the disease are not fully understood, although serious abnormalities in blood and urine levels of various hormones have been clearly identified.

The research protocol was designed to evaluate a new drug called Nafarelin, which is administered by nasal spray twice daily. Preliminary evidence suggested that it might reduce hormonal abnormalities and many symptoms associated with the disease. The design of the study required that each subject participate for five months and involved three stages. At the outset, subjects would enter the hospital for three days of general testing and baseline measurement of hormone production. During the first day, subjects would receive complete physical and pelvic examinations. They would also have blood withdrawn from an indwelling catheter every ten minutes for twenty-four hours to measure the serum levels of various hormones. On the second and third days, three additional tests were scheduled to assess hormone production, requiring seventeen additional blood samples. There was also an ultrasound evaluation of the ovaries scheduled for the second day, and a twenty-four-hour urine specimen was to be collected each day.

At the start of their next menstrual cycle, subjects were to begin using the drug daily for two months. The drug is intended to produce hormone changes, and possible side effects include vaginal bleeding, changes in menstrual cycle, hot flashes, breast tenderness, and mood changes. During this period, blood sampling was required on fifteen days and involved forty separate venipunctures.

Following completion of therapy, each subject would repeat the three days of testing performed at the outset of the study. After this assessment, subjects would return once a week for eight weeks, providing one blood sample (via venipuncture) to track the return of baseline hormone levels.

The protocol called for the treatment of fifteen patients with confirmed PCOD and ten normal control subjects. Because the patients were to receive extensive evaluation of their disease and a potentially effective treatment free of charge, they would not be compensated. The control subjects would be paid $750 and would be recruited from patients at the university's gynecology clinic.

The biochemist emphasized that the protocol was well designed, and she underscored the importance of using the complex schedule for blood sampling to provide accurate longitudinal measurements of hormones whose blood levels may fluctuate considerably over time. She noted that the reliability of the results of many previous investigations of PCOD had been seriously weakened by the practice of drawing too limited a number of blood samples.

Rather, her concerns focused on the plan to pay control subjects $750 and to recruit these volunteers from the university clinic. In her view, one form of undue inducement involves enticing prospective subjects to participate in a study that they consider seriously contrary to their interest in avoiding harm and discomfort, but which they enter only to receive the payment offered. She maintained that compensation should primarily serve to reimburse subjects for lost work time, transportation costs, and other inconveniences but should not be so attractive as to involve persons in studies that they would otherwise decline to enter because of significant risks or discomforts.

She believed that the study's compensation plan did not meet these requirements. First, the schedule of procedures was so rigorous that she believed no woman would consider it consistent with her interests to participate as a control subject, even if she were satisfactorily reimbursed for her personal expenses. Second, the plan for recruiting subjects involved inviting patients at the university gynecology clinic, who are almost exclusively very poor or unemployed. She maintained that this was probably the only group of women who could be convinced to undergo the procedures involved in the study and that they would agree to participate only because they could desperately use the $750 payment. Thus, the net result was that subjects would be induced to participate only to receive the compensation and in spite of the significant discomforts involved—in her view a paradigm example of one form of undue inducement.

An ethicist suggested that there were other moral commitments endangered by the plan for recruiting subjects. The principle of justice requires that the burdens of involvement in clinical research be fairly distributed among different segments of the population. If women who were not poor or unemployed were unlikely to participate, then the net result was that only economically disadvantaged women would bear the burdens of participation in the study. Thus, he thought that the inducement was undue not only because it took advantage of the decision-making weaknesses of prospective subjects but also because it would violate the requirements of social justice.

However, the chairperson of the committee took considerable exception to the reviewer's assessment of the compensation issue. He said that one goal of federal research regulations is to ensure that persons are able to make informed decisions, based on their own values and interests, about participation in studies. He maintained that disallowing clinic patients as normal control subjects would constitute a paternalistic violation of this goal. The reviewer was proposing that clinic patients not be allowed to make their own decisions about involvement, so that they might be protected from the discomforts and inconveniences of participation in the study.

Moreover, he questioned the assumption that participation as a normal control would be contrary to the interests of most subjects. He pointed out that although the study involved an unusually large number of nontherapeutic procedures for control subjects, none carried more than minimal risk and most involved only minor discomforts. Subjects who are not bothered by procedures such as venipunctures might not consider them a serious burden and might regard $750 as good payment for being involved. Moreover, the reviewer seemed to assume that none of the prospective subjects would have altruistic commitments and that their decisions would be based solely on the desire for reimbursement. But interest in promoting the welfare of others might provide sufficient motivation for some subjects.

Another committee member suggested a different perspective on the justice issue. He agreed that poor or unemployed clinic patients would be the only persons choosing to participate. But this would provide people who most needed the money with the greatest opportunity to earn it. Rather than discriminating against poor subjects by imposing unfair burdens, the study provided an opportunity to earn badly needed money.

In responding to these criticisms, the ethicist claimed that the socioeconomic status of most clinic patients results in their being unduly susceptible to financial inducements to act in ways contrary to their self-perceived interest in avoiding harm and discomfort. In effect, they are operating with an impaired decision-making capacity. Respect for them as persons would normally require provision of the opportunity to decide for themselves about participation. However, respect for persons also requires that appropriate safeguards be provided for those who are less than fully autonomous, as suggested in the federal regulations.

The committee lawyer recommended that the impasse might be resolved by requiring the investigators to draw their control subjects from patients of private-practice gynecologists in the city. These patients would typically have much higher incomes than the clinic patients and therefore would be less susceptible to the financial inducement. However, a committee member from the department of obstetrics and gynecology indicated that this requirement would make execution of the study much more administratively burdensome, would increase its costs, and might seriously lengthen the time required to complete it. He did not think that the concerns raised merited these additional costs.

4.6 Nontherapeutic Research Procedures Involving Children

In treating childhood cancer, the use of chemotherapies in combination provides the best therapy for patients with metastatic disease at diagnosis. Development of multiple drug regimens requires the determination of several variables, including (1) which drugs to use in combination, (2) the appropriate dosages, (3) whether they should be administered simultaneously or sequentially, (4) the optimal time interval between administrations, and (5) the number of times the pattern needs to be repeated. Historically, these questions have been addressed by comparing outcomes of different regimens in securing remissions of the disease, prolonging life, and achieving disease-free survival. But this method has had limited results. Although "empirical" manipulation of variables 1 through 5 has improved clinical outcomes, these improvements have now reached a plateau in several types of childhood cancer. Moreover, exhaustive controlled manipulation of the variables to determine optimal treatment requires a very large number of both subjects and clinical trials for each tumor type. Since only six thousand to eight thousand children contract childhood cancers each year in the United States, this investigative approach is not feasible.

A solution involves the development of a theory about how tumor cells proliferate and how chemotherapy can be optimally employed to destroy them. One branch of this theory involves cell kinetics—knowledge concerning the manner in which tumor cells proliferate before and after alteration by chemotherapy. Cell-kinetic studies have already yielded important information concerning the effect of cancer chemotherapy on tumor cells. For example, many drugs have been found to affect tumor cells in a specific stage of the cell cycle.[11] These drugs have also been shown to affect tumor cells in different ways. Some irreparably damage tumor cells, others cause a buildup of cells at a particular point in the cell cycle by blocking their progression through that stage (synchronization), and still other drugs cause nondividing cells to enter the division process where they are more sensitive to lethal drug action (recruitment). Finally, it has been determined that the duration of the cell-kinetic effects of drugs varies.

This information can be applied to treatment design in a couple of ways. First, cell-kinetic information may suggest what antitumor drugs to combine and what interval to allow between their administration. For example, drug A may block tumor cells at one stage in the cell cycle for forty-eight hours, causing a buildup of cells at that point. If drug B kills tumor cells in the next stage of the cell division process, it might be given forty-eight hours after the first to maximally destroy the synchronized group of cells entering that phase. Second, cell-kinetic information may be useful in predicting which patients will not respond to treatment. That is, the drugs may not have their usual cell-kinetic effects during their initial dose in patients who eventually fail to achieve remission. This would allow an early change to drugs that might be more effective.

The final study reviewed by the institutional review board was of the tumor cell kinetics of two drugs, ARA-C and VM-26, being used to induce remission of acute lymphocytic leukemia.[12] The investigators had three objectives: to examine the specific impact of these drugs on tumor cells, to clarify the optimal time interval between repeat administrations of the drugs, and to determine whether the absence of a cell-kinetic effect during the first dose correlates with treatment failure. If useful information were obtained, more effective scheduling of the drugs might be possible. If treatment failure could be predicted, future patients could be changed more quickly to other chemotherapies.

However, the development of cell-kinetic information requires the use of serial, nontherapeutic procedures to obtain accessible tumor cells. These cells must be examined at frequent intervals after the administration of chemotherapy. The plan in this study required that bone marrow samples be obtained when the first drug was given and then eight, forty-eight, and seventy-two hours after its administration. Except for the first bone marrow aspiration (required as a baseline to monitor the patient's progress in therapy), the procedures were nontherapeutic.

Bone marrow samples were to be obtained by aspiration from the posterior crest of the pelvic bone. A needle is inserted through the skin and into the marrow cavity of the pelvic bone, and a small sample of marrow is withdrawn using a syringe. Although a local anesthetic is injected into the skin and the membrane covering the bone, the bone itself cannot be anesthetized. The subject may feel pain as the aspiration needle passes through the bone into the marrow cavity. He or she also usually experiences pain when suction is applied to remove the marrow. The extent of pain is highly variable, from minor discomfort to rather intense pain, and is affected by the subject's degree of tenseness and anxiety. There is also a small risk of infection and excessive bleeding in leukemia patients who have an unusually low number of white blood cells and platelets. Finally, leukemic marrow can be densely packed and difficult to aspirate. In this case, the aspiration needle may have to be reinserted at a different spot. The procedure can be completed within two minutes.

Following presentation of the protocol, the chairperson of the committee reviewed federal research regulations regarding the use of nontherapeutic procedures with children. She noted that they freely allow procedures that involve no more than "minimal risk"—defined as an anticipated risk of harm whose probability and magnitude are not greater than those ordinarily encountered in daily life or during the performance of routine physical or psychological exams. However, when risks exceed the minimal level, special requirements must be met before nontherapeutic procedures can be used. (1) The risk involved must represent only a minor increase over minimal risk. (2) The procedures must present experiences to subjects that are reasonably similar to those they have had during treatment. (3) The procedures must be likely to yield generalizable knowledge about the subjects' disorder that is vitally important for understanding or ameliorating the disease.

These rules were developed by the National Commission for the Protection of Human Subjects of Biomedical and Behavioral Research. The commission maintained that research using minimal-risk, nontherapeutic procedures with children is morally permissible because, by definition, minimal-risk procedures expose them to no more risk than other daily activities. Thus, the duty to protect children from harm would not be violated by such research. However, the commission was much more reluctant to allow nonbeneficial procedures that create special risks of harm. But it recognized that vitally important knowledge for ameliorating specific childhood diseases might be gained from studies employing nontherapeutic procedures with more than minimal risks. Consequently, it endorsed their use when the three conditions specified above are met. The chairperson suggested that the protocol be reviewed under these rules, because serial bone marrow aspirations involve a degree of harm beyond that encountered in everyday experience.

A lively debate about the protocol ensued. A physician-researcher claimed that the special conditions were met. He noted that the bone marrow aspirations would be performed only by experienced physicians, so that the risk of any problem other than physical discomfort was small. In addition, he argued that because children with acute lymphocytic leukemia must occasionally undergo bone marrow aspirations, the procedures would be commensurate with their current experiences. Finally, he suggested that the development of cell-kinetic knowledge is an important way to improve chemotherapy for leukemia.

But a child-psychologist argued that the physician's judgment of potential harm focused only on physical harms and failed to consider subjective experiences of anxiety and fear. She pointed out that some children are "terrified" by invasive procedures, even those as benign as venipunctures. If one considers these psychological harms, risks might far exceed a "minor increase over minimal risk" for particular children. She also pointed out that satisfaction of the "commensurability" condition does not ensure that psychological harms will not occur. If a child is made extremely anxious by a procedure, having undergone it a few previous times is unlikely to make a psychological difference. Finally, she emphasized that many children are suffering from acute complications of their disease, such as malaise, fever, joint pain, infection, and bleeding, or the side effects of therapy, such as nausea and vomiting. These problems may exacerbate the psychological stress of medical procedures.

A basic scientist questioned whether the study would contribute knowledge "vitally important" in improving treatment for acute lymphocytic leukemia. He maintained that knowledge about the cell cycle specificity of the drugs and the duration of their cell-kinetic effects might allow minor manipulations of the treatment schedule but would not lead to major improvements in rates of disease remission. He also pointed out that although it might become possible to predict nonresponders to therapy using cell-kinetic information, there is little effective "second-line" therapy for acute lymphocytic leukemia to which treatment could be changed.

The lawyer on the committee found the regulations inadequate because they make no provision for disallowing the involvement of younger children who object to the procedures (hospital policy required securing assent only from children older than twelve). He expressed deep moral concern about performing bone marrow aspirations on children who verbally or nonverbally might resist involvement. Presumably, these children would also be those for whom such procedures are particularly frightening or painful. Even allowing for such objections, he feared that less aggressive children might be too reticent to voice their objection to parents or physicians. Similarly, children suffering from acute symptoms of their disease might be too weakened to express their concerns.

Another scientist attempted to address these various problems. He suggested that his colleague who judged the study as unable to produce "vitally important knowledge" was assigning too strict a meaning to the phrase—making it equivalent to "breakthrough knowledge." Even very good studies are typically able to make only piecemeal improvements in treatment. He judged that the study could meet the latter criterion. He also suggested that the committee could be confident that the physician-investigators would not involve children who had typically exhibited serious distress when undergoing bone marrow aspirations. Just as a practical matter, it would be too difficult to complete four marrow aspirations on these children within the designated period of time.

But the lawyer was not satisfied. Even granting the "good intentions" of investigators, he was concerned about children who would feel compelled to go along with the procedures or who would not object only because they did not understand that the procedures were not related to their treatment.

At this point, the chairperson summarized the panel's options: (1) disapprove the study; (2) approve it in its present form; (3) require that the investigators reduce the number of procedures or forgo the study; or (4) approve the study but require some special provisions for selecting the subjects, in order to ensure that the study would not include subjects who were highly distressed by the procedures. (For example, screening interviews with a psychologist might be used.)

4.7 Discomfort from Repeated Nontherapeutic Research Procedures Involving Competent Adults

The institutional review board reviewed a protocol designed to determine the advantages of buffered over regular aspirin in providing protection to stomach linings. Although it is an effective analgesic, aspirin may cause exacerbations of peptic ulcers, stomach distress and heartburn, and gastrointestinal bleeding. Evidence suggests that aspirin interacts with the stomach lining in a way that breaks down the resistance of the mucosal surfaces to stomach acid. Thus, an important question is whether aspirin containing antacid or "buffering" ingredients will significantly decrease the impact of acid on mucosal linings when aspirin is ingested. Previous studies have been poorly designed and inconclusive in their results.

The researchers proposed to use healthy, competent adult subjects without previous history of gastrointestinal disease. Four different medications were to be compared: two forms of buffered aspirin (differing in the amount of buffering ingredients), Alka Seltzer (differing in the type of its buffering ingredient), and plain aspirin. Each subject would take one drug for a three-day period (twenty-four tablets) and then be switched to the second, third, and fourth drugs in subsequent three-day trial periods. The effects of each drug on the stomach lining were to be determined by direct visual inspection of the stomach lining utilizing a procedure known as endoscopy. After each endoscopy, the investigating physician was to rate the condition of the stomach mucosa, using a scale that distinguishes four different conditions of the lining (ranging from "completely normal" to "ulcerated"). During each three-day trial period, subjects would undergo three endoscopies: before beginning the drug, halfway through the trial period, and after the three-day period was completed. Trial periods would be separated by a seven-day break designed to rest the stomach lining. Thus, twelve endoscopies would be performed on each subject over a total study period lasting at least thirty-three days.

Endoscopy requires the passage of a flexible fiberoptic tube through the mouth and into the gastrointestinal tract. The tube may range from 8 to 12 mm in diameter (the thickness of an adult thumb) and between 90 and 115 cm in length. An image of a particular section of the gastrointestinal lining is transmitted along the fiberoptic tube to an eyepiece. Beginning approximately one hour before the procedure, subjects are given sedative medication but are not anesthetized. Immediately before the procedure, a modest amount of topical anesthesia is applied to the pharyngeal surface to reduce gagging and initial discomfort associated with passage of the tube. The subject is positioned on his or her left side, and the tube is directed into the stomach as the subject makes swallowing motions. During visual examination of the stomach, air is pumped into it to permit a general survey of the lining. The examination may last from fifteen to thirty minutes.

The amount of pain and discomfort associated with the procedure varies. Especially anxious subjects experience more discomfort than others. The majority of persons gag during the period of twenty to forty-five seconds in which the tube is passed into the stomach. Sometimes, the amount of gagging requires that the subject receive additional sedation and that the procedure be restarted. When the air is pumped into the stomach, a bloated feeling usually occurs. However, actual risks are small. One survey identified a complication rate of 1.3 per 1000 examinations. In 211,400 endoscopies, there were 228 medication reactions, 70 perforations, 63 episodes of bleeding, and 129 instances of cardiopulmonary failure. The risk of death is estimated at 1 in 5000 procedures, but it occurs almost exclusively in seriously debilitated patients with life-threatening problems such as heart disease.

During the deliberations of the review board, several viewpoints were aired. One person expressed concern about approving any study that requires performing twelve nontherapeutic procedures as uncomfortable as endoscopies. While not questioning the scientific importance or design of the study, she maintained that the extent of discomfort exceeded the limit that should be set for medical investigations employing nontherapeutic procedures.

A second panel member examined the protocol from the standpoint of informed consent. He could not imagine any subject who would knowingly and willingly choose to undergo twelve nontherapeutic endoscopies. Indeed, if subjects agreed to enter the study, one could assume from this fact alone that they did not understand the nontherapeutic character of the procedures, the degree of discomfort, or the number of procedures involved. Even if some subjects could be recruited, the chance of securing the thirty persons required for statistical analysis of results seemed utterly remote.

But another committee member rejected these arguments. In his view, the requirement for informed consent is based on respect for the capacity of persons to make decisions based on their own values and interests. If we really respect this capacity, we ought to give potential research subjects the opportunity to say whether or not they wish to enter the study. Failure to provide this opportunity would be paternalistic, with the board members deciding for prospective subjects whether the discomforts were an acceptable "cost" of involvement.

This board member also insisted that the risk/benefit ratio of the study could not be determined independently by the committee. This assessment, he asserted, is relative to the value persons place on involvement in scientific research and the degree of discomfort associated with the research procedures. Persons with differing values regarding participation in research and differing degrees of tolerance for medical procedures might make very different assessments of the risk/benefit ratio.

A final participant in the debate drew a distinction between risks and discomforts. He noted that federal regulations require that the institutional review board be able to make the judgment that "risks to subjects are reasonable in relation to anticipated benefits." As the figures show, actual risks from endoscopies are very slight. On the other hand, buffered aspirin is widely used on the assumption that it protects stomach linings, making the question of its genuine effectiveness clinically important. Thus, the risk/benefit ratio seemed quite reasonable. By contrast, board members not favoring approval were focusing on "discomforts." He suggested that the board did not need to worry about this concern, provided it was satisfied on the matter of risks. He moved for the protocol's approval.

As discussion continued, the panel members distinguished at least five possible ways of taking action: (1) approve the protocol as it stands; (2) approve the study but require that the middle endoscopy in each three-day trial period be eliminated (reducing the total endoscopies to eight for each subject); (3) approve the study only with extensive revision in its design, allowing each subject to receive only one drug and undergo only three endoscopies; (4) approve the protocol as designed but require monitoring of informed consent by each subject (e.g., through postinterview assessment of each subject's level of comprehension of the study's purposes and procedures, or through the presence of an auditor during each interview); or (5) disapprove the protocol altogether.

4.8 Physicians' Treatment Preferences and Recruitment of Subjects for a Randomized Clinical Trial

Dr. B. was a university obstetrician considering a research study on the best method of delivering babies having a breech presentation.[13] Although the breech position occurs in only 3 to 4 percent of births, such cases are troublesome because vaginal delivery involves risks for the breech fetus. Because the fetal umbilicus passes through the cervix (lower part of uterus) before the head, the umbilical cord is compressed between the cervix and head. Delivery must proceed without delay in order to avoid hypoxia (lack of oxygen) resulting from cord compression. However, because the fetus's head is the largest part of its body,[14] there is a risk that the head will be entrapped by a pelvis wide enough to allow passage of the lower body but not the head.[15] Hypoxia caused by an entrapped head can result in brain damage or death. Additional risks include trauma to the brain, spinal cord, or skeleton when the obstetrician applies traction to deliver the fetus. Cesarean section avoids these dangers but involves risks for the mother. A mortality rate of 30.9 per 100,000 cesarean sections, compared to 2.7 per 100,000 vaginal deliveries, was reported by Evrard and Gold.[16] A study by Rubin and colleagues revealed a death rate from cesarean section of 59.3 per 100,000 in comparison to 9.7 per 100,000 vaginal deliveries.[17] Other complications of cesarean section include infection, injuries to the urinary tract, and hemorrhage requiring transfusion. In rare cases a hysterectomy might be necessary to control uterine bleeding. In a recent study, Bowes and colleagues found significant nonfatal maternal complications in 21 percent of cesarean sections, compared to 4 percent of vaginal deliveries.[18] Thus, decisions about the method of delivery of breech fetuses involve balancing the risks to fetus and mother. Uncertainty about the frequency of fetal injuries in vaginal breech deliveries makes these decisions even more difficult.

According to Dr. B.'s proposal, patients at the university hospital who begin labor with the fetus in the breech position would be asked to participate in a randomized clinical trial (RCT). The study would focus on premature deliveries because the frequency of breech presentation is much higher for this group. Patients would be randomized to either cesarean section or a trial of labor. The trial-of-labor group would deliver vaginally unless an unforeseen complication required cesarean section. Patients would be eligible for the study only if their labor could not be arrested with drugs or there was a medical reason not to halt labor.[19] Also, patients for whom there was an independent medical reason to perform cesarean section would be excluded. The outcomes for women and fetuses in the vaginal and cesarean section groups would be compared for statistically significant differences in complication rates.

The study would be of considerable interest because it could influence current practice and provide a scientific basis for decision making. Currently, most obstetricians recommend cesarean section when the fetus is breech. The main reasons are to avoid risks to the fetus and prevent malpractice litigation arising from a poor outcome for the fetus. Given this common practice, a legal defense of vaginal delivery would be difficult. However, the practice of usually recommending cesarean section lacks a solid scientific basis. The type of research that could ascertain whether cesarean sections produce significant benefits for breech fetuses is a prospective[20] randomized study, such as the one being considered. Such a study has never been performed for premature breech deliveries,[21] and it is possible that a poor outcome because of vaginal delivery is rare.

Ethical issues regarding Dr. B.'s proposed study were discussed at length in a protocol development meeting. A colleague claimed that every experienced obstetrician knows from clinical practice that vaginal delivery increases risks to the breech fetus. Although their probability is unknown, their magnitude is so great that they justify cesarean section. Moreover, he noted that several retrospective studies provide evidence that vaginal delivery has an unfavorable balance of risks and benefits for the breech fetus. For example, Goldenberg and Nelson reviewed the records of all singleton (not twins, etc.) fetuses weighing 500 to 2500 grams

(1.1 to 5.5 pounds) born at Yale New Haven Hospital from September 1970 through August 1975.[22] Excluding major congenital anomalies and fetal deaths before admission, the vaginal deliveries consisted of 118 breech and 946 vertex fetuses. The mortality rate during hospitalization was 43.2 percent for the breech group, compared to 10.7 percent for vertex. Among those weighing 1000 to 1499 grams (2.2 to 3.3 pounds), 80 percent of the breech infants were in distress, compared to 37 percent of the vertex infants.[23] Another study was conducted by Bowes and colleagues at the University of Colorado Medical Center.[24] They reviewed the records of all singleton breech fetuses weighing more than 500 grams born from July 1970 through June 1977. The neonatal death rate, covering twenty-eight days after birth and excluding major congenital anomalies and Rh disease, was 68 percent among fifty-seven fetuses delivered vaginally, compared to 25 percent for twelve delivered by cesarean section. This difference was statistically significant. Thus, Dr. B.'s colleague thought it likely that a trial of labor is unfavorable for the fetus, compared to cesarean section, and that randomizing fetuses to the trial-of-labor group would violate the principle "Do no harm." Although physicians on staff might cooperate in enlisting their patients for the study, in regular practice they would surely recommend cesarean section.

An ethicist in the working group suggested that disagreement about the trial-of-labor approach raised an important ethical question about whether staff physicians should share their treatment preferences with prospective subjects. He noted that physicians have an obligation to protect the welfare of their patients, which requires provision of a recommendation regarding optimal treatment. If physicians who have a definite treatment preference failed to convey this information, they would be violating the obligation to serve the welfare of their patients.

He said that the same conclusion followed from the obligation to secure informed consent. The informed consent doctrine requires disclosure of information that reasonable persons would consider relevant to treatment decisions. If the treatment preference of one's physician is an item of information a reasonable person would consider relevant to the decision about entering a randomized trial, then there is an obligation to provide this information. Moreover, there would be serious impediments in the ability of prospective subjects to make an informed decision, underscoring the importance of having the assistance of a trusted physician-advisor in deciding about participation. For example, patients in labor are often afraid of pain, of having a deformed baby, and of death itself. These fears and the pain of labor can interfere with the ability to assimilate information. The proposed study would involve women who have a sudden complication that can result in death or serious handicap of the baby. Such circumstances can increase the degree to which affective factors impair consent. Another impediment is the limited time to make a decision. With labor progressing, a vaginal delivery is expected unless a prompt decision is made to perform a cesarean section. The pressure of time creates stress that can impair the patient's ability to absorb information about a randomized clinical trial.

However, another obstetrical colleague of Dr. B. disputed these objections.

First, he rejected the claim that there was satisfactory evidence to consider trial-of-labor less safe for fetuses with a breech presentation. He noted that some retrospective studies have supported vaginal delivery. For example, in one review of the medical records of breech fetuses weighing more than 2000 grams (4.4 pounds), 209 were delivered vaginally and 125 by cesarean section. There were no deaths in the vaginal group, and the one death in the cesarean section group was unrelated to the breech position. The authors concluded that breech fetuses weighing more than 2000 grams should not be routinely delivered by cesarean section.[25] More importantly, the colleague argued, retrospective studies have shortcomings in scientific design. They assume that the control and study groups are equivalent in regard to all important variables except the treatment being investigated or that the data can be corrected for differences. He said that the fallibility of this assumption is illustrated by Goldenberg and Nelson's study. The groups they compared, vaginal breech and vertex deliveries, are not equivalent because certain factors affecting outcome occur more frequently in breech than vertex cases, such as prolapsed cord,[26] prematurity, and low birth weight. The appropriate comparison is between breech fetuses delivered vaginally and those delivered electively by cesarean section. The comparison groups in the study by Bowes and colleagues were also inequivalent. The average birth weight of the vaginal group was 953 grams (2.1 pounds); it was 1165 grams (2.6 pounds) for the cesarean section group. The higher survival rate in the latter group was probably caused in part by the greater size and maturity of those babies. Also, the vaginal deliveries occurred from 1970 to 1974, whereas most of the cesarean sections occurred from 1975 to 1977. The authors stated that survival improved sharply during the latter period because of more aggressive resuscitation and treatment. The colleague pointed out that equivalence can be questioned in any retrospective study, because of the possibility of bias in selection of subjects and assignment of treatment to subjects. Furthermore, attempts to correct the data can be challenged because they assume that all variables affecting prognosis are known. Even if all variables were known, important data concerning them might be missing from the records being reviewed. Randomization of prospective subjects eliminates bias in the selection of subjects and assignment of treatment, and it tends to provide treatment groups that are equivalent with respect to variables affecting prognosis, regardless of whether they are known. Thus, the assertion that trial-of-labor has a less favorable balance of risks and benefits to the fetus was based on inadequate scientific data.

Second, in the absence of a sound scientific basis for preferring cesarean delivery for premature fetuses in the breech position, he asserted that it was permissible for participating physicians to not convey their treatment preferences when recruiting subjects. He pointed out that it is common for physicians involved in randomized clinical trials to have considered opinions about which treatment will prove to be optimal. Nevertheless, they must be willing to suspend clinical practice based on these opinions until adequate scientific data are collected. Otherwise, it would not be possible to complete randomized clinical trials in a timely fashion and to secure the important medical knowledge they routinely yield.

A nurse-midwife also supported the proposed study. She agreed that there were obstacles to informed consent but believed that the patient could overcome them with assistance from her physician and nurse. Fear could be reduced by preparing the patient for labor and giving reassurance. Helpful preparation might include breathing exercises, arranging to have a labor coach, and an explanation of what to expect in labor and delivery. A handout in advance could describe the RCT, explaining that the patient would be asked to enter the study if her fetus was in the breech position during labor. It might also state that a patient refusing to enter the study would simply undergo the procedure recommended by her obstetrician—usually a cesarean section. Indeed, the nurse-midwife thought that an important reason for conducting the study was that the current practice of recommending cesarean section tends to place decision making more in the hands of the physician than the patient. She suggested that the results of the study might enhance the ability of women to make decisions in such cases by providing sound information. Also, there has been growing concern that unnecessary cesarean sections are performed. Current practice concerning the breech fetus may be contributing to this problem.

4.9 Parental Preferences and a Child's Involvement in a Randomized Clinical Trial

C.R. was a thirty-month-old child whose family resided in a small town fifty miles from the medical center. Her father was an auto mechanic. Her mother stayed at home, caring for C.R., two brothers, and a sister. C.R. had been well until two weeks before her hospitalization. At that time, her mother noticed that several mosquito bites on her limbs were intermittently oozing blood. Over the next three days she suffered from a persistent low-grade fever and malaise. The pediatrician thought she had tonsillitis and prescribed antibiotics. After improving for several days, she again became feverish and pale and bled frequently from the sores on her arms and legs. The pediatrician then referred the family to a children's medical center.

Her initial physical exam confirmed the presence of numerous hemorrhagic skin lesions, as well as swelling in her liver and spleen. Analysis of C.R.'s blood revealed that her hemoglobin content (which measures the blood's oxygen-carrying capacity) was quite low (5.9 gm/dl) and that her white blood cell count was very high (56,000 per cubic milliliter). Aspiration of her bone marrow established a diagnosis of acute lymphocytic leukemia, a cancer involving uncontrolled proliferation of abnormal white blood cells. Examination of her cerebrospinal fluid showed no evidence of leukemia in her central nervous system.

Thirty years ago childhood acute lymphocytic leukemia was rapidly and uniformly fatal. Extensive research has now produced treatment regimens that achieve initial complete remission in more than 90 percent of children whose disease, like C.R.'s, involves good prognostic signs.[27] Nevertheless, at least 50 percent eventually die from the disease or its complications. As a result, identification of safer and more effective therapy continues to be a primary research objective.

There is a standard format for treatment. The initial phase, called remission induction, lasts about four weeks and involves the use of various cancer drugs to destroy leukemic cells in the blood and bone marrow. The second phase involves prophylaxis of the central nervous system with drugs and/or radiation to remove undetected leukemic cells from the cerebrospinal fluid and the areas in which it circulates around the spinal cord and brain. This phase of treatment lasts two or three weeks. Finally, a maintenance phase of therapy, lasting thirty months, is undertaken to secure long-term disease remission by destroying remaining pockets of leukemic cells.

C.R.'s parents consented to her inclusion in a clinical investigation. One aspect of this study focused on central nervous system (CNS) prophylaxis, examining the comparative benefits and risks of two new approaches. One treatment involved administration of the drug methotrexate, given intravenously, orally, and intrathecally (injected into the space around the spinal cord which contains cerebrospinal fluid). The other involved administration of both cranial radiation (1800 rads) and intrathecal methotrexate.[28] Subjects were randomly distributed between these two treatments.

The induction phase of C.R.'s treatment went smoothly, and she achieved complete remission of her disease within three weeks. As this phase of therapy ended, she was randomized to receive the CNS prophylaxis using both methotrexate and cranial radiation. However, her mother expressed serious reservations about cranial radiation. She was deeply worried about the effects of radiation on her child's brain and how it might alter her behavior and intellectual development. Although this risk had been discussed during the initial consent process, it became a special concern of C.R.'s mother after she had several discussions in the clinic waiting area with the parents of a child who had experienced difficulties in school after receiving cranial radiation five years earlier. These parents also related stories about numerous other children with behavioral and academic problems apparently related to radiation therapy.

There was some basis for the fears Mrs. R. expressed. In one study, a comprehensive set of neuropsychological tests was administered to thirty-seven long-term survivors of acute lymphocytic leukemia.[29] On measures of academic achievement, the thirty patients less than eight years of age at diagnosis obtained test scores approximately one standard deviation below the general population mean. Fourteen of these thirty patients exhibited memory deficits and excessive distractibility which may have interfered with academic progress. These patients had received 2400 rads of craniospinal radiation or cranial radiation combined with intrathecal methotrexate. In another study, seventeen of thirty-two patients in remission had abnormal findings on CT scan representing degenerative changes in their cerebrums.[30] Abnormalities involving decreased reflexes, motor weakness, and altered vibratory sensations were also found in nineteen of thirty-two patients. All patients with abnormal findings had received CNS prophylaxis involving at least 2000 rads of cranial radiation and intrathecal chemotherapy. In both studies, control groups similarly tested exhibited only a few isolated abnormalities.

The physician leading the investigation discussed these problems at length with C.R.'s mother. He confirmed that one motivation for testing a CNS prophylaxis using only methotrexate was concern about the side effects of combining radiation and chemotherapy. However, he explained that the randomization of patients between therapies was based on a lack of knowledge about which therapy had the best risk/benefit ratio. First, CNS prophylaxis using radiation and intrathecal methotrexate had become the treatment of choice, reducing the risk of CNS relapse to less than 10 percent for patients achieving complete remission during induction therapy.[31] It was very uncertain that CNS prophylaxis with chemotherapy alone would achieve the same benefits. Second, using methotrexate alone for CNS prophylaxis might also have serious consequences for intellectual and neurological functioning. Finally, the present study involved a lower dosage of radiation (1800 rads) than that used in previous investigations. There was evidence that this dosage might substantially reduce the risks of cerebral damage. Despite these explanations, C.R.'s mother would still not agree to her inclusion in the arm of the trial requiring cranial radiation.

Because it was the third case in recent weeks in which randomization to the radiation arm of the trial had been refused, considerable debate was provoked at the weekly staff conference about how to deal with families who prefer an alternative treatment. One staff member suggested that there was little they could do except accommodate these preferences. Regulations of the Department of Health and Human Services specify that "participation is voluntary" and that "the subject may discontinue participation at any time without penalty or loss of benefits to which the subject is otherwise entitled."[32] Thus, the investigator would have to accept the mother's refusal if careful explanation of the medical facts failed to secure her cooperation.

There are good reasons for the federal regulations. First, when more than one treatment is medically acceptable, patients and guardians should be free to choose the option most compatible with their values and beliefs. Second, the initial agreement of a subject or guardian to participate in a study may not be adequately informed or free. Risks are often poorly understood or discounted until they materialize during treatment. Persons may also feel pressure when investigators ask them to participate in studies, especially if the illness is life-threatening and they are not familiar with other sources of treatment. These problems with the initial consent are eased by providing persons with an opportunity to reconsider their involvement. Finally, participation in research is usually viewed as an act of altruism undertaken at the discretion of the participant for the benefit of society.

But the investigator who had spoken with C.R.'s mother had a different view. To begin with, he viewed the child's participation in the study as a straightforward quid pro quo. In exchange for her participation, she was receiving a treatment that knowledgeable investigators believed might be safer and more effective than previously used central nervous system therapies. Moreover, treatment was being provided in a setting where staff members were highly skilled in providing the most effective supportive care for complications of the disease and side effects of the therapy. As a result, it was misleading to view the mother's permission as an act of altruism. Rather, in choosing not to allow the child's continued involvement, she was seeking the special benefits of treatment at the research center while failing to fulfill her end of the bargain. Second, he pointed out that the primary purpose of the institution was to accumulate knowledge useful in treating childhood diseases. Continued treatment of the child at the center would not contribute to this objective. Moreover, it would draw personnel and resources away from patients whose treatment could be combined with their enrollment in clinical studies. Lastly, insisting on the child's continued involvement would not violate the obligation to promote the child's well-being, because there was no basis for claiming that the radiation arm of the protocol was less effective or safe than alternative therapies.

As a result, he believed that it was appropriate to take a different approach with the mother. First, she should be told again that randomization of her child to radiation treatment would not compromise her welfare. Second, it would be emphasized that in failing to allow the child's continued participation in the trial she was breaking her end of the bargain to cooperate in research activities in exchange for high-quality care. Third, she should be told that, because the purpose of the institution was to conduct clinical investigations, the hospital had no obligation to continue treating the child if she were no longer included in the protocol. If the mother's refusal persisted, the patient would be transferred to a practitioner in the community. Thus, continued treatment at the research center should not be considered a benefit to which the family "was otherwise entitled."

Another staff member felt strongly that it was inappropriate to discontinue caring for the child. Although granting that the primary function of the institution was to carry out pediatric research, she believed that referral of the patient to a practitioner in the community would border on abandonment. She pointed out that families of children facing potentially fatal illness endure a heavy burden of emotional suffering. They form a strong attachment to the staff whose knowledge and skills provide hope for saving their child's life. Although adequate care could be provided elsewhere, this move would only increase their sense of insecurity and exacerbate their emotional distress. Nevertheless, she agreed that the investigator should be able to freely state his opinion in his discussions with the mother.

But the first staff member was uncomfortable with both approaches. He pointed out that federal regulations are built on the premise that participation in research is voluntary. If staff members were free to tell the parents that referral for care in the community would result from failure to continue in the protocol, this would play forcefully on their insecurity and anxiety. Similarly, telling the mother that she was reneging on the "bargain" would apply substantial pressure, especially in light of her susceptible position. Thus, either approach would cause the mother's permission to be less than adequately voluntary. Moreover, he felt that if the mother accepted randomization as a result of such pressure, it might undermine her confidence that the attending physician was interested in respecting her values and beliefs. Finally, he thought that the institution had an obligation to provide compassionate care to children even if they could not be included in current protocols, because the hospital had a role in promoting the existence of a community that responds to the needs of its most vulnerable members.

However, the investigator did not view these concerns as decisive. He pointed out that the insecurity and anxiety of the family, as well as the authority of the physician, are factors operating in any consent situation involving research with children who have life-endangering illnesses. If these factors undermine the voluntariness of the consent that might result from further discussions with the mother, they also create serious doubts about the voluntariness of any parent's initial decision to permit treatment of their child's life-threatening illness in a research protocol. The investigator also doubted that it would promote the welfare of the mother to merely concede her irrational belief. In addition, he rejected the idea that part of the institution's mission was to routinely tailor research therapies to the preferences of patients or their families. If this became a common practice, clinical studies could not be completed in a timely fashion. He believed that this consequence would be a more serious violation of the hospital's role in the community.

4.10 Compensating Research Injuries

Clinical studies have shown that adriamycin is an effective drug for inducing remissions in various cancers. An example is its usefulness in treating children with osteosarcoma (a form of bone cancer). Before the 1970s, children whose disease at diagnosis had not spread beyond its original site in a limb were treated by amputation alone. Unfortunately, most later experienced spread of the tumor to their lungs, so that no more than 5 to 20 percent achieved long-term disease-free survival. However, in the early 1970s, the introduction of adriamycin and other drugs altered the general approach to the treatment of osteosarcoma. Experienced investigators believed that most patients had undetected disease in their lungs at diagnosis (micrometastases), which later spread and resulted in dismal survival rates. If chemotherapy were given after amputation of the affected limb and before the appearance of overt disease in the lungs (adjuvant chemotherapy), it might be possible to destroy undetected pockets of tumor cells. Initials tests with adjuvant chemotherapy indicated that long-term disease-free survival rates could be improved to 40 to 60 percent of all patients without evidence of lung disease at diagnosis. At this time, numerous clinical investigations were under way to identify the most effective combination of drugs to use in adjuvant chemotherapy, and adriamycin was being used in many protocols.

Unfortunately, adriamycin can damage the muscle wall of the heart, sometimes resulting in fatal congestive heart failure.[33] Early studies of cardiac function in adults receiving adriamycin suggested that the total cumulative dose should be no more than 550 milligrams per square meter of body surface in most patients and 450 mg per square meter in patients receiving concurrent cyclophosphamide (another cancer drug) or previous radiation to the area of the heart. However, there were difficulties in applying these guidelines to children. One was that some children experienced congestive heart failure at much lower dosages of the drug. Another problem was that setting a maximum dosage might deprive some children of additional adriamycin needed to eradicate remaining pockets of tumor, even though they had not suffered cardiac damage. Resolution of these problems required the development of sensitive clinical tests and criteria for determining when children might be developing congestive heart failure.

The final research study reviewed at the meeting of the institutional review board involved the development of means to monitor adriamycin-induced cardiac toxicity in children. One objective was to compare the adequacy of various diagnostic tests in detecting the early stages of congestive heart failure, such as chest X ray, electrocardiogram, phonocardiogram, and echocardiogram.[34] The other objective was to develop better standards for determining when these tests indicate congestive heart failure, by comparing test findings with pathological damage to the heart found at autopsy in children who die from the spread of their cancers. Because the knowledge might be very helpful in caring for future patients, and because the diagnostic tests involved minimal-risk, noninvasive procedures, the study was approved.

Following the review of protocols, the chairperson asked committee members whether they should submit a policy opinion regarding compensation for injured research subjects to the President's Commission for the Study of Ethical Problems in Medicine and Biomedical and Behavioral Research, because the latter group was considering proposals for a federal compensation program. She noted that proposed schemes differed sharply on whether individual investigators, research institutions, or the federal government should bear financial responsibility for a compensation program, but each scheme would provide compensation for research injuries not caused by negligence. She pointed out that proposals also differed regarding the appropriate elements of compensation. Some plans would restrict compensation to the cost of treatment for research injuries, but other proposals would include compensation for economic damages (such as lost wages) and for pain and suffering. Finally, she noted that most proposals would cover injuries resulting from both therapeutic and nontherapeutic research procedures.

The university lawyer suggested that there was a straightforward case supporting a federal compensation program. Pediatric cancer research is a publicly financed enterprise, designed to promote public welfare by improving treatment for future cancer patients. Patients who are harmed by investigative therapies, such as children who suffer adriamycin-induced cardiac damage, incur injuries while contributing to the public goals served by research. The principle of justice requires that we distribute the benefits and burdens of social policies in a way that equalizes the opportunity of each person for a good life. Injuries to these patients impair their ability to have a good life; therefore, society should redress their injuries by providing compensation.

But this position generated serious objections. A clinical investigator pointed out that cancer therapy carries serious and unavoidable risks, and patients and their families recognize and accept these risks when giving informed consent to enter research studies. She suggested that studies investigating the use of adriamycin provided a good example. Adriamycin was currently being used in therapeutic research protocols for a variety of pediatric tumors at the university. Every consent form explained that it could cause serious heart damage and that patients would be closely monitored. Moreover, the consent forms explicitly stated, in accordance with federal regulations, that compensation was not available for injuries suffered during research studies.[35] Because patients and their families give informed consent to receive potentially dangerous therapies without the promise of compensation, it was not clear why society owed them compensation when unavoidable or nonnegligent cardiac damge occurred.

Another investigator noted that the lawyer's view assumed that cancer patients receiving research therapies were placed at special risk for the benefit of society. By contrast, he claimed that they were being given a special opportunity in the face of potentially fatal illness. First, research treatment often constitutes the best therapeutic option. For example, in the case of osteosarcoma, conventional therapy for patients whose disease had not spread beyond the affected limb at diagnosis (amputation only) produced no better than a 20 percent chance for long-term disease-free survival. Research studies using adjuvant chemotherapies such as adriamycin were achieving disease-free survival rates of 40 to 60 percent. Second, each new study builds on previous research results, and its treatment plan is constructed to improve on the effectiveness of previous research therapies. Third, he emphasized that comprehensive supportive care, both medical and psychosocial, is better in cancer research settings than in community hospitals. Cancer research centers have specialized diagnostic and laboratory equipment. Medical specialists highly experienced in cancer therapy can closely collaborate in the care of individual patients. Psychologists and social workers familiar with the unique problems of cancer patients and their families are available.

A medical ethicist suggested that these were not decisive objections. Although persons can voluntarily agree to accept risks without the promise of compensation, there are concerns about the quality of consent given by children and their parents in the pediatric cancer setting. Severe emotional distress reduces the ability of families to appreciate all the implications of the treatment plan when giving consent. Persons do not give substantial weight in their deliberations to low-probability risks, even though injuries may be substantial if they materialize. Moreover, he pointed out that discussion of special benefits is not relevant to injuries received in research studies involving nontherapeutic procedures. These studies are intended to increase medical knowledge but use procedures not intended to benefit the children who are subjects. Finally, he suggested that the concept of social justice is not the only basis for supporting a federal compensation program. For example, public support for medical research might be enhanced if the public is aware that compensation is available for research injuries.

The chairperson of the committee suggested that, whatever the theoretical arguments, there were many practical problems with compensation schemes. She noted that there is little evidence that serious injuries frequently result from nontherapeutic procedures. Most involve only minimal risk, such as the diagnostic tests to be used in the study monitoring the cardiac status of children receiving adriamycin. She also pointed out that it is often difficult to distinguish clinically between injuries caused by investigative cancer therapies and the disease itself. For example, a patient with tumor in his bone marrow may have a reduced ability to stop bleeding or to ward off serious infections as a result of either tumor or cancer chemotherapy; both may impair the development of blood cells in the bone marrow. Consequently, it might be clinically difficult to identify "compensable injuries." Finally, she was worried that investigators might be afraid to try innovative therapies if they were forced to worry about the increased costs of insurance if compensable injuries often occurred.

The committee could not reach immediate agreement, and further discussion was postponed. The chairperson asked her colleagues to give additional thought to the question of what federal policy, if any, should be adopted concerning compensation of subjects for nonnegligent research injuries.

Commentary

Medical research involving human subjects refers to a class of activities using medical procedures in a way designed to produce generalizable knowledge.[36] The fundamental moral issue posed by these activities results from conflicting values. On one hand, we seek to enhance the general welfare of society by expanding our body of generalizable medical knowledge. On the other hand, the design, procedures, or circumstances involved in research studies may necessitate some compromise of the moral interests—that is, the rights and welfare—of human subjects. These moral interests fall into three categories: the interest in exercising the capacity for autonomous choice, the interest in avoiding harm, and the interest in fair treatment. Thus, key issues concern the extent to which subjects' moral interests falling in each category may be compromised in pursuing the social good of expanded medical knowledge.[37]

The cases presented illustrate the issues clustered around each category of moral interests. For example, respect for personal autonomy demands that investigators secure the informed consent of subjects before their participation in research. Cases 4.1 through 4.4 explore ways in which the conduct of studies may necessitate alteration of the informed consent requirement. Similarly, procedures utilized in some studies may expose subjects to risks of harm. Cases 4.5 through 4.9 examine the acceptable limits within which investigators may infringe on the interests of subjects in avoiding harm. Finally, the interest of persons in fair treatment requires that the burdens of participation in research be fairly distributed among potential subjects. Cases 4.5, 4.6, and 4.10 raise questions about the degree to which the burdens of research may be imposed on persons who are disadvantaged by physical illness, age, or social status.

Moral frameworks for addressing issues of research ethics fall into three categories, distinguishable according to the types of considerations used to determine acceptable limitations on the moral interests of subjects.[38] The first approach might be called the *social benefit* view. It would allow limitations on the moral interests of subjects to be determined entirely by their impact in fostering or impeding medical research. If particular limitations would promote the expansion of medical knowledge (without offsetting negative consequences), then these limitations ought to be established. Carried to its logical conclusion, it would permit unacceptable violations of the rights and welfare of individuals. This approach is clearly inadequate, and we do not examine it further.

A second strategy might be labeled the *subject-oriented* approach. It would define the protected moral interests of research subjects apart from consideration of the social goods resulting from expanded medical knowledge. Using our general conceptual understanding of respect for autonomy, protection from harm, and fair treatment, this approach would derive basic requirements for consent, limitation of risk, and fair treatment of subjects. Permissible research would be restricted to studies satisfying these prior moral requirements.[39]

A final strategy is the *balancing* approach. This would determine specific moral requirements for the conduct of human research by balancing the moral interests of human subjects and the social benefits of clinical research. Unlike the social benefit view, this approach assigns significance to the moral interests of subjects that is not entirely dependent on whether recognition of these interests in medical research would promote the general welfare of society. Unlike the subject-oriented approach, it would allow determination of the protections afforded the moral interests of human subjects to be influenced by consideration of how specific requirements might foreclose or permit realization of the social benefits derived from research activities. Thus, a balancing strategy integrates both the social benefits of medical research and the moral interests of subjects in determining rules for the conduct of human research.

Despite extensive scholarly debate, important questions remain unresolved. In examining issues related to each category of moral interests identified above, we compare and contrast positions articulated by proponents of the subject-oriented and balancing approaches. This review leads naturally to consideration of the deeper philosophical assumptions underlying these different approaches.

Problems Related to Consent

Every important code of research ethics acknowledges the moral importance of informed consent. The opportunity to give informed consent is a mechanism for protecting the moral interest of subjects in exercising autonomous choice, which involves deliberating about and acting on their own values and interests. Exercise of personal autonomy requires that at least three conditions be satisfied. Persons must have access to the information needed to make their choices. They must also rationally assess this information within the framework of their own values and interests. Finally, they must be free to carry out the decisions reached in deliberation. The essential elements of an adequately informed consent—information, comprehension and voluntariness—provide these conditions.[40]

Moral problems related to informed consent are generated by features of the consent situation or research design that limit the quality of information, comprehension, or voluntariness involved in the subject's choice. Subject-oriented and balancing approaches assess these situations in very different ways. A subject-oriented view would set limits on the use of subjects by spelling out the implications of respect for autonomous choice. The potential social benefits of research are not considered an appropriate basis for modifying these requirements. By contrast, the balancing approach would develop specific consent requirements by considering both the autonomy interests of subjects and the social benefits of medical research. The fulcrum of this balancing process is usually the degree of risk at which subjects will be placed. Specifically, partial fulfillment of conditions for an adequately informed consent is permitted if (1) it is necessary to achieve research objectives, and (2) it will not significantly compromise the welfare of subjects. On the other hand, if risks associated with the research may seriously affect subjects' welfare, then the conditions for adequately informed consent must be strictly observed.

The information condition requires disclosure of facts that a reasonable person in the subject's position would want to know in deciding about participation. Cases 4.1 and 4.2 illustrate how execution of research projects may require limiting the information provided. In case 4.1, investigators were assessing the usefulness of a four-question interview for detecting persons suffering from alcoholism. However, it was necessary that subjects not understand the purpose of these questions, because this knowledge might cause them to give less than candid answers. In case 4.2, a randomized clinical trial was comparing the efficacy and safety of two treatments for osteosarcoma in patients with no evidence of widespread disease at diagnosis. Early results suggested that patients receiving amputation alone were experiencing spread of their disease more frequently than patients undergoing chemotherapy after amputation. Some investigators thought that preliminary results should be disclosed to prospective subjects.

A subject-oriented view requires strict observance of the information condition. It would generally prohibit deceptive nondisclosure of pertinent information, because subjects are deprived of "their right to decide freely and rationally how to invest their time and persons."[41] For example, investigators in case 4.1 should disclose the study's purpose, because reasonable persons would want to know that their alcohol use was being probed. However, this type of approach might not rule out studies in which prospective subjects are asked to accept nondisclosure of pertinent information.

Similar conclusions obtain regarding disclosure of preliminary research results. Assuming that reasonable persons with a life-threatening disease would want to know treatment trends, even if they are not statistically significant, disclosure should be required. However, the proponent of a subject-oriented view would likely hold it impermissible to ask subjects to consent to nondisclosure in case 4.2. Persons suffering from a life-threatening disease might consider any information about efficacy and safety of treatment highly germane. Consequently, it might be argued, prospective subjects would consent to nondisclosure only if they did not appreciate the possible significance of this information for their decision.[42]

By contrast, a balancing approach would permit nondisclosure of information if it is necessary to achieve research objectives and subjects will not be placed at significant risk. In case 4.1, adequate assessment of the four-question interview requires that subjects be deceived about the study's purpose. Assuming that the confidentiality of subjects is carefully protected, their involvement will not impose significant risk. Thus, a balancing view would allow this study.[43] Similarly, nondisclosure of preliminary research results in case 4.2 would be permissible. Because the differences between treatment arms have not achieved statistical significance, there is insufficient evidence that randomization to the "less favorable" treatment imposes significant risks. Moreover, it is reasonable to assume that recruitment of a sufficient number of subjects to the amputation-only treatment would not be possible if preliminary results were disclosed.

The comprehension condition requires that subjects understand the facts of the situation and are able to rationally assess this information relative to their own values and interests. In case 4.3, the only remaining treatment option for an adolescent girl with an incurable tumor involved participation in the study of a new cancer drug. Because her parents were denying the terminal nature of her illness, it was unclear whether they could fully appreciate the low probability of benefit from the drug or carefully assess their daughter's participation in the study relative to her current needs.[44]

For a subject-oriented approach, valid consent must include adequate comprehension of the consequences of involvement. Because there are serious doubts that the parents adequately appreciate the low probability of benefit, investigators should not seek the participation of their daughter in the trial. By contrast, a balancing strategy may permit less than fully adequate comprehension when the latter is unavoidable and participation in research will not seriously compromise the subject's welfare. In phase I cancer trials, prospective subjects are usually influenced by powerful emotional factors as they struggle to deal with incurable disease. In this respect, some compromise in comprehension is unavoidable. In addition, phase I drugs are administered on the assumption that "there is a chance of remission of disease."[45] Taking into account this possible therapeutic benefit, it can be argued that the subject's welfare is not compromised.[46] Thus, a balancing approach might allow acceptance of the parents' consent.

The third condition for adequate consent is voluntariness of the subject's choice. It requires that the subject's decision reflect his or her own life plans, rather than being induced by external factors. In case 4.5, a study was proposed to assess a new treatment for polycystic ovarian disease, and its design required intensive assessment of hormone production. For their participation, control subjects would receive $750 in payment. An IRB member expressed concern that the amount of compensation offered to normal control subjects might lead them to undergo considerable discomforts and inconveniences they would not consider compatible with their own values and interests, except for the monetary rewards involved. Her concern was intensified by the fact that normal controls would be recruited from the university gynecology clinic, most of whose patients are either very poor or unemployed.

A subject-oriented approach requires that the subject's decision to participate represent an adequately voluntary choice. One mechanism for ensuring that the decision reflects the subject's values and interests involves appealing exclusively to the subject's willingness to accept risks or inconveniences for the benefit of society. This means that payments offered should be restricted to fair compensation for the time expended and inconveniences endured by the subject. But payment should not be so high as to provide an independent motive for participation.[47] In the present case, the level of compensation might be lowered to reduce the likelihood that such independent motives were operative.

A balancing strategy may yield a different analysis of monetary inducements. According to this approach, appealing to the interest of persons in receiving payment when necessary to secure their participation may not per se constitute an unacceptable compromise on voluntariness of choice. Payments for research participation may be set at levels necessary to secure the required number of subjects, provided that subjects will not be placed at significant risk of harm.[48] In case 4.5, participation might have resulted in considerable discomforts and inconveniences but involved only minor risks. As a result, a balancing approach might uphold the compensation amount established, even though prospective subjects could decide to participate only to secure payment for their services.

Problems Related to the Risk of Harm

Codes and commentaries on research ethics also devote considerable attention to the welfare interests of human subjects. The welfare of research subjects can be safeguarded in several ways. First, protecting their well-being involves not exposing subjects to the risk of harm without their consent. However, as signified by the *volenti non fit injuria* maxim, the restriction may be waived when persons consent to involvement in risk-bearing activities. This waiver requires that subjects knowingly and willingly accept participation in research that carries the risk of harm.

Second, protection of welfare interests involves preventing harms to research subjects that may be unnecessary or otherwise inappropriate in light of the goals of the research. One requirement here is that human subjects not be used when research objectives can be achieved without their involvement. Another requirement is that investigators employ the least risky procedures consistent with sound design of their research. Moreover, the risks of harm to which subjects are exposed must be reasonable in relation to the anticipated benefits of the research.

Third, the protection of welfare interests requires that physicians relieve the harms caused by disease when providing therapy in the research setting. This requirement reflects the special obligation of physicians to serve their patient's well-being. In the context of research, this means that the risk of therapeutic research procedures must be justified by the expectation of benefits to the subject, independently of the social benefits of the research itself. It also means that therapeutic procedures utilized must have a risk/benefit ratio that is at least as advantageous for the subject as any alternative treatment acceptable to the subject.[49]

The basic thrust of these requirements is to reduce the risk of incremental harm to subjects, harm whose probability and/or magnitude is greater than what is necessary to protect their welfare. One way of isolating incremental harm utilizes the distinction between therapeutic and nontherapeutic research procedures. Therapeutic research procedures are intended to benefit subjects, as well as to contribute to achievement of research objectives. Administering chemotherapies to cancer patients to determine their efficacy and safety involves therapeutic research procedures. By contrast, nontherapeutic research procedures are only intended to contribute to achievement of study objectives. For example, performance of extra venipunctures to study the breakdown and distribution of cancer chemotherapy in the body involves nontherapeutic research procedures. Nontherapeutic procedures are not intended to benefit subjects; therefore, any associated risks to which subjects would not otherwise be exposed are incremental. Therapeutic research procedures may also carry a risk of incremental harm if they are not at least as likely as other alternatives to be efficacious or safe in treating a patient's disease. Thus, in examining issues related to the welfare interests of human subjects, we must consider both nontherapeutic and therapeutic research procedures.

Moral problems related to the welfare of human subjects arise in situations where the subject's limited capacity to consent or the design of the research project requires modifications in the protective conditions described. A subject-oriented view would not allow pursuit of the social benefits of medical research to modify these requirements. This means that investigators may not expose subjects to risks of incremental harm when performing either therapeutic or nontherapeutic procedures, unless they give adequately informed consent. Investigators must also prevent any unnecessary exposure of subjects to risks of incremental harm. Moreover, therapeutic research procedures must not be used that provide less than optimal treatment. By contrast, a balancing approach would formulate specific restrictions on the exposure of subjects to incremental risks by considering both the welfare interests of subjects and the expected social benefits of medical research. Again, the fulcrum of this balancing process is usually the degree of risk to which subjects might be exposed. Partial fulfillment of the conditions for protecting the welfare of subjects might be permitted if it is necessary to achieve research objectives and the well-being of subjects will not be significantly compromised.

There are important differences in the practical implications of these approaches. The first relates to studies whose execution involves modification of the requirement that only consenting subjects be exposed to incremental risk. In case 4.6, the research proposal involved an investigation of the impact of two anticancer drugs on leukemia cells. Its design required that subjects undergo three nontherapeutic bone marrow aspirations. Because the study involved children with acute lymphocytic leukemia, many would not be able to consent.

For a subject-oriented view, the permissibility of using nontherapeutic research procedures with subjects unable to consent would depend on whether or not they would be exposed to the risk of incremental harm. The identification of nontherapeutic procedures that do not involve the risk of incremental harm relies on the concept of "minimal risk." The insight underlying this concept is that there are always risks associated with our daily activities and that research procedures with a similar level of risk do not increase the risks to which persons are already exposed.[50] Thus, the use of minimal-risk, nontherapeutic procedures is permissible because they create no incremental risks for nonconsenting subjects.[51]

Federal regulations define minimal risk as the probability and magnitude of harm that is "ordinarily encountered in daily life or during the performance of routine physical or psychological examinations or tests."[52] Examples of minimal-risk procedures include routine immunizations, minor changes in diet, venipunctures, and physical examinations. For the proponent of a subject-oriented approach who accepts this description of minimal risk, use of nontherapeutic procedures with subjects unable to consent must involve no more risk than these common procedures. Because the performance of multiple bone marrow aspirations in case 4.6 clearly exceeded this level, their use with children unable to consent would be impermissible.

By contrast, a balancing approach would establish limits of risk by weighing both the social benefits of medical research and requirements for protecting the welfare of subjects. This balance is usually achieved by allowing the use of nontherapeutic procedures involving incremental risk if it is necessary to achieve research objectives and the welfare of subjects will not be significantly compromised. This approach is reflected in the current federal regulations. The regulations prohibit the exposure of children to significant risks by specifying that nontherapeutic procedures involving more than minimal risk may be used only if there is only a minor increase over minimal risk and the interventions are likely to be familiar to children with the disorder being studied. In addition, the regulations specify that the study must be necessary to produce knowledge about the subject's disorder that is vitally important.[53] In case 4.6, the research procedures involve more than minimal risk, but they do not usually pose significant risk of harm to the welfare of child subjects.[54] Moreover, the use of bone marrow aspirations involves procedures with which children with leukemia are already familiar. If successful, the study may yield knowledge that is very useful in designing future regimens for treating the disease. Thus, the proponent of a balancing approach who accepts the specific conditions formulated in the federal regulations would consider the study in case 4.6 to be morally permissible.

The second area of difference between the two approaches concerns studies whose execution involves modification of the principle to minimize harms to which subjects are exposed. An example is provided by protocols in which competent adult subjects are asked to undergo nontherapeutic research procedures involving a substantial amount of discomfort but no serious risks to their welfare. In case 4.7, investigators proposed to evaluate the effectiveness of buffering agents in reducing the tendency of aspirin to intensify irritation of stomach linings by gastric acid. The design of the study required subjects to undergo twelve nontherapeutic endoscopies to assess the impact of four medications on the condition of the stomach lining. Although the risks of serious medical complications are remote, endoscopy may cause considerable gagging and discomfort when the tube is passed into the stomach, and a bloated feeling occurs when air is pumped into the stomach to enhance visualization of its linings.

For a subject-oriented approach, the acceptability of this study might be challenged on two counts. First, strict observance of the conditions for protecting the welfare of subjects requires their consent to the imposition of the risk of incremental harm. A proponent of a subject-oriented position might question the possibility that any prospective subject would knowingly and willingly undergo twelve endoscopies unrelated to the provision of medical benefits. Second, conditions for protecting subjects' welfare interests include the requirement that risks of incremental harm should be reasonable in relation to anticipated social benefits. A proponent of a subject-oriented approach might insist that the number of nontherapeutic procedures be reduced. Otherwise, the magnitude of the discomforts subjects would endure is unreasonable in relation to the limited social benefits of the knowledge gained.

But use of a balancing approach might not make approval of this study contingent on the assessment of whether the incremental harm is reasonable in relation to the anticipated social benefits. First, even though subjects may experience considerable discomforts, there is only a remote chance of significant harm. Second, the performance of numerous endoscopies is necessary to secure the information sought regarding the comparative changes produced by the drugs on the lining of the stomach. Thus, it might be morally permissible to waive the protective condition requiring assessment of the harm/benefit ratio.[55]

A third area of disagreement between the two approaches involves studies whose design requires modification in the protective condition that investigators not provide less than optimal treatment when providing therapy in the research setting. In case 4.8, the investigator is considering a randomized clinical trial to compare the therapeutic efficacy and safety of two approaches to premature delivery of fetuses in the breech position. The usual practice is to perform a cesarean section, but the investigator maintained that careful analysis of the literature does not justify the common view that vaginal delivery significantly increases risks to the fetus. However, some obstetricians whose patients would be eligible for participation in the trial strongly preferred cesarean section, based on their previous clinical experiences.

Proponents of subject-oriented and balancing approaches would specify different requirements for involving subjects in randomized clinical trials. A subject-oriented approach would require investigators to strictly observe the duty to not provide less than optimal treatment. One regular component of care is the provision of a recommendation regarding the treatment alternative the physician believes offers the most favorable risk/benefit ratio for the patient. This suggests that physicians who believe that the treatment arms of a randomized clinical trial are not equally favorable should not recommend participation to their patients.

Use of a balancing strategy may lead to less stringent conditions for involvement of subjects in randomized clinical trials. Protections for welfare interests may be modified if it is necessary to achieve research objectives and the welfare of subjects will not be significantly compromised. Modification of the requirement that physicians make treatment recommendations may satisfy both conditions. First, requiring physicians to make treatment recommendations can seriously impair efforts to accrue enough subjects who accept randomization, because they are more likely to want the treatment preferred by their physician. Second, withholding a recommendation will not significantly compromise the welfare of subjects, because randomized clinical trials are not justified unless investigators can honestly state that there is no scientifically validated reason for preferring one of the treatments being compared. Thus, a balancing approach may allow investigators to seek participation of subjects in the randomized clinical trial without sharing their treatment preferences.

Problems Related to Fair Treatment

The interest of subjects in fair treatment received little attention in the early codes and commentaries on research ethics. This lacuna was addressed by the national commission, which identified justice as a fundamental moral principle regulating human research and examined its implications for the protection of human subjects.[56]

Justice requires that benefits and burdens of cooperative social endeavors be distributed in ways that protect the equal opportunity of all persons to pursue their life plans. For example, the judicial system is a cooperative social activity. Justice requires that its benefits (e.g., the protections afforded by legal rights) and its burdens (e.g., the responsibility for serving on juries) be distributed in a way that gives each citizen an equal opportunity to pursue his or her life plans. Similarly, medical research is a cooperative social endeavor subject to the requirements of distributive justice. The potential burdens associated with research participation are controlled by mechanisms—such as informed consent—designed to protect the interests of subjects in exercising autonomous choice and avoiding harm. Thus, fair distribution of the burdens of research participation requires that these protective mechanisms be implemented in a manner ensuring that all subjects are equally protected.

However, preservation of equal opportunity may require that some classes of subjects be treated differently from others in the distribution of protective mechanisms. For example, monitoring the consent process may be necessary to ensure that subjects with limited comprehension (e.g., retarded persons) knowledgeably choose to participate in research. Similarly, special limits on incremental risk may be necessary to prevent seriously ill subjects from incurring substantially more harm than healthy subjects. Thus, fair distribution will involve different levels of protection for different classes of subjects.

Subject-oriented and balancing approaches will assign different weight to fair treatment in the conduct of research. A subject-oriented approach will emphasize distribution of protective mechanisms in a manner that strictly preserves the equal opportunity of all subjects. By contrast, a balancing approach may permit restrictions dictated by justice to be modified if it is necessary to achieve research objectives and the welfare of subjects is not thereby significantly compromised. These contrasting approaches lead to different conclusions on a variety of justice-related issues, such as the use of socially disadvantaged populations, the limits of risk appropriate for seriously ill subjects, and the scope of compensation programs for injured subjects.

Problems related to the use of disadvantaged persons are illustrated by case 4.5. As described earlier, normal control subjects would undergo extensive testing and receive the trial medication, being paid $750 for their participation. Most would be poor or unemployed women. The key justice-related issue is whether economically disadvantaged subjects need special protections to prevent constraints on autonomous choice caused by undue inducement.

A subject-oriented approach emphasizes that protections for autonomous choice should be distributed in ways that protect equally the ability of all subjects to deliberate about and act on their life plans. Because economically indigent persons are especially vulnerable to monetary inducements, they should be provided with stronger protections than might be provided for more economically fortunate subjects. In case 4.5, investigators might reduce the amount of compensation offered, thereby relieving the excessive vulnerability of economically disadvantaged women. Or they might seek subjects from gynecologists serving more economically prosperous patients.

Use of a balancing strategy may permit modification of these requirements under two conditions. First, the modification must be necessary to achieve research objectives. For example, it may not be administratively feasible to coordinate the accrual of subjects from multiple private gynecology practices. It may also not be possible to secure a sufficient number of subjects if the payment is substantially reduced. Second, modification in the requirements of justice must not significantly compromise subjects' welfare. In the present case, subjects would be asked to endure substantial inconveniences and discomforts, but their welfare would not be significantly impaired. Thus, a balancing approach may permit modification in the requirements of justice if genuinely necessary for carrying out this study.

A second area of controversy regarding fair treatment concerns the limits of incremental risk to which seriously ill subjects may be exposed. The basic requirements of fair treatment for the seriously ill in medical research seem straightforward. Because serious illness is accompanied by numerous impairments (pain, suffering, disability, etc.), seriously ill patients are less able than their healthier counterparts to pursue their life plans. Provision of equal opportunity requires that they be exposed to fewer risks of harm than healthier persons.

For example, one condition for protecting the welfare of human subjects requires that they not be exposed to the risk of incremental harm without their consent. For subjects unable to consent, this requirement implies that nontherapeutic procedures must involve no more than minimal risk. If justice requires that seriously ill persons should incur a lesser degree of risk than other subjects, then the use of nontherapeutic procedures with seriously ill subjects unable to consent must involve no more than this same level of minimal risk.[57] Thus, in case 4.6 the performance of three nontherapeutic bone marrow aspirations, whose level of risk is more than minimal, is prohibited because the subjects are seriously ill children unable to consent.[58] Because a subject-oriented position would demand strict observance of requirements for fair treatment, it would prohibit this study.

By contrast, a balancing approach might permit a waiver of this rule if it is necessary to achieve research objectives and the welfare of subjects will not be significantly compromised. First, there must be important knowledge about diseases or their treatment that cannot be obtained except through the use of nontherapeutic research procedures involving some risk of incremental harm (i.e., more than minimal risk).[59] Second, restrictions on the use of nontherapeutic procedures involving more than minimal risk must be formulated to prevent significant risks to the welfare of subjects. For example, the restrictions might require that the procedures (1) involve only a minor increase over minimal risk and (2) present experiences familiar to subjects. When these conditions are satisfied, the balancing view would permit nontherapeutic procedures involving more than minimal risk, even with seriously ill subjects unable to consent.[60] Thus, the strict requirements of justice might be waived in case 4.6, provided that the procedures used are necessary to secure important knowledge and satisfy the conditions for protecting subjects against significant risks.

Another area of controversy regarding fair treatment involves compensation for injured research subjects. The problem is illustrated by case 4.10. In the 1970s, cancer researchers investigated the usefulness of various drugs in preventing the spread of osteosarcoma (a bone cancer) beyond its site of origin in a child's arm or leg. One very promising drug was adriamycin, but subsequent clinical experience revealed that large cumulative doses may cause congestive heart failure. Investigators were not able to foresee this serious side effect, so the harm caused to patients was not the result of negligence. The moral issue is whether there is an obligation to compensate subjects who incur injuries not caused by negligence.

A subject-oriented approach again involves a straightforward application of the notion of fair treatment. Harms incurred by research subjects are burdens resulting from participation in a cooperative social endeavor. They render injured subjects less able to pursue their life plans than noninjured subjects or persons who do not participate in research. Provision of compensation constitutes a useful mechanism for redressing the inequality caused by their injuries.[61] Thus, a subject-oriented view would favor the establishment of compensation programs for injured subjects.

Proponents of a balancing approach do not reject compensation for research injuries per se but rather question its appropriateness for injuries sustained in research involving therapeutic procedures. Again, the modification is based on its necessity for achieving research objectives and the absence of serious negative consequences for the welfare of subjects. First, there is concern that the costs of a program of providing compensation for injuries resulting from therapeutic research procedures might drain money from the limited funds available for research.[62] Second, it is claimed that the absence of compensation for injuries resulting from research therapies does not seriously compromise the welfare of subjects, because the risk of harm is offset by special advantages associated with participation in the research. These advantages are especially evident in research on catastrophic diseases such as cancer. Often, the treatment being evaluated represents the best option for dealing with a life-threatening illness, because standard treatments are either ineffective or nonexistent. Moreover, nursing care is often more intensive and specialized in the research setting. Finally, the research center often provides access to a variety of specialists and services for diagnosis, monitoring, and rehabilitation unavailable in the general hospital. Thus, even if a subject sustains injury from a therapeutic research procedure, it may have constituted the option for treatment having the best overall harm/benefit ratio.[63] The use of adriamycin in treating osteosarcoma in children provides a good example. With the introduction of chemotherapy, disease-free survival rates increased from 20 to 50 percent. Although some children suffered from adriamycin-induced congestive heart failure, its use significantly improved "cure" rates. Thus, the proponent of a balancing approach might limit compensation to injuries caused by nontherapeutic research procedures. This restriction would protect the funds necessary for some types of research while reflecting the fact that reception of research therapy often constitutes a special opportunity for the subject even if injury ultimately results.

Society, Subjects, and Medical Research

Subject-oriented and balancing approaches yield systematically different conclusions regarding the moral restrictions that should circumscribe the conduct of medical research. These differences reflect profoundly dissimilar views about the role of society in sponsoring cooperative activities, the expectations placed on its members, and the importance of medical research as a societal venture.

The subject-oriented approach emphasizes strict observance of rules protecting the moral interests of human subjects. This approach reflects three basic assumptions. First, the basic role of society is to implement norms of behavior that protect its members from violation of their moral interests by other persons. Society may provide support for activities that serve the interests of many of its members (e.g., medical research leading to reduced disability from heart disease), but its primary function is to protect persons when they are engaged in social interactions. Second, society can expect of its members that they will observe these basic rules for protecting the moral interests of each person. But except for cooperative ventures instrumental in the preservation of society itself (e.g., participation in military defense), society should not require that its members participate in any particular kinds of social activities. Third, although medical research may produce highly significant improvements in the welfare of members of society, it is not ordinarily essential to the preservation of society.

These basic assumptions lead to the conclusion that the benefits of medical research should be treated by society as highly desirable but morally optional. Because the growth of medical knowledge is not necessary for the preservation of society itself, society should not require participation of its members in research activities. Society might support medical research that will substantially benefit its members, but its basic function is to safeguard the moral interests of persons in exercising autonomous choice, avoiding harm, and receiving fair treatment. Thus, society should require strict respect for these moral interests in the conduct of clinical research.

A balancing view starts from a very different set of assumptions. First, society has the general function of providing the essential conditions its members need to pursue their life plans. These conditions include protection against exploitation by others, but they also involve provision of the essential goods persons must have to pursue their life plans, such as adequate housing, nutrition, and education. Second, because provision of essential resources to all members of society can only be secured through social cooperation, all individuals are expected to assist in their production. Constraints on the moral interests of individuals (e.g., imposition of taxes effecting a redistribution of resources) may be necessary in order to provide all persons with essential goods. However, limitations of basic moral interests may not deprive persons of conditions essential to pursuit of their own life plans. Third, the essential resources persons need to pursue their life plans include adequate health care. Because the growth of medical knowledge plays a critical role in improving the quality of existing medical care, the conduct of medical research should be considered an essential component in providing adequate medical care to the members of society.

These assumptions suggest a different approach to the use of human subjects. Because expansion of medical knowledge is a means for developing an essential social resource, society should formally sponsor clinical investigation. Society should also set expectations for the involvement of its members in clinical research, because the latter is not possible without substantial public involvement. Protections for the moral interests of subjects may undergo limited modification if necessary in the conduct of research activities, provided that their welfare is not significantly compromised.

The differences between these two approaches to the regulation of human research turns on the wisdom of modifying protections for the basic moral interests of individuals in order to enhance the welfare of other persons. From a societal standpoint, the crucial issue concerns which manner of regulating our social relationships will most effectively support the activities of all members of society. Underlying the respective answers is the assignment of different weight or importance to prominent features of social interactions. One consideration is the extent to which persons misuse those who are more vulnerable than themselves. If the frequency with which researchers might exploit subjects is given overriding weight, then the result is a disinclination to depart from the strict requirements of the subject-oriented approach. On the other hand, confidence that socially approved modifications in basic moral protections will be sensitively and rigorously observed by medical researchers would provide support for a balancing approach. A second consideration is the perceived dependency of persons on one another for basic goods or resources. If particular emphasis is placed on the fact that many persons are highly dependent on others for goods or resources essential to pursuit of their life plans, then modification of basic moral interests of individuals to enhance the welfare of others may be a socially attractive policy. By contrast, confidence that persons are satisfactorily able to pursue their life plans if provided with basic protections for their moral interests constitutes a basis for resisting any modification in subject-oriented restrictions. A third factor concerns the degree of compatibility between the values and interests of particular individuals and the needs of other members of society. If particular focus is placed on the ways in which the interests of individuals may diverge from the needs of other members of society, then the restrictions of a subject-oriented approach may be considered critical to the protection of the values and interests of each person. However, if some interest in the general welfare of others is considered essential to the personal fulfillment of each individual, limited modification in the requirements of a subject-oriented view may be viewed as thoroughly consonant with each person's life plans. Thus, the conflicting approaches to the use of human subjects may at their root reflect different estimations of the moral significance of vulnerability, interdependence, and sociability in human relationships.

Notes

1. When investigators compare two treatments, they study only a small sample from the total population of persons with the disease. Even if a difference between treatments is found, it may be the result of chance selection of an unusual sample that does not represent the entire population. The confidence level is a statistically determined probability that the difference found in the sample holds for the entire population.

2. This refers to 110 mg of AMSA per square meter of the patient's body surface area. Thus, the dosage is adjusted according to the size of the pediatric patient.
3. Blunt trauma refers to a wound or injury caused by external force, such as might occur in motor vehicle accidents.
4. Diminished blood flow to the liver is part of a general physiological response to trauma that includes diversion of blood from visceral organs to parts of the body whose functions are more important to survival.
5. Molecules of a drug can become bound to protein molecules in the blood. It is widely believed that the pharmacologic effect of a drug is better correlated with its free (not bound to proteins) rather than its total (free plus bound) concentration in the blood.
6. The ISS and TS are scales that grade the severity of injury. See Susan P. Baker et al., "The Injury Severity Score: A Method for Describing Patients with Multiple Injuries and Evaluating Emergency Care," *Journal of Trauma* 14 (1974): 187–96; and Howard R. Champion et al., "Trauma Score," *Critical Care Medicine* 9 (1981): 672–76.
7. This notation refers to 1 mg of lidocaine per kg of patient body weight.
8. Carski and colleagues discuss four cases of allergic reactions to indocyanine green reported to its manufacturer, including one fatality. Two patients had no previous allergies, and none had a history of allergy to iodine. However, the low incidence of adverse reactions is indicated by the estimate that more than two hundred forty thousand procedures using indocyanine green were performed in the period during which these reports were submitted. See Theodore R. Carski et al. (letter), "Adverse Reactions after Administration of Indocyanine Green," *Journal of the American Medical Association* 240 (1978): 635.
9. See *Code of Federal Regulations* 45, sec. 46.116.
10. For discussions of deferred consent, see Norman Fost and John Robertson, "Deferring Consent with Incompetent Patients in an Intensive Care Unit," *IRB: A Review of Human Subjects Research* 2 (August–September 1980): 5–6; Tom L. Beauchamp, "The Ambiguities of 'Deferred Consent'" *IRB: A Review of Human Subjects Research* 2 (August–September 1980): 6–8.
11. The life cycle of dividing cells (or cell cycle) covers the period from the formation of two identical, immature cells to their own subsequent division into daughter cells. However, not all newly formed cells enter this cycle. Some differentiate into fully mature cells and ultimately die. Others enter a resting phase, remaining dormant until stimulated to divide or to differentiate into mature cells.
12. Acute lymphocytic leukemia is a form of cancer involving uncontrolled replication of lymphocytes, a type of white blood cell. Their production in overwhelming numbers interferes with the normal function of other blood cells, making the patient highly susceptible to hemorrhage and infection. Untreated, the disease is usually fatal within six months.
13. Presentation refers to the part of the fetus presenting itself at the cervical opening. Normally, the top of the head presents, referred to as vertex presentation. In breech presentation the feet or buttocks present (and emerge from the uterus first in a vaginal delivery).
14. For a term fetus the abdomen can be larger than the head. Because the abdomen is more compressible than the head, however, it can assume a smaller diameter during birth. For premature fetuses the head is larger than the abdomen.
15. If the fetus is premature, the woman's pelvis is usually large enough to allow passage of the fetal head. In such cases, however, there is a risk that the head will be

entrapped by a cervix that is dilated enough to permit passage of the lower body but not the head.
16. John R. Evrard and Edwin M. Gold, "Cesarean Section and Maternal Mortality in Rhode Island," *Obstetrics and Gynecology* 50 (1977): 594–97.
17. George L. Rubin et al., "Maternal Death after Cesarean Section in Georgia," *American Journal of Obstetrics and Gynecology* 139 (1981): 681–85.
18. Watson A. Bowes, Jr., et al., "Breech Delivery: Evaluation of the Method of Delivery on Perinatal Results and Maternal Morbidity," *American Journal of Obstetrics and Gynecology* 135 (1979): 965–70.
19. Other things being equal, fetal health is promoted by halting premature labor, thereby permitting additional fetal development. In some cases, however, allowing delivery to proceed is better for the fetus. For example, if the amniotic membranes have ruptured, there is a risk of fetal infection by microorganisms normally present in the vagina. When tests in such cases indicate that the fetus has mature lungs, it is sometimes considered medically reasonable to allow labor to continue.
20. A prospective study accumulates data about patients as they are being treated. In contrast, a retrospective study examines the records of previous patients.
21. An RCT involving delivery of term frank (both legs flexed at the hips and extended at the knees) breech fetuses has been reported. The investigators concluded that routine cesarean section should not be performed for term frank breech. See Joseph V. Collea et al., "The Randomized Management of Term Frank Breech Presentation: Vaginal Delivery vs. Cesarean Section," *American Journal of Obstetrics and Gynecology* 131 (1978): 186–93.
22. Robert L. Goldenberg and Kathleen G. Nelson, "The Premature Breech," *American Journal of Obstetrics and Gynecology* 127 (1977): 240–44.
23. In this context, distress refers to an Apgar score less than 7 at one or five minutes after birth. The score is based on an assessment of heart rate, degree of respiratory effort, muscle tone, cry response, and skin color, on a scale of 1 to 10. A low score indicates asphyxia or other compromise to the infant's cardiopulmonary system.
24. Bowes et al., "Breech Delivery."
25. I. Mann and Janice M. Gallant, "Modern Management of the Breech Delivery," *American Journal of Obstetrics and Gynecology* 134 (1979): 611–14.
26. A prolapsed cord emerges through the cervix before delivery of the fetus. Asphyxia or fetal death can occur as a result of compression of the cord between the fetus and the cervix.
27. Patients with acute lymphocytic leukemia can be divided into "standard risk" and "high risk" groups at diagnosis. In the research study discussed, standard-risk patients were defined as having no demonstrable central nervous system disease, no chest mass, an initial white blood cell count less than 100,000 per cubic milliliter, and lymphoblast cells negative for surface immunoglobulin and E-rosette formation (interaction with red blood cells from sheep). These factors were used to distinguish patients with a good prognosis for long-term, disease-free survival from those with a less favorable prognosis, the latter requiring more aggressive therapy. C.R.'s diagnostic evaluation placed her in the standard-risk group.
28. A rad is a unit of measurement of the absorbed dose of ionizing radiation. It corresponds to an energy transfer of 100 ergs per gram for any absorbing material. Its actual biological effect depends on the type of tissue exposed to the radiation and the type of radiation delivered.
29. John Goff, H. R. Anderson, and Peter Cooper, "Distractibility and Memory Deficits

in Long-Term Survivors of Acute Lymphoblastic Leukemia," *Developmental and Behavioral Pediatrics* 1 (1980): 158–63.
30. Nili Peylan-Ramu et al., "Abnormal CT Scans of the Brain in Asymptomatic Children with Acute Lymphocytic Leukemia after Prophylactic Treatment of the Central Nervous System with Radiation and Intrathecal Chemotherapy," *New England Journal of Medicine* 298 (1978): 815–18.
31. Before the time when CNS prophylaxis was used, the initial site of relapse for more than 50 percent of patients was the central nervous system. Marrow relapse and eventual death would follow for most of these patients. Thus, effective prevention of CNS disease is essential to long-term, disease-free survival.
32. *Code of Federal Regulations* 45, sec. 46.116a.
33. Congestive heart failure is caused by heart disease or injury and characterized by shortness of breath and retention of fluid (edema). Fluid congestion may occur in the lungs or the peripheral circulation or both, depending on whether the heart failure is left-sided, right-sided, or general.
34. Each of these diagnostic procedures is used to identify specific pathological features of heart structure and function. Chest X ray permits demonstration of abnormal heart size and shape. An electrocardiogram provides a graphic representation of electrical impulses in the heart. Analysis of the pattern of electrical impulses may suggest specific abnormalities in heart function. A phonocardiogram is a graphic display of heart sounds and murmurs as recorded from chest wall microphones. It provides information about the precise timing of cardiac events. An echocardiogram uses ultrasound techniques to make graphic recordings of the position and motion of the walls and internal structures of the heart. It provides information regarding the size of heart chambers, the thickness of heart walls, and the competence of valves.
35. Federal research regulations issued by the Department of Health and Human Services specify that the elements of informed consent must include "an explanation as to whether any compensation and an explanation as to whether any medical treatments are available if injury occurs and, if so, what they consist of, or where further information may be obtained." See U.S. Department of Health and Human Services, "Public Health Service: Human Research Subjects," *Federal Register* (1981): 8390, sec. 46.116.
36. See Robert Levine, *Ethics and Regulation of Clinical Research*, 2d ed. (Baltimore and Munich: Urban and Schwarzenberg, 1986), p. 3.
37. In this respect, our position differs from that of Wikler, who maintains that the basic moral issue is "the possibility of subjects being injured or hurt." See Daniel Wikler, "The Central Ethical Problem in Human Experimentation and Three Solutions," *Clinical Research* 26 (1978): 380–83. We maintain that there are three separate types of moral issues, corresponding to the distinct categories of relevant moral interests.
38. See James Childress, *Priorities in Biomedical Ethics* (Philadelphia: Westminster Press, 1981), pp. 53–55.
39. A pure subject-oriented view may not be reached in the bioethics literature. Most proponents would allow that if the very existence of society is threatened by some disease and medical research may prevent its catastrophic consequences, then it is permissible to compromise the moral interests of prospective subjects (e.g., by conscripting participants) if necessary to carry out the research. For example, see Hans Jonas, "Philosophical Reflections on Experimenting with Human Subjects," in Paul Freund, ed., *Experimentation with Human Subjects* (New York: George Braziller, 1969), pp. 11–13. However, for the range of "everyday" instances of

medical research, the subject-oriented view as defined here represents a distinct philosophical approach to the ethics of human-subjects research.

40. This division of the elements of informed consent is identified by the National Commission for the Protection of Human Subjects of Biomedical and Behavioral Research, *The Belmont Report: Ethical Principles and Guidelines for the Protection of Human Subjects of Research* (Washington, D.C.: U.S. Government Printing Office, 1978), pp. 10–14.
41. Diana Baumrind, "IRBs and Social Science Research: The Costs of Deception," *IRB: A Review of Human Subjects Research* 1 (October 1979): 2.
42. Alternative solutions to the problem of disclosing preliminary results are examined in Robert Veatch's article "Longitudinal Studies, Sequential Design, and Grant Renewals: What to Do with Preliminary Data," *IRB: A Review of Human Subjects Research* 1 (June–July 1979): 1–3.
43. Current federal regulations reflect a variant of a balancing approach. The regulations specify that incomplete disclosure is permissible when (1) the research involves no more than minimal risk, (2) the waiver will not adversely affect the rights or welfare of subjects, (3) the research could not practically be carried out without the waiver, and (4) whenever appropriate, the subjects will be provided with additional pertinent information after participation. See *Code of Federal Regulations* 45, sec. 46.116.
44. Obviously, the present case deals with permission to use a child rather than consent by a subject. However, similar affective factors may impair understanding and rational assessment in both surrogate decision makers and prospective subjects.
45. See Mortimer Lipsett, "On the Nature and Ethics of Phase I Clinical Trials of Cancer Chemotherapies," *Journal of the American Medical Association* 248 (1982): 941–42.
46. However, the "therapeutic intent" of phase I trials has been challenged. See Terrence Ackerman and Carson Strong, "Ethics of Phase I Clinical Trials" (letter), *Journal of the American Medical Association* 249 (1983): 883; and the President's Commission for the Study of Ethical Problems in Medicine and Biomedical and Behavioral Research, *Implementing Human Research Regulations* (Washington, D.C.: U.S. Government Printing Office, 1983), pp. 41–43.
47. Lisa Newton proposes a similar policy for restricting monetary inducements in "Inducement, Due and Otherwise," *IRB: A Review of Human Subjects Research* 4 (March 1982): 4–6. However, Newton maintains that this policy should not be used to ensure the voluntariness of subject consent, because it is unjustifiably paternalistic to restrict payment levels to protect persons from weakness of the will. Rather, she supports this policy as a means of recruiting subjects who are maximally motivated to understand the information required for an adequate consent.
48. Ruth Macklin develops several objections to this approach to subject compensation. See "'Due' and 'Undue' Inducements: On Paying Money to Research Subjects," *IRB: A Review of Human Subjects Research* 3 (May 1981): 1–6.
49. See Levine, *Ethics and Regulation,* p. 62.
50. The formulation of this insight derives from Ross Mitchell. See "The Child and Experimental Medicine," *British Medical Journal* (1964): 721–27.
51. Numerous authors adopt this approach, although the maximal level of risk permitted with subjects unable to consent is variously defined as "minimal risk," "no discernible risk," "negligible risk," and so on. The most prominent statement of this position is offered by Richard McCormick in "Proxy Consent in the Experimental Situation," *Perspectives in Biology and Medicine* 18 (1974): 2–20. However, a very

different subject-oriented position is formulated by Paul Ramsey, who maintains that the use of nontherapeutic research procedures with children is wrong because they are used without their consent for reasons unrelated to their own welfare, even if they are not harmed. See Paul Ramsey, *The Patient as Person* (New Haven: Yale University Press, 1970), pp. 1–58. The fundamental problem with Ramsey's view is his use of the principle of respect for personal autonomy to clarify duties toward children who lack the capacity for autonomous choice.

52. See *Code of Federal Regulations* 45, sec. 46.102. For a critique of the usefulness of the concept of minimal risk in evaluating human research, see Loretta Kopelman, "Estimating Risk in Human Research," *Clinical Research* 29 (1981): 1–8.
53. See *Code of Federal Regulations* 45, sec. 46.406.
54. However, in some cases, marrow aspiration may pose more than a "minor increase" in risk. Some subjects experience much anxiety and fear when undergoing a marrow aspiration (with a corresponding increase in pain and discomfort). Assuming that potential psychological harm is a component of risk assessment, these persons are exposed to the risk of substantial harm. Thus, a proponent of a balancing strategy must allow that subjects unable to consent be evaluated on an individual basis in determining the permissibility of their involvement.
55. The report of the national commission on the role of institutional review boards supports a balancing approach, suggesting that if "the prospective subjects are normal adults, the primary responsibility of the IRB should be to assure that sufficient information will be disclosed in the informed consent process." See National Commission for the Protection of Human Subjects of Biomedical and Behavioral Research, *Institutional Review Boards: Report and Recommendations* (Washington, D.C.: U.S. Government Printing Office, 1978), pp. 24–25. By contrast, current federal regulations (*Code of Federal Regulations* 45, sec. 46.111) require that IRBs assess the reasonableness of the risks in relation to the anticipated benefits of the research.
56. See National Commission, *Belmont Report*, pp. 8–10, 18–20.
57. The strict implication of the fair treatment principle is that seriously ill subjects unable to consent should be exposed to less than minimal risk. However, if minimal risk is equivalent to the unavoidable risk involved in ordinary daily life, it is not possible to expose subjects to less than minimal risk.
58. This line of argument is developed by Commissioner Robert Turtle in his opinion dissenting from the recommendations of the national commission regarding research with children. See National Commission for the Protection of Human Subjects of Biomedical and Behavioral Research, *Report and Recommendations: Research Involving Children* (Washington, D.C.: U.S. Government Printing Office, 1977), pp. 146–53.
59. For a brief overview of the usefulness of nontherapeutic procedures having more than minimal risk in research on childhood cancer, see Terrence Ackerman, "Moral Duties of Investigators toward Sick Children," *IRB: A Review of Human Subjects Research* 3 (June–July 1981): 1–5.
60. This specification of the factors justifying the use of nontherapeutic procedures having more than minimal risk is similar to the national commission's recommendations on research with children. See National Commission, *Report and Recommendations: Research Involving Children*, pp. 7–10.
61. See James Childress, "Compensating Injured Research Subjects: I. The Moral Argument," *Hastings Center Report* 6 (December 1976): 21–27.

62. Available information suggests that most research-related injuries involve therapeutic procedures. In one survey, 10.8 percent of subjects involved in "therapeutic research" were reported injured, compared to only 0.8 percent of subjects involved in "nontherapeutic research." Sixty-five percent of all injuries reported in therapeutic research involved the administration of cancer chemotherapies. See Philippe Cardon et al., "Injuries to Research Subjects," *New England Journal of Medicine* 295 (1976): 650–54.
63. See Terrence Ackerman and Alvin Mauer, "Compensation and Cancer Research," *New England Journal of Medicine* 305 (1981): 760–63.

5
Physicians, Third Parties, and Society

5.1 Request for Surgery the Physician Considers Unnecessary

A twenty-four-year-old woman made an appointment to see her obstetrician-gynecologist after she missed a period. A pregnancy test proved positive. The patient had married after graduating from college and now worked for a local newspaper. Her husband was a college graduate employed at a nearby manufacturing company. This was her first pregnancy, and she was quite excited. However, she was also apprehensive; she had genital herpes and was worried about transmitting the disease to her fetus.

Genital herpes is caused by the herpes simplex virus and is transmitted through sexual activity and by contaminated hands. The symptoms include pain, tenderness, or an itching sensation around the penis or vulva, sometimes accompanied by headache, fever, or a generally ill feeling. Blisters appear in the genital area and may form inside the vagina and on the cervix. They eventually rupture, forming open sores that are extremely painful and last one to three weeks. After the blisters subside the virus remains in the body in a dormant stage and can later reactivate. About half of the people who get genital herpes have recurrences that may be spaced weeks or months apart. Recurrences are usually less severe and eventually cease altogether. It is believed that transmission of the disease only occurs during active infections, so sexual activity can be resumed after a symptomatic episode. There is no cure, but drugs are available to relieve the symptoms.

The patient had contracted herpes in an extramarital encounter about six months earlier and had experienced one recurrence. She had not told her husband that she had herpes, and she avoided intercourse during periods of active infection by telling him she had "female problems" which her doctor was treating.

The major risk to a fetus is in acquiring the disease during delivery. If the mother has an active infection, the fetus can become contaminated during its passage through the cervix and vagina. If her amniotic membranes have been ruptured for a considerable time before the birth, the virus can also spread upward from the cervix and infect the fetus. According to one author, approximately 40 percent of women who have an active infection at the time of vaginal delivery transmit the disease to the fetus.[1]

Herpes simplex infection of the newborn is not a genital disease and is much more serious than genital herpes in adults. The mortality rate for infected newborns has been reported to be approximately 62 percent. Among survivors, about 46 percent have handicaps in varying degrees, usually consisting of psychomotor impairment or eye damage.[2] The disease can involve either localized or disseminated infection. The most common sites of local infection are the brain, eye, skin, and oral cavity. Among these, brain involvement has the worst prognosis in terms of survival and handicaps. The possible consequences include microcephaly (small head size), hydrocephaly (excess accumulation of cerebrospinal fluid in the brain), porencephalic cysts (regions in which there is an absence of brain tissue), and varying degrees of motor retardation. Infected eyes can result in corneal scarring, cataracts, inflammation of the retina, and blindness. The more frequent clinical course is disseminated infection, in which the virus spreads to internal organs through the blood. The most commonly affected organs are the liver and adrenal glands, although many other organs can be affected, including the lungs, heart, and intestines. Widespread cell destruction occurs in the affected organs, and the disseminated form has a worse prognosis for survival than the localized form.

The patient's apprehensiveness was caused by the fact that she knew about the seriousness of neonatal herpes infections. She also knew that neonatal herpes can be prevented by performing a cesarean section, thereby avoiding fetal contact with the virus during delivery. She told the obstetrician that she definitely wanted to have a cesarean section.

The physician explained that a cesarean section is medically indicated in certain cases but is often not necessary. A widely accepted approach is to monitor the mother closely for evidence of active infection and perform a cesarean section only if there is such evidence. In this manner, neonatal herpes can be prevented when there is active infection, and unnecessary cesarean sections can be avoided. There are significant risks to the mother associated with cesarean section, including a death rate of 3 to 9 per 10,000 operations.[3] Additional complications include infection of the abdominal wound, bleeding requiring blood transfusions, or uncontrollable bleeding necessitating a therapeutic hysterectomy. Thus, it is desirable to avoid a cesarean section unless there are compelling reasons for performing one.

The monitoring consists of weekly swabbing of the cervix and vulva and making cultures of the swabbed material. Growth of herpes virus in the culture is evidence of active infection. Several studies have reported the results of such an approach. In managing fifty-eight pregnancies, Grossman and colleagues performed weekly cultures beginning at thirty-six weeks gestational age and continuing until delivery.[4] When a patient went into labor, the results of her most recent culture determined the preferred method of delivery. If that culture was positive or if she had clinical signs of infection such as pain, itching, or blisters, a cesarean section was performed. If the culture was negative and there were no clinical signs of infection, a vaginal delivery was recommended. This approach permitted twenty-five vaginal deliveries with no cases of neonatal herpes infection.

In following a similar approach for eighty-three pregnancies, Harger and colleagues found that among those cultures that were positive, 92 percent could be declared positive by the end of four days of culture incubation.[5] They recommended vaginal delivery if the two most recent cultures were negative and had been prepared at least four days before the onset of labor and if there were no clinical signs of infection. Fifty-six infants were delivered vaginally with no cases of neonatal herpes. Similar methods resulted in fifty-four vaginal deliveries reported by Vontver and colleagues[6] and eighty-eight vaginal deliveries attended by Boehm and colleagues[7] with no instances of neonatal herpes.

The obstetrician emphasized that this approach was widely accepted and recommended it to the patient. She listened carefully and seemed to understand what was being proposed. She then asked the obstetrician if this method was "100 percent certain" of preventing neonatal herpes infections. The doctor replied that he could not guarantee that the infant would be protected but that the chance of its becoming infected was very low and there were no reported cases of neonatal herpes using this method. Upon hearing this, the patient continued to maintain that she wanted a cesarean section. She stated that she wanted to do everything possible to protect her baby and was willing to assume the risks of cesarean section in order to protect her fetus. She said that she felt so guilty about having herpes—and thereby subjecting her baby to risk—that she could not bear the thought of the baby getting the disease.

Her insistence on having a cesarean section troubled the physician. Following her wishes could result in performing an operation that, in his view, was medically contraindicated. His options included the following: (1) agree to perform a cesarean section; (2) refuse to take the approach the patient wanted and suggest that she may want to seek another obstetrician; (3) try to persuade the patient during her pregnancy to accept his approach, but if she remains adamant then follow her wishes; or (4) neither agree nor disagree with the patient, and simply follow the approach he had recommended.

In deciding what to do, there were several considerations. Respect for parental authority was an obvious factor. The woman had a responsibility to protect the well-being of her child, and her request for a cesarean section constituted a decision concerning how to carry out that responsibility. There was a possibility that the approach recommended by the physician would result in the infection of her infant, although the probability appeared low. For example, there could be virus present on the surface of the cervix, vagina, or vulva that might not be detected by culture. This could occur either because the virus was not picked up by the swab or because the culture would eventually become positive but had not done so at the time of delivery. Also, active infection in the mother might begin immediately after her last culture was taken. Therefore, her request reflected a decision to increase the risk to herself in order to decrease the risk to her fetus. This involved a value choice concerning risk taking rather than a strictly medical matter. It could be argued that turning down her request in order to protect her from the risks of a cesarean section would be paternalistic. On the other hand, it was possible that her wishes were greatly influenced by her feelings of guilt—and perhaps by fear of discovery by her husband. Perhaps the guilt was preventing her from appreciating the physician's point of view. Paternalism might be justified if her guilt and apprehensiveness were serious encumbrances to a well-thought-out decision.

Another factor was concern for patient well-being. The physician had an obligation to consider the well-being of both mother and fetus. His professional responsibility to protect the well-being of his patients requires, it could be argued, that he minimize the overall risk to mother and fetus. This view lends support to option 2 or 4.

In addition, several considerations suggest that physicians who are asked to deviate from medical standards have a right to refuse. First, respect for autonomy involves acknowledging their freedom to not violate their own ethical convictions, which may include the commitment to act in accord with professional standards. Second, this right seems to be required if doctors have a role responsibility to practice according to standards of the profession.

Another factor was the physician's own well-being. If he refused to follow the mother's wishes, she delivered vaginally, and the infant became infected, then he could be sued by the mother to recover damages for any harm that might occur. Also, if he refused her request he might lose her as a patient, a possibility that did not please him because he was trying to build up his clientele. These considerations would support option 1 or 3.

5.2 Providing Free Care

Weekly pediatric grand rounds examined the issue of whether private pediatricians have an obligation to provide care when families are unable to pay. The case involved J.D., a six-and-a-half-year-old boy who had been under Dr. B.'s care since three months of age. He was the only child of parents who had separated two years earlier. J.D. and his mother lived with his maternal grandparents. Mrs. D.'s divorced sister also lived in the home with her twenty-two-year-old son, who had Down's syndrome and was moderately retarded.

During his first four years as Dr. B.'s patient, charges for J.D.'s pediatric care were promptly paid. However, four successive billings for a balance of sixty-eight dollars were subsequently left unpaid. At this point, a letter was sent to the mother by Dr. B.'s business manager indicating that the account would be submitted to a collection agency unless payment were promptly received. The letter also stated that once the account was submitted to the collection agency, the office would "cease to provide pediatric services until the balance is paid in full" and would "not permit credit for any future services rendered." The existing balance was finally paid about six weeks after the mother received a notice from the collection agency.

About one year later, the family's account showed a balance of seventy-nine dollars, and four successive billings again went unanswered. Although this bill was also sent to the collection agency, no payment was received. The account had remained in arrears for sixteen months, with no payments received, when J.D.'s mother phoned to tell Dr. B. that the cousin with whom they were living had contracted hepatitis B. The cousin's physician had informed family members that it was probably a highly contagious strain of the virus, because blood tests had determined that the cousin was positive for the hepatitis B virus surface antigen (HBsAg) and the hepatitis B virus e antigen (HBeAg).[8] Discussion with the mother also revealed that J.D. was frequently in close casual contact with the cousin; both were cared for at home by the grandparents when J.D. was not at school. Moreover, the retarded cousin had very poor personal hygiene skills and frequently suffered from bowel incontinence. This information heightened Dr. B.'s concern about J.D.'s risk of being infected, because the virus can be found in most body fluids and can be transmitted through physical contact.

Acute hepatitis B is a serious viral infection of the liver. Although it is rarely fatal in children beyond infancy and most completely recover, 10 percent of patients develop chronic liver disease. The course of the illness is often long and difficult. Its initial phase, lasting one to two weeks, may involve a variety of systemic symptoms. These include loss of appetite, nausea and vomiting, extreme fatigue, muscle and joint pain, headache, inflammation of the throat and nasal passages, cough, and sensitivity to light. A temperature above 100 degrees is often present. The second phase involves the onset of jaundice.[9] Usually the initial symptoms subside in young children, but this phase can be marked by exacerbation of some original symptoms. The liver becomes large and tender, and patients experience pain and discomfort under their lower right ribs. Some patients also have swollen glands in the neck (cervical adenopathy). This phase may last from several days to a month, although its average duration in children is about ten days. During the recovery phase, which may last from two to twelve weeks, the constitutional symptoms disappear, but some enlargement of the liver and abnormalities of its biochemical function may persist.

There is no specific treatment. Hospitalization is sometimes necessary to establish the diagnosis, and patients who experience persistent vomiting may also require intravenous feeding to maintain adequate nutrition and hydration. Restricted physical activity and substantial bed rest are necessary during the acute stages of the infection.

Persons exposed to hepatitis B can receive a prophylaxis, hepatitis B immune globulin (HBIG). This drug provides high levels of antibodies against the virus. Clinical studies have shown that it may prevent the disease in 75 percent of previously exposed persons. It is given in two injections, one immediately following exposure and one a month later.

J.D.'s mother asked Dr. B. if he would administer the prophylaxis. Dr. B. told her that the drug would cost about one hundred sixty-five dollars. He said that he was very reluctant to provide it, because her account had been delinquent for sixteen months and he did not want to incur an additional unreimbursed expenditure. Mrs. D. explained that she had only a modest clerical job, the income from which hardly covered her own living expenses. Her husband, a machine operator at a local factory, was responsible for giving her money to cover J.D.'s needs. However, he frequently failed to give her money, and she had paid the previous bill out of her own pocket. She did not currently have the money for the HBIG, and she did not think that she could get it from J.D.'s father.

Dr. B. offered to perform the blood tests needed to determine whether J.D. should receive the prophylaxis. These tests indicated that the child was not yet infected and could therefore benefit from the drug. Although the health department would administer it free of charge, the parents would have to pay for the drug. Thus, Dr. B. faced the decision of whether to purchase the drug and administer it without the guarantee of payment.

The first commentator on the case was a private pediatrician. He maintained that persons have a moral right to secure their well-being by selecting an occupation, securing the skills and resources necessary to practice it, and disposing of these skills and resources as desired. This moral right implies that private physicians should be free to serve only persons willing to pay for their services. He added that this right is recognized in the American Medical Association's Principles of Medical Ethics, which maintain that "A physician shall, in the provision of appropriate patient care, except in emergencies, be free to choose whom to serve."

He admitted that once a physician has entered a therapeutic relationship, he or she may not abandon the patient. However, failure of the patient or family to act in accord with the implicit terms of the relationship, which require full payment for the doctor's services, relieves the physician of the obligation to continue the relationship. Moreover, Dr. B. had clearly informed the family in writing that further services would not be rendered until previous charges were paid.

He concluded that Dr. B. did not have a moral obligation to provide the immunization to J.D. without the promise of prompt compensation. Doing so would be morally praiseworthy, but failure to provide the immunization would not be morally blameworthy because it exceeded the requirements of moral duty. Nevertheless, Dr. B. should direct the family to other community resources if available.

The other commentator, a professor of medical ethics, took a significantly different view. His analysis started with three factual claims. First, he noted that medical knowledge and skills are socially produced resources. Society heavily underwrites the costs of medical education and research. In addition, medical knowledge and skills are developed through social cooperation, involving collaborative efforts of scientists, medical educators, research subjects, and teaching subjects. Second, medical care is a primary good to which all persons must have access in order to optimally pursue their life plans. Finally, he noted that the social status of physicians is comparatively high in terms of income, prestige, and authority.

He next formulated an interpretation of social justice. He asserted that justice requires that primary social goods be distributed in ways that equalize the opportunity of all persons to pursue their life plans. Moreover, persons who lack these essential goods, through no fault of their own, should receive special assistance from society in securing them.

Applying these considerations to the problem of free care, he noted that physicians often encounter disadvantaged persons who cannot secure medical care through the usual social programs (such as Medicaid) established to satisfy the requirements of justice. Obviously, physicians have the professional skills necessary to satisfy these needs. Moreover, because they receive comparatively high social and economic rewards, it is not unfair to require that they provide some services free of charge. Consequently, physicians should be considered an essential component in society's "safety net" for assisting persons who cannot secure necessary medical care. In cases such as J.D.'s when the patient bears no fault for being unable to pay for medical care, the physician has a moral obligation to provide it without the promise of compensation. Dr. B. should administer the immunization to the child.

The presentations generated considerable debate among those present. A private pediatrician suggested that the ethicist's view involved unacceptable consequences. If a physician is required to provide free care whenever a patient or family is unable to pay, he or she might suffer a substantial reduction in income. She asserted that it would be unfair to expect the average pediatrician to forgo 20 to 40 percent of his or her potential income to provide free care. Nevertheless, in some areas of the local community this might be the result if private pediatricians regularly gave free care.

The ethics professor agreed that the private physician could not be expected to provide free care whenever it is needed. He suggested that the obligation be considered "imperfect," an obligation not owed to any specific person as a right, which may be discharged at the discretion of the physician in a limited number of cases. However, he noted that this concession only required modification of his conclusion. It did not undermine his analysis of the physician's obligation as rooted in social justice.

But a resident challenged the view that justice requires provision of free care by the physician. He pointed out that the same reasoning can be extended to other essential goods, such as adequate food, clothing, and housing. If the physician must provide medical care to patients otherwise unable to secure it, then grocers, clothing retailers, and apartment owners should also be expected to provide a certain percentage of free services. Assignment of this obligation only to the physician is patently unfair; each of these other occupations also provides essential goods.

Another private pediatrician identified a more subtle injustice. He pointed out that although many pediatricians already perform a substantial amount of uncompensated community service, some do not participate in these activities. If pediatricians have an obligation to provide free care only "at their discretion," the inevitable result would be that some pediatricians would bear far more of the responsibility than others. Thus, the burden would be unfairly distributed.

However, another resident rejected the view that providing the immunization to J.D. was merely an "imperfect obligation." He claimed that each person has a duty to prevent serious harm to others when it can be done without great sacrifice. He suggested that the loss of one hundred sixty-five dollars might not be a significant sacrifice, given the typically large income of physicians. Moreover, this duty becomes stronger as the likelihood and magnitude of the harm facing the patient increases. He pointed out that hepatitis B can be a long and difficult illness and that it does occasionally result in chronic liver disease or loss of life. Moreover, J.D. was at high risk for contracting the infection. Because there was a significant risk of serious harm, he believed Dr. B. had a moral obligation to administer the immunization and should be held morally blameworthy if he failed to provide it.

5.3 Risk of Litigation as a Factor in Decision Making

The patient was a twenty-eight-year-old woman at term in her second pregnancy. She came to the hospital in labor, with regular contractions and her cervix dilated 3 centimeters. When the obstetrician examined her in the labor room, he discovered that the fetus had a breech presentation.[10] An ultrasound examination was performed, confirming a frank breech presentation.[11] Based on the ultrasound, the fetus was estimated to weigh approximately seven and a half pounds.[12] No congenital anomalies detectable by ultrasound could be seen. The obstetrician gave the patient a drug to temporarily arrest her contractions and attempted external version (turning the fetus in utero to a vertex presentation).[13] This attempt was not successful. Therefore, a decision would soon have to be made whether to perform a cesarean section or attempt a trial of labor. The latter approach would involve an attempt to deliver vaginally, with cesarean section being performed only if a complication developed, such as fetal distress.[14]

During the past several decades, cesarean section had become widely preferred among obstetricians in delivering breech fetuses, for several reasons. First, there had been concern that vaginal delivery involves increased risk for breech fetuses, compared to cesarean section. One problem is that the fetus's head emerges from the uterus after its body. The fetal head can become entrapped behind a pelvic opening that allows passage of the body but not the larger head.[15] Because the fetal umbilicus emerges from the uterus before the head, it becomes compressed between the entrapped head and the wall of the birth canal. If compression persists, cerebral anoxia (lack of oxygen) resulting in fetal death or brain damage can occur. Another source of risk is a higher incidence of prolapsed umbilical cord[16] in breech presentation, compared to vertex. A prolapsed cord can also become compressed between fetus and mother, resulting in anoxia. Other injuries can include trauma to the head, spinal cord, skeleton, or visceral organs caused by traction applied by the obstetrician in order to deliver the fetus. Risks of spinal cord injury resulting in death or paralysis are particularly great if the head is hyperextended (tilted back). Another impairment that can occur is brachial plexus palsy, consisting of arm paralysis caused by stretching or tearing of the brachial plexus (nerves from neck to arms) caused by lateral force on the head.

Second, vaginal delivery of the breech fetus had become risky for obstetricians. Recent years had seen a large increase in the number of lawsuits. These had included a number of suits involving breech fetuses who, it was claimed, were injured because vaginal delivery was recommended by the obstetrician. Moreover, some suits had resulted in large settlements in favor of the plaintiffs.

Because of these two factors, many obstetricians began routinely recommending cesarean section in all breech cases to avoid the risks of head entrapment and cord prolapse. Although there had been no well-designed scientific studies comparing cesarean section and trial of labor for breech fetuses, articles appeared in the obstetrics literature advocating cesarean section. The cesarean section rate in the United States for breech fetuses increased from 11.6 percent in 1970 to 60.1 percent in 1978.[17] Cesarean section for breech became a standard that was widely accepted.

More recently, several studies had supported the view that a trial of labor for the term breech in selected cases constitutes better care than routine cesarean section. Particularly noteworthy was a study in which patients at term were randomized to cesarean section or trial of labor.[18] Patients eligible for the study had a singleton (not twins, etc.) frank breech fetus with estimated weight between 2500 g (approximately 5 pounds 8 ounces) and 3800 g (approximately 8 pounds 6 ounces). Frank breech was chosen because head entrapment is unlikely when both legs are flexed at the hips; the legs and hips have a combined diameter greater than the head. Patients for whom there was an independent medical reason to perform cesarean section were excluded. Patients randomized to trial of labor underwent measurement of the pelvic opening using X rays. Cesarean section was recommended for those whose pelvis was considered too small. Cesarean section was also performed when complications that threatened the well-being of the fetus arose during trial of labor. A total of 60 fetuses were delivered vaginally; 148 were delivered by cesarean section. There were no deaths in either group, excluding fetuses with congenital anomalies. The only notable difference in infant morbidity consisted of two cases of brachial plexus palsy in the vaginally-delivered group. One of the injuries was completely resolved at five days of age. The other had improved considerably at twenty-eight days of age, but whether it fully resolved was unknown, because the infant was lost to follow-up.[19] The authors attributed both injuries to the lack of experience in breech delivery of the residents who delivered the infants. Maternal complications in the two groups were also compared. Postpartum morbidity, such as infection or blood loss requiring transfusion, occurred for 49.3 percent of women who underwent cesarean section but only 6.7 percent of those who delivered vaginally. The authors concluded that vaginal delivery is reasonable in selected cases of term frank breech presentation.[20]

Several conditions that, according to this study, are necessary for a safe trial of labor were met in this case. First, the presentation was frank rather than complete or footling breech.[21] Second, the fetal weight was in the acceptable range. Third, the size of the pelvic opening was considered adequate; the patient's first baby had weighed eight pounds twelve ounces—considerably larger than the present one—and had been delivered vaginally. Fourth, there were no other indications for cesarean section. Fifth, the obstetrician had obtained considerable experience and was reasonably skilled in delivering breech fetuses. Moreover, if hyperextension of the fetal head were identified by X ray[22] or other complications developed, cesarean section could be performed.

The options available to the obstetrician included the following: (1) discuss both approaches with the patient, including risks and benefits to her and the fetus, and ask which approach she prefers; (2) discuss both approaches and recommend trial of labor; or (3) discuss both approaches and recommend prompt cesarean section.

Concern for patient autonomy appeared to support option 1, which attempted to minimize physician influence. However, there were factors that could impair the patient's ability to make a considered decision. One was the woman's lack of familiarity with the medical pros and cons. Moreover, patients in labor are frequently afraid of pain, being injured, having a defective baby, or even dying. Such fears and the pain of labor can sometimes interfere with the ability to assimilate information about treatment options. Another obstacle was the limited time for deliberation, because of the progress of labor, which can create stress that further impairs the ability to absorb information and make a well-thought-out decision.

Concern for the pregnant woman's well-being supported option 2, because vaginal delivery would avoid the maternal risks of cesarean section. These risks include, in addition to infections and hemorrhage, occasional injuries to the urinary tract and, in a small percentage of cases, performance of hysterectomy to control uterine bleeding. Furthermore, there is a small but elevated risk of maternal death, compared to vaginal delivery.[23] Maternal well-being is also usually promoted by protecting the well-being of the fetus. The view that option 2 would preserve fetal well-being was supported by the recent studies indicating that trial of labor does not increase fetal risks provided that certain conditions are present. Thus, the interests of the woman in avoiding risks to herself and the fetus, coupled with factors that could diminish the autonomy of any decision she might make by herself, supported option 2.

On the other hand, several considerations favored option 3. First, even when candidates for trial of labor are carefully selected, there is a small chance of serious injury to the fetus associated with breech presentation. Some would hold, therefore, that promotion of fetal well-being justifies routine cesarean section, despite a significant increase in maternal complications. Second, vaginal delivery involved greater risks of legal liability for the physician. Unfortunate events can occasionally occur during trial of labor that are beyond an obstetrician's ability to control. Abruptio placenta (premature separation of the placenta from the uterus) might occur, causing rapid fetal hemorrhage. The umbilical cord might be wrapped around the fetus's neck, causing cord compression and death. Any fetal birth injury could result in a lawsuit, even if it were beyond the ability of a competent obstetrician to control the events causing the injury, for a plaintiff might argue that cesarean section would have prevented the harm.

Concern to avoid lawsuits is based on the serious harm they can cause to physicians. Even if the plaintiff does not win, being sued causes emotional stress and can threaten a physician's reputation among colleagues and patients. Meetings with lawyers and court appearances result in significant time lost from practice. There are also financial costs resulting from legal fees, diminished practice time, and occasional loss of patients because of damaged reputation. The total impact of these factors is sometimes so serious that a physician's health is adversely affected as well.

It might be argued that option 1 would also protect the physician from the type of lawsuit in question. However, if the patient chose vaginal delivery and a fetal birth injury occurred, it could later be argued that impediments to decision making had diminished her capacity to consent. Thus, option 3 would better insulate the physician from such suits than option 1. If sued, the obstetrician could cite the published studies in his defense. However, most obstetricians continued to routinely perform cesarean section in these cases, a fact that would make a legal defense difficult.

5.4 Pressures to Provide Customary Care

A forty-one-year-old man was taken to a county hospital after he shot himself in the head. The bullet had entered at the right temple and exited at the left frontal area. The patient was comatose and was immediately put on a ventilator. The physicians' initial assessment was that his condition was terminal. Therefore, surgery was not attempted, and vital signs were not monitored except for blood pressure, which was normal.

According to the family, he had been depressed following his recent medical discharge from the army for severe cirrhosis caused by heavy alcohol abuse. He had been informed by army doctors that he would probably die from the cirrhosis within a few years unless he completely stopped drinking. He also learned that he might die even if he did stop. (The five-year survival rate for cirrhosis patients who abstain from alcohol and have good diets is approximately 60 percent.) After being discharged, the patient had continued to drink heavily. He was unmarried, and his family consisted of his parents and a brother. The patient had recently told his family that he simply wanted "to go ahead and die." His brother said that the patient had been drinking heavily the day he shot himself.

Two days passed, and the doctors realized that the patient might survive longer than expected. When the family was informed of this they requested that he be transferred to the regional veterans hospital, because he was eligible for government-funded medical care. Upon admission to the VA hospital he was still comatose. He could move his arms and legs but responded only to deeply painful stimuli. It was decided to undertake exploratory surgery. Widespread brain damage was found, and bone particles and dead tissue were removed from the path of the bullet. After the operation, the patient was taken to the ICU.

Following surgery, his body continued to assume the posture of a decerebrate individual. He could move his legs but did not respond to commands. There were also roving eye movements which may occur with brain damage and involve no awareness or visual perception. An EEG was abnormal but not completely flat. The EEG report stated that the tracing was consistent with absence of function in the cortex, the part of the brain controlling thought, speech, and consciousness. A CT scan showed widespread cortical damage as well. The patient's pupils showed midposition dilatation and were reactive to light. Other reflexes controlled by the lower brain, such as the doll's-eye movement[24] and the ciliospinal reflex,[25] were present. Thus, the brain stem appeared to be intact, which meant that the patient was not legally dead. Although the patient could breathe spontaneously, he continued to require respirator assistance in order to maintain normal blood levels of oxygen.

After eight days the patient was moved to a ward, where he continued to require ventilatory support. The day before he left the ICU his temperature rose to 101 degrees, and he continued to have temperature spikes each day for the next several days. He was being fed through a nasogastric tube.

On the tenth day following the injury there still had been no improvement in the patient's neurological status. According to the medical literature concerning unconscious head trauma patients, the failure to improve by this time strongly suggested that he was not going to regain consciousness. Additional evidence was provided by the massive cortical brain damage revealed by the surgery, CT scans, and EEG. The diagnosis was persistent vegetative state.

The attending physician discussed the prognosis with the intern who was taking care of the patient. The attending physician believed that the patient would eventually die from a complication such as pneumonia or urinary tract infection. It could not be predicted how long he would remain alive—it might be for one more day or many years. Cases have been reported in which patients in persistent vegetative state lived for twenty years or more, but it seemed unlikely that a patient with cirrhosis would survive that long. The attending physician and intern agreed that no heroic measures should be taken.

At this point the patient's temperature had spiked for three consecutive days, indicating an infection. The source of the infection was not yet known, but soon the intern would have to decide whether to treat it. He asked the attending physician whether he thought treatment should be provided. However, the attending physician wanted the intern to decide for himself, because he believed that wrestling with such questions is an important part of medical training.

According to the family, the patient had never stated his wishes concerning life-support treatment. The intern considered whether the patient's wishes could be inferred from his behavior. The patient's stated desire to die suggested that he would want lifesaving treatments withheld. However, whether his statement reflected an autonomous, considered wish would depend on the extent to which he was depressed, whether he was under the influence of alcohol, and how well he understood his prospects concerning future quality of life. His suicide attempt might also be construed as evidence that he would now want lifesaving treatment withheld, but he had apparently been drinking heavily the day he shot himself.

The intern discussed the patient's prognosis with the family. They had been visiting regularly and understood that it was highly unlikely that he would regain consciousness. The intern suggested that no heroic measures should be attempted, and the family indicated their agreement that "life-prolonging" measures not be used. There was no discussion concerning which procedures should be considered heroic or life-prolonging, except that the family and intern agreed to withhold antibiotics. Withdrawing other life-support measures such as nasogastric tube feedings and the respirator was not explicitly discussed.

The next day the patient again ran a fever, and the intern seriously considered reversing the decision to withhold antibiotics. He explained to a colleague that as a junior member of the medical staff, he was concerned about what the older physicians would think of his performance. He sensed that withholding antibiotics would be much more controversial than giving them. He said that if he were an older, established physician, he would probably feel more confident about withholding the antibiotics.

He mentioned the view of a senior physician with whom he had previously worked. One day during rounds that physician had asserted firmly that antibiotics could not be considered heroic treatment because they involved little risk to the patient, were usually relatively inexpensive, and required little effort to administer. He remembered hearing other physicians and nurses express the view that antibiotics are "ordinary" means and that there is a professional obligation to give such treatment if it is likely to control the infection. Similar considerations applied to tube feedings, which many regard as ordinary means of supportive care. In addition, many doctors would regard withdrawal of tube feedings or the respirator to be illegal, based on a belief that there is a legal distinction between stopping a treatment and failing to initiate it. (In fact, the law does not make this distinction.) Moreover, there is a potential for legal liability in withholding treatments that are widely viewed as ordinary. In a recent California case, for example, two physicians had been charged with murder after fluids and feedings were withheld from a comatose patient.[26] The district attorney argued that fluids and feedings are "ordinary" means and that, therefore, there is a legal obligation to provide them. Although the charges were dismissed by an appellate court, a different conclusion might be reached by courts in the local jurisdiction, if faced with a similar case.

On the other hand, the decision to withhold antibiotics was supported by several considerations. The main one was that the antibiotics were unlikely to benefit the patient. Some might claim that life itself has intrinsic value and should always be maintained, but the fact that the patient was irreversibly unconscious made it implausible to suppose that he would benefit from continued life. Some would even consider prolonging life in such circumstances to be contrary to the patient's interests, in the sense that it demeans the person the patient used to be. Another aspect of patient benefit was the degree of comfort that would be provided by the treatments, particularly the antibiotics and tube feedings. Would a fever or lack of food produce an unpleasant sensation for the patient? No one knew with certainty, and some might say this lack of certainty is grounds for treating. Nevertheless, because there appeared to be a complete lack of awareness, it was quite unlikely that there would be discomfort.

An additional concern was the cost of care, which could be substantial with long-term survival. Because the cost would be incurred by the government, it could be asked whether there are better ways to spend public funds.

Another consideration was the interests of the family. Prolonged survival of a comatose relative can take a severe emotional toll on the family. Death of the patient might permit the grieving process of the family members to progress toward resolution. Also, the family had requested that antibiotics be withheld. It could be argued that the family's decision should be overridden if it caused harm to the patient, but such harm did not appear likely in this case because the patient was irreversibly unconscious.

5.5 Confidentiality and Child Abuse

F.W., a forty-two-year-old man, was referred to a special treatment unit by his lawyer for psychological evaluation before trial on charges of engaging in sexual acts with adolescent boys and for possible initiation of remedial treatment. The unit specialized in the evaluation and treatment of sexual offenders. At the beginning of the evaluation, the patient signed a document promising him confidentiality regarding any information related in the interviews.

F.W. was raised by his mother and stepfather and reported that he was abused by his stepfather. After high school, he served in the Navy. Following discharge, he had a stable work history in the music industry and ran a successful recording studio on the West Coast. He had been married five times and had two children. He was separated from his fifth wife to whom he had been married for seven years. He described her as a "cold woman" and stated that their sex life had never been satisfactory.

The patient's first sexual experience was at the age of eight and involved childhood sex play with other boys. At age fifteen, he became sexually involved with a twenty-five-year-old man and spent the summer with him. He found this to be a satisfying experience. Since that time, he reported approximately one or two homosexual experiences per year with adult males. He reported that since adolescence he had also had sexual experiences with approximately thirty women and had not had any specific sexual dysfunction until the past three months, when he had experienced impotence with adult women. Over the last fifteen years, he had had increasing sexual interaction with adolescent boys. He reported that he had never used force and that these experiences had been "voluntary on the part of the boys." Testing in the sexual physiology laboratory indicated that his maximum sexual arousal was to young boys in the twelve- to-fifteen-year-old range. He also showed arousal to adult males in addition to moderate arousal to adult females. Thus, he was bisexual, with an excessive deviant arousal to young boys.

Personality assessment determined that he was currently very depressed and having difficulty coping. Test results suggested that those problems represented a stress reaction primarily caused by his current legal difficulties, rather than being related to his homosexual activities as such. In fact, he revealed that he did not consider his interactions with adolescent boys to be a problem except for the resulting legal difficulties. He also refused to acknowledge that this behavior might cause psychological harm to the young men involved. He insisted that his legal problems simply represented the repressiveness of society and its inability to allow "alternative life-styles." In general, he appeared to be a very manipulative person not concerned about the effects of his behavior on others.

During the interview with the staff psychiatrist, he freely admitted that he was currently involved in what he described as a "love relationship" with a thirteen-year-old boy. He claimed that this relationship was occurring with the knowledge of the boy's parents, although it was not clear that they recognized the sexual nature of the relationship. The patient frequently stayed overnight at the boy's home and also took him on trips. He apparently spent substantial sums of money buying presents for both the boy and his parents. In the course of the discussion, he even stated the name of the boy and revealed the location of the parents' home. He said that he had no intention of breaking off the relationship, denied that it might be harming the boy, and insisted that the interviewer simply failed to understand the "specialness" of the relationship.

This information posed a difficult dilemma for the psychiatrist. A promise had been made assuring the patient of strict confidentiality concerning the information revealed. Confidentiality is so crucial to the conduct of medical care, especially in a sexual treatment unit, that the therapist was not inclined to disregard it. Nevertheless, the patient was involved in an ongoing relationship that could seriously disrupt the adolescent's psychosexual development, resulting in lifelong impairment of his ability to engage in loving relationships. Prevention of serious and irreversible harm to the boy required discontinuation of the relationship and provision of appropriate psychotherapy. Thus, the physician felt a strong concern for the well-being of the boy. Although similar activities were frequently revealed by patients treated in his unit, the information usually referred to past acts, often did not concern ongoing relationships, and rarely included the names and addresses of the children involved.

Other factors also needed to be considered. One was the well-being of the patient. Reporting the case to the child welfare authorities would undoubtedly exacerbate his legal difficulties. Moreover, the failure to maintain confidentiality would probably preclude the initiation of treatment for the patient's sexual deviance. The therapist did have doubts, however, about the prospects for resolving the patient's sexual problems. Until he accepted responsibility for his actions, substantial progress could not be made in changing the patient's sexual behavior.

Finally, as director of the unit, the therapist was deeply troubled by the potential impact of the failure to maintain confidentiality on the effectiveness of the unit as a community resource. Patients were often referred by lawyers, because many encountered legal difficulties as a result of their sexual activities. Moreover, there was only a small cadre of lawyers in the large metropolitan area served by the treatment unit who accepted or specialized in defending sexual offenders. If the therapist reported this patient to the child welfare authorities, word might quickly spread among the lawyers that the therapists in the unit were not to be trusted. Referral of patients by these lawyers might drop off dramatically. Thus, the general welfare of the community as it might be affected by a decline in the number of patients treated was also at stake.

The psychiatrist determined several possible courses of action: (1) maintain strict confidentiality; (2) threaten the patient with notification of the child welfare agency (just a bluff), using the threat as a lever to get him into therapy; (3) report the case to the child welfare authorities; (4) speak privately with the parents of the boy, pursuing the legal route only if unsuccessful in getting them to break off the relationship; (5) ask the lawyer to apply pressure to the patient to break off the relationship; or (6) make persuasive efforts to get the patient into therapy, using initial sessions to convince him that he should end the relationship.

5.6 Rejection of a Consultant's Advice

C.P., an eighty-two-year-old man, was brought to the hospital after a monthlong bout with nausea, vomiting, and alternating periods of constipation and diarrhea. Although he had experienced abdominal pain and weight loss for about a year, X-ray studies of his gastrointestinal tract ten months and two months before admission had not revealed any disease. His wife and son reported that he had also suffered periods of mental confusion in recent weeks. His medical history included irregular heartbeat (cardiac arrhythmia) and mild Parkinson's disease, a slowly progressive disorder of the central nervous system which causes tremors, rigidity of muscles, and slowness of movement. But until recent weeks he had remained self-sufficient, chopping wood for his fireplace and caring for his fruit and vegetable garden.

A diagnostic workup revealed serious chemical abnormalities. His hemoglobin level was below normal, indicating a reduction in the blood's oxygen-carrying capacity (anemia). He had excessive calcium in his bloodstream, as well as excessive amounts of urea nitrogen, uric acid, and creatinine, waste materials normally removed from the blood by the kidneys. His urine output was greatly reduced (less than 600 ml per day), and excessive amounts of protein were found in his urine.

The symptoms and laboratory results suggested the possibility of multiple myeloma, complicated by acute kidney failure. Multiple myeloma is a cancer involving unregulated multiplication in the bone marrow of plasma cells, a type of blood cell that produces antibodies. Because the tumor cells release large amounts of protein that interfere with urine formation, the disease often results in renal failure. Further tests of bone marrow, blood, and urine confirmed both aspects of the diagnosis. A complete X-ray series also revealed several cancerous lesions in the patient's skull and ribs, sites in which patches of tumor frequently develop.

Multiple myeloma is invariably fatal, although some patients live for years. Prediction of length of survival is very difficult. A hematology consultant thought C.P. might survive up to eighteen months if his disease responded to chemotherapy. He recommended chemotherapy with melphalan and prednisone, and the treatment was initiated.

However, the daily increases in the urea nitrogen and creatinine in the patient's blood suggested that he could only survive a few more days without aggressive treatment for the kidney disease. The attending physician requested a consultation by a nephrologist (kidney specialist), who confirmed the seriousness of the kidney failure. He did not believe that they could wait for the cancer chemotherapy to relieve it. (A positive response to chemotherapy may gradually resolve the kidney failure by reducing the number of cancer cells secreting the proteins that impair kidney function.) Rather, he suggested that the patient undergo regular hemodialysis. If this treatment did not restore satisfactory renal function, then plasmapheresis might be tried.

Hemodialysis is a process in which waste products resulting from inadequate kidney function are removed from the blood. Blood is delivered continuously from the patient's arm into the dialysis machine and returned after cleansing. The dialysis procedure lasts four to six hours, and most patients require treatment three times per week. Plasmapheresis is a procedure in which the blood is also delivered from the patient's arm into a machine. However, the machine removes the plasma from the blood (it is the plasma that contains the harmful proteins) and replaces it with fresh plasma. Although the procedure has only been used experimentally in a few cases of multiple myeloma, preliminary results suggest that it may remove ten times the amount of harmful protein eliminated by hemodialysis. In the experiments, the procedure has been performed about once per week.

However, the attending physician was opposed to acting on the consultant's recommendations. He believed that the acute renal failure should be managed conservatively with dietary restrictions and intravenous medications. He had several reasons for this view. First, given the extent of the cancer, the degree of kidney failure, and the general condition and age of his patient, he believed that the patient would not survive more than a few months, even with abatement of his renal failure. Second, death caused by renal failure would probably involve less pain and suffering than death from cancer. Thus, he ordered conservative management for the kidney failure and continuation of the chemotherapy and entered a do-not-resuscitate note in the patient's chart.

The consulting nephrologist was appalled. He thought the patient had a right to decide whether he preferred more aggressive therapy. Although the consultant suggested to the attending physician that the patient should make the decision, the recommendation met with resistance. The attending physician expressed concern that dialysis might compromise the patient's quality of life. Emotional distress can result from dependence on the machine and changes in body function. Because dialysis patients receive medications to keep their blood from clotting, brain hemorrhages can occur, and dramatic shifts in body chemistry caused by dialysis can produce seizures. Moreover, even if successful, it might only keep the patient alive long enough to undergo severe pain that develops as skeletal lesions caused by the multiple myeloma spread. Finally, the attending physician regarded lightly the hope that plasmapheresis might help. The evidence from the medical literature regarding its usefulness was only anecdotal; besides, it had only been used with much younger myeloma patients.

The consultant replied that the dialysis might not compromise the patient's well-being. Whether serious physical or emotional side effects would occur was a matter of conjecture. The impact on quality of life could not be determined without the patient's own assessment of his degree of suffering and remaining capacity for meaningful life. It seemed reasonable to at least try dialysis. The patient could later decline further aggressive care if his life became intolerable. Moreover, conservative management of his kidney failure hardly seemed to promote his well-being; he was likely to die shortly without more aggressive treatment.

However, these remarks did not alter the attending physician's view. At this point the nephrologist considered whether he should talk directly with the patient. He knew that this would violate the hospital's rules of etiquette, which required that recommendations be made only to the attending physician. However, professional etiquette seemed less important than his obligations to the patient. Besides, the patient, not the attending physician, was paying for the consultant's involvement in the case.

However, the appropriateness of speaking directly with the patient about more aggressive care was not clear-cut. C.P. might become very confused, especially if the attending physician then gave the patient a strongly negative appraisal of this option. C.P. had no more than a fourth-grade education, making an explanation of the medical situation difficult. The likelihood that he would be able to sort matters out was further constrained by his increasingly frequent periods of mental confusion, resulting from kidney failure and the excess calcium in his blood.

The intervention might also intensify the patient's suffering. The conflicting opinions were bound to create substantial anxiety and erode C.P.'s faith in his attending physician. If his kidneys were already irreversibly damaged, the intervention might only make his final days more difficult. There was also the obvious danger that the patient's interests would get submerged in a struggle between the physicians about the handling of the case.

The established system for making consultant's recommendations assigned to the attending physician the obligation of evaluating conflicting information and presenting a treatment plan to the patient. There were good reasons for this approach. Not only does it spare the patient from having to sort out technical points of dispute, but it also allows the attending physician, who is presumed to know the patient better than others, to tailor the information and advice to the needs and interests of the patient. It was hard to make an exception to such a generally sound approach.

Finally, the consultant knew that his colleagues carefully observed the rules of etiquette regulating consulting relationships. As a staff member accepting consultations from attending physicians, he believed that he was making a tacit promise to observe these rules. Speaking to the patient would require breaking this promise.

5.7 Abortion Resulting in a Live Birth

The patient was thirty-eight years old and was childless following two miscarriages. Now she was pregnant again, and she and her husband were hopeful that things would go well. Because of her age, there was an increased risk of having a fetus with Down's syndrome, so her obstetrician recommended an amniocentesis. The procedure was carried out when she was fifteen weeks into her pregnancy. Unfortunately, examination of fetal cell chromosomes in the amniotic fluid indicated that the fetus had Klinefelter syndrome. This is a condition in which the sex chromosome configuration is XXY, resulting in a male who typically has dull mentality, long legs, small penis, and infertility associated with small testes and low testosterone production. The average IQ is ten to fifteen points below that of their normal siblings, with about 15 to 20 percent of affected persons having an IQ below 80. There is also a tendency to have behavioral problems, including immaturity, shyness, poor judgment, and unrealistically boastful and assertive behavior.

The patient was counseled concerning this syndrome, and the options were discussed with her, including the possibility of an abortion. She felt ambivalent about an abortion, because the defects associated with Klinefelter syndrome are relatively moderate. Some affected individuals have normal intelligence and a quality of life quite acceptable to them. However, the degree of retardation could not be predicted, so she and her husband agreed that she would have the abortion.

She was then counseled concerning the abortion procedure. In particular, the doctor told her that if the fetus should happen to be born alive following the abortion, then he would be required by hospital policy to call a pediatrician from the hospital's intensive care nursery. This policy was based on the state's abortion law, one section of which specified the physician's duty to possibly viable infants born alive during an abortion:

The rights to medical treatment of an infant prematurely born alive in the course of an abortion shall be the same as the rights of an infant of similar medical status prematurely born spontaneously. Any person who performs or induces an abortion of such an infant shall exercise that degree of professional skill, care, and diligence in accordance with good medical practice necessary to preserve the life and health of such infant prematurely born alive in the course of an abortion except that if it can be determined, through amniocentesis or medical observation, that the fetus is severely malformed, the use of extraneous life support measures need not be attempted.

Any person who violates the provisions of this section shall be guilty of a felony.

One issue raised by such statutes concerns what is medically indicated for preserving the lives of infants born alive during an induced abortion. Their medical condition may not be the same as infants born after spontaneous premature labor. Their expulsion from the uterus may be more traumatic, and the chemicals used may have harmful effects on the fetus. The uncertainty about what is medically indicated and the legal risks in failing to treat support an approach of "erring in the direction of life." The legal risks are underscored by a recent case in which an obstetrician was charged with murder for failing to provide medical care for a premature infant born alive in the course of an abortion.[27] Also, the term *severely malformed* was not defined in the statute, so there was room for legal debate about whether a fetus with Klinefelter syndrome would fall into that category. Consequently, it was the hospital's policy that all infants born alive in the course of an abortion be taken to the intensive care nursery.

The next day an abortion was performed using prostaglandin vaginal suppositories, which cause uterine contractions. A male infant was subsequently delivered having a slow heartbeat and weighing 270 grams (9.5 ounces). A pediatrician was called, and the infant was promptly carried to the intensive care nursery. The pediatrician's assessment was that the infant was so premature that no treatment could possibly save his life. He was wrapped in a blanket for warmth. A heartbeat continued for a short period of time, and then the infant expired.

The obstetrician informed the mother of the infant's outcome. Later, a hospital clerk brought a birth certificate to the physician for his signature. He informed the clerk that he would not sign the certificate because he felt it was inappropriate in the case of an induced abortion. He knew that if he signed it, the certificate would then be taken to the mother for her signature. He was concerned about the psychological effects of presenting her with a birth certificate.

A recent study has indicated that there is considerable emotional trauma to parents in abortions for genetic abnormalities, compared to abortions for social reasons.[28] The psychological effects include a relatively high incidence of post-abortion depression among both mothers and fathers. The differences may be caused in part by the fact that abortion for genetic indications is usually the termination of a desired pregnancy, whereas abortion for social reasons is typically a solution to an unwanted pregnancy. Abortion for genetic reasons involves loss of the healthy child who was hoped for, and it is frequently accompanied by parental grief, anger, guilt, and disappointment. That such abortions are typically performed relatively late in pregnancy may add to the emotional trauma. (The necessity of a late abortion is based on the requirement of a sixteen-week-gestational-size uterus for a successful amniocentesis and up to a four-week period for cell culture and analysis.) The further into pregnancy, the greater the opportunity for the mother to identify with the fetus, feel it moving inside her, and become emotionally attached to it.

Such abortions are perceived by parents as more than just the loss of a wanted pregnancy, however. First, the parental role in the cause of death may have psychological effects. Some parents, for example, have reported greater depression following an abortion for genetic reasons than occurred with a previous stillbirth. Second, there is often a sense of guilt and shame associated with genetic disease. The self-esteem of parents may be shattered when it rests on societal and personal values giving high priority to the ability to create a normal, healthy child.

The doctor promptly consulted a physician colleague and learned that a birth certificate was required by law. Specifically, the state statute concerning vital records requires a birth certificate for each live birth and defines *live birth* as applying to any "product of conception" which, irrespective of the duration of the pregnancy, shows signs of life upon expulsion or extraction from its mother. A physician who fails to sign a birth certificate can be found guilty of a misdemeanor and be fined not more than fifty dollars or be imprisoned for not more than a year, or both. The chief administrator of the hospital also has a legal obligation to see that the certificate is prepared and can be punished in the same way for failure to do so. Such laws are important for several reasons, such as the usefulness of birth certificates in generating vital statistics regarding birth rates and infant mortality rates.

The obstetrician realized that in his experience the law was not faithfully obeyed in many hospitals. In some cases an abortus with a heartbeat was simply not sent to the nursery, and thus the hospital administration was not aware that a live birth had occurred. In other cases there may be confusion over the legal definition of live birth.

The physician faced a difficult question. Should he sign the birth certificate? He recognized the importance of vital statistics, but it seemed to him that a birth certificate in cases such as this one could result in misleading statistics. The infant mortality rate might be artificially raised by including deaths resulting from induced abortions. He was also especially concerned about the well-being of the mother. To fill out a birth certificate would relabel what had occurred. Rather than reinforcing the view that this was an abortion of a fetus with a chromosomal anomaly, this might emphasize in the patient's mind that she and her husband had killed their baby. The result might be an intense feeling of guilt or a serious depression. Thus, obeying the law would probably not directly benefit others and might very well harm the patient.

On the other hand, the physician believed that we have a moral obligation to obey the law, because our system of laws as a whole promotes the good of society. According to a utilitarian argument, an act of disobedience might weaken the respect for law on the part of the violator and others who are aware of the violation, resulting in a greater harm in the long run than would be caused by obeying the law.

In future cases he might avoid being put in such a situation. He could refrain from calling a pediatrician when the infant was too small to survive. In this way, hospital officials would be unlikely to become aware of the live birth, and a birth certificate would not be prepared. However, this would pose a risk to the physician of criminal prosecution; someone who knew what happened might report it to the local prosecutor. Another approach would be to use intraamniotic injections of saline instead of prostaglandins to induce abortions. A saline solution is more likely to kill the fetus before expulsion. According to one review article, the expulsion of a fetus with signs of life occurs in 1 percent or less of saline-induced abortions, compared to about 7 percent of prostaglandin abortions; the risk of maternal mortality is about the same for the two agents.[29] A third alternative would be to counsel the patient ahead of time concerning the possibility of there being a birth certificate. This approach, however, would not eliminate the possibility of psychological harm to the mother in cases in which a birth certificate is presented for her signature.

5.8 Costly Nutrition for a Terminal Patient

The patient was a forty-three-year-old woman who had seen a doctor one and a half years earlier because of vaginal bleeding between periods. At that time a standard workup was performed, including a fractional D&C.[30] Tissue from her uterus was examined by a pathologist and found to be cancerous. The diagnosis was adenocarcinoma of the uterus,[31] and the extent of disease based on clinical evidence was stage II.[32] The patient received standard treatment, which began with external and intracavitary radiation.[33] This was followed by surgical removal of her uterus, ovaries, and fallopian tubes and biopsies of appropriate lymph nodes. Examination of the dissected tissue revealed that the tumor had spread to the pelvic lymph nodes and the right ovary. In addition, there was tumor at the edge of the surgical specimen where the incision had been made through the upper part of the vagina. Because the cancer had spread to her vagina, a decision was made to also use chemotherapy.

After six weeks the patient refused further chemotherapy, complaining that the drugs made her feel sick. She continued to obtain pain medication at the clinic where she had first received treatment but did not seek further chemotherapy. The cancer continued to grow, and one year after the initial diagnosis she went to the emergency room because of pain in her abdomen and vomiting. She was diagnosed as having a bowel obstruction from tumor compressing her intestines.

The patient agreed to chemotherapy for shrinking the tumor before surgical correction of the bowel obstruction. In the meantime, a nasoenteric-decompression tube[34] was used to pump gastric secretions from her intestine, thereby preventing vomiting and rupture of the intestine. In order to provide nourishment, total parenteral nutrition (TPN, also known as hyperalimentation) was begun. This involves insertion of a catheter into the right subclavian vein, through which a liquid containing the total nutritional needs of the patient can be delivered directly into the bloodstream. The nutrient is a specially prepared solution containing specified proportions of protein, carbohydrates, fat, vitamins, and minerals.

After three weeks of chemotherapy some medical problems arose which delayed surgery. One was acute renal failure, characterized by a decreased urine output and a rise in creatinine and urea nitrogen in the blood.[35] Investigation revealed hydronephrosis of the left kidney caused by an obstruction of the left ureter by tumor.[36] A nephrostomy tube was inserted, leading from the kidney to the surface of the patient's flank. This permitted urine to pass from the kidney to a collection bag attached to the patient's leg, and the patient's kidney function soon recovered. Another problem was septicemia caused by the hyperalimentation line.[37] This was treated successfully by removing the hyperalimentation catheter and administering antibiotics.

Soon afterward, the small bowel obstruction was surgically treated by means of a loop jejunostomy,[38] which permitted the portion of the intestine between the stomach and the site of obstruction to be put into use again. During the recovery period the patient's fluid output (urine and fluid from the stoma) was much greater than the amount of fluid being taken in by mouth. Because the patient was having difficulty maintaining sufficient input, TPN was begun again.

Because of the grave nature of her illness, the patient arranged to be transferred to a distant city near her family. The patient was single, and her family included her mother, a twenty-six-year-old son, and a niece. For a short period the patient stayed at her mother's home, where she continued to receive hyperalimentation. The TPN had been continued to ensure good nutrition during the move. However, it was soon necessary to take the patient to a local hospital because of increased pain in her lower abdomen and general malaise.

Within a few days after admission, the attending physician decided that it might be appropriate to provide nutrition by some other means. The special nutrient solution used in TPN is very expensive, in this case costing approximately one hundred seventy-five dollars per day. In addition, the provision of TPN by central venous catheterization is a relatively invasive procedure which has risks of infection and septicemia. Removal and reinsertion of the catheter can cause pneumothorax, arterial puncture, or air embolus.[39] The physician recommended a gastrostomy, an operation to insert a feeding tube directly into the patient's stomach. Pureed food could be provided through the tube, eliminating the need for TPN. The patient agreed to this procedure, but it was canceled when her physician observed tumor growing through the scar from the previous abdominal surgery. In addition, the patient's entire abdomen was firm, indicating that there was tumor throughout. The amount of fluid and fecal matter draining into the jejunostomy bag had also decreased markedly over the past several days, indicating that another obstruction had occurred. These findings suggested that the tumor was widely disseminated through the jejunum and that there probably was not enough tissue intact to adequately digest food. It was likely, therefore, that feeding by gastrostomy tube would not be effective.

The patient understood that her condition was terminal. Occasionally she was rather depressed over her illness and her separation from the out-of-state home where she had lived for twenty years. Whenever discussions turned to the fatal nature of her disease, she became tense and anxious. She maintained hope that God would cure her, which appeared to play an important role in her attempt to cope with the situation. Her physician suggested that she could either stay in the hospital or return to her mother's home, where care by a visiting hospice nurse could be arranged. She said she preferred to remain in the hospital because she could not manage her personal toilet by herself. Apparently she felt it would invade her privacy too much to have her close relatives assist in her bodily hygiene. Another question discussed was whether resuscitation should be performed if she suffered a cardiac arrest. The patient stated that she did not want to be resuscitated or have other "heroic" measures carried out in such circumstances.

At that point the question of continuing the TPN came to a head among the staff. One physician suggested that they discontinue it. He pointed out that TPN is a costly and sophisticated technology normally reserved for patients with a reasonable chance of recovery. Thus, it might be considered a "heroic" procedure in this case. Because the patient wanted no extraordinary means to sustain her life, he did not think it consistent to continue hyperalimentation.

The staff considered various options. One approach would be to present to the patient the alternatives of continuing or forgoing TPN. It would be explained that because there was no other way to feed her, withholding TPN would result in her death within a short period. The physician would emphasize that her wishes would decide the matter. The pros and cons would be discussed with her, attempting to avoid bias or persuasion. This approach gives priority to patient autonomy and reflects the view that patients have a right to refuse procedures necessary to maintain life, even the provision of nutrition. In support of this approach, it could be argued that the physician's duty to respect the patient's autonomy should take priority over concern about costs. It could also be pointed out that because the patient had been permitted to choose between home care and continued hospitalization, even though hospital care is much more expensive, she should be allowed to make a similar decision concerning TPN.

Another course of action would be to recommend to the patient that TPN be discontinued. Several considerations supported this approach. First, if the patient died within a relatively short period, she would be spared considerable pain and suffering associated with the progression of her cancer. Second, it might add to the emotional suffering of the patient's family to have the dying process prolonged by continued use of TPN. Third, the high cost of TPN was cause for concern. The patient was in a public hospital, and the taxpayers would ultimately pay any portion of her bill the patient could not cover. The rising cost of health care had become a public policy issue that was affecting the traditional attitude

Physicians, Third Parties, and Society 211

that no expense is to be spared to prolong life. The concern had been illustrated by a recent report that approximately 22 percent of all Medicare expenditures are incurred for dying patients during the terminal phase of illness, although they constitute only 5 percent of all Medicare patients.[40]

A third option would be to simply continue the TPN without raising the issue with the patient. In support of this approach, it can be argued that it is wrong to allow someone to die by discontinuing nutrition and hydration. Providing food and water has symbolic meaning as an expression of care and concern, and withholding it may be interpreted as showing a lack of concern for the patient. According to another argument, withholding nourishment differs from withholding other life-prolonging medical procedures, such as respirator therapy. In withholding respiratory support, one allows the patient to die from the disease. Death by starvation, however, is caused by the physician's action. This makes withholding nourishment morally indistinguishable from active killing of patients by lethal injection, which is widely considered to be morally wrong. A defender of the third option might also claim that efforts to reduce costs should be directed toward persuading the patient to receive care at home rather than discontinuing TPN. On this view, there should be further discussions with her concerning the advantages of home hospice care.

5.9 Cost Factors in the Choice of Treatment for Kidney Stone Disease

T.K. was a retired seventy-one-year-old man whose sole income was the monthly social security payments he and his wife received. They had no health insurance other than their Medicare benefits. He was brought to the hospital after having intermittent pain in his back and abdomen on the left side for about three weeks. In the last several days his pain had become intense, and he was constantly nauseated. Because the patient had a twenty-year history of kidney stone disease, diagnostic assessment focused on the likelihood that he had formed another stone. X-ray and intravenous studies of his urinary tract revealed a calcified stone, approximately 1.5 cm in diameter, located in the pelvis of the left kidney. There was no evidence that the flow of urine had become seriously obstructed.

Kidney stones are masses of crystals embedded in a protein matrix that provides cohesion and structure. They may vary in size from microscopic crystals to large masses that fill the space in the kidney where urine is collected. They are caused by failure of the kidney to maintain excreted materials in solution. This breakdown may result from abnormally high levels of excreted materials (such as calcium), decreased amounts of water in the urine, or reduction in the level of substances that inhibit stone formation. Kidney stones may develop in or migrate to areas in the urinary tract where they obstruct the flow of urine. The movement of stones and the development of obstructions can cause severe pain, bleeding, and infection, as well as permanent kidney damage.

Perhaps 80 percent of kidney stones are small enough for persons to pass in their urine. However, the urologist thought it would be unlikely that T.K. would pass this stone spontaneously, because it was larger than one centimeter in diameter. Moreover, it was already causing severe symptoms. If the growth or movement of the stone produced a serious urinary tract obstruction, these symptoms would worsen. Therefore, the urologist believed that a medical procedure to remove the stone was presently indicated.

There were two treatment approaches that might be used. One procedure was percutaneous nephrolithotomy (PN). After the patient is given general or regional anesthesia, a needle is passed through the patient's side into the kidney, using X-ray guidance to determine proper placement. The tract is then dilated using successively wider catheters. Finally, a nephroscope is passed through the tract into the renal pelvis. The nephroscope allows the stone to be visualized and permits the passage of forceps or a stone basket that can be used to extract it. When the stone is initially too large to be extracted through the nephroscope, ultrasonic or electrohydraulic probes can be placed in contact with the stone. The energy from these probes disrupts the stone's matrix and shatters it into manageable fragments. The second procedure is extracorporeal shock-wave lithotripsy (ESWL). Under general or regional anesthesia, the patient is partially immersed in a large tub filled with degasified and demineralized water. A high-voltage underwater generator transmits a focused, high-energy shock wave through the water. Because the body tissue has a density similar to water, the wave travels through the tissue until it strikes the stone, shattering it into smaller fragments. Provision of 300 to 1800 shock waves (depending on stone size) is usually sufficient to reduce the stone to powder or sandlike particles, which can be passed spontaneously in the urine. Thus, unlike percutaneous nephrolithotomy, ESWL does not require invasive surgical maneuvers.

For stones in the pelvis of the kidney that are one to two centimeters in diameter, the two treatment approaches have a comparable likelihood of success. For example, in one large series, 91 percent of patients with renal pelvic stones less than two centimeters in diameter were free of residual stone fragments three months after ESWL.[41] Similarly, in patients undergoing PN, more than 90 percent are free of residual stone fragments as demonstrated by X ray after the procedure.[42] Moreover, the procedures have a similar incidence of complications requiring secondary procedures. In both cases, the main problem involves residual stone fragments causing pain and obstruction as they move down the urinary tract. When ESWL is performed, some stone fragments may not be reduced to a passable size. Similarly, when stones must be fractured during PN, it may not be possible to visualize and remove all fragments. However, patients undergoing ESWL and PN have a similar incidence of stone fragments requiring secondary urological procedures—somewhat less than 10 percent of patients receiving these treatments.[43] In the case of T.K., the location of his stone and its relatively small size suggested a high likelihood of success and a low probability of complications.

On the other hand, considerations related to the postoperative course did not weigh so evenly. Both procedures involve the usual postoperative nausea and vomiting related to anesthesia. Patients undergoing either treatment also have bloody urine for twenty-four to forty-eight hours after the procedure. However, postoperative pain is considerably less with ESWL. In one study, only 30 percent of patients required postoperative analgesia.[44] In another study, 36 percent had no pain and 31 percent only minor pain with stones one to two centimeters in diameter.[45] By contrast, a study of three hundred patients undergoing PN revealed that patients needed an average of 9.9 doses of narcotic medication to provide pain control during the first five days after the procedure.[46] There is also the discomfort of a catheter inserted into the kidney, which remains in place for at least three days to drain fluid and blood that may collect in the area from which the stone has been removed. In addition, whereas the average hospital stay for patients treated with ESWL is a little more than two days, patients treated with PN have an average hospital stay of more than five days.[47] ESWL patients can also resume normal activities almost immediately after leaving the hospital; normal time to resumption of daily activities is about one week with PN.[48]

However, as head of the urology service at the public hospital, the physician considered other factors that might bear on the choice of treatment. At a recent meeting, the medical director had revealed that the hospital, which treats a large percentage of indigent patients, was losing about eight hundred thousand dollars per month. The service chiefs were advised to impress upon staff physicians the need to be cautious in ordering clinical procedures. Moreover, the urologist had recently received data analyzing hospital costs and reimbursements for urological procedures during the preceding year. The average costs of providing ESWL to patients was $4100, and Medicare reimbursement was only $2300—a net loss of $1800 per patient. The average hospital costs for patients undergoing PN was $8731 per patient. However, with Medicare reimbursement of $7976 for patients more than seventy years of age, the hospital lost only about $755 per patient. Thus, the hospital could reduce losses by more than $1,000 per patient by performing PN rather than ESWL for patients older than seventy.

The urologist believed that there were several reasons why it might be appropriate to recommend the procedure less advantageous to the patient. First, the public hospital faced a severe financial crisis, precipitated by the increasing percentage of indigent patients and recent cutbacks in state and federal funding for health care. The hospital faced the prospect of serious reductions in number of personnel and the scope and quality of medical services. Second, the urologist recognized that physicians determine a high percentage of patient care expenditures and that his colleagues often failed to carefully consider the rationale for ordering tests and procedures. Thus, more conservative clinical practice might provide substantial savings for the hospital. Third, PN was comparable to ESWL in terms of the likelihood of success and the low incidence of complications. If he opted for PN, he would not be providing a less effective treatment. Finally, the urologist recognized that his facility, as the local hospital serving persons unable to pay, might not always be able to offer optimal care. Given the current fiscal restraints, provision of minimally adequate care to all indigent patients might require that some receive less than optimal treatment. Without more satisfactory public financing for indigent health care, compromises in quality seemed inevitable.

On the other hand, there were strong reasons for not choosing PN. The urologist was committed to doing what was best for his patient. He knew that postoperative pain and discomfort is less severe and the period of hospitalization and disability less lengthy with ESWL. Another consideration was that adequately informed consent requires that the major reasons for and against treatment options be discussed with the patient. Acknowledgment of the financial reasons for recommending PN might be awkward for the urologist and upsetting to the patient. However, if he failed to discuss the option of undergoing ESWL, the requirements of informed consent would not be met. A third factor was his awareness that some colleagues routinely used ESWL in this type of uncomplicated case. Although they might be ignoring their fiscal responsibilities, it seemed unfair to deny his patient a treatment option available to other patients. Finally, the physician was aware that the cost analyses provided only average figures regarding the costs incurred by the hospital for the procedures. In any individual case, the hospital's costs for a patient undergoing PN might be much greater than the average expenditure and, therefore, the hospital's loss after reimbursement by Medicare might exceed the average loss incurred when providing ESWL. There was no assurance that the use of PN rather than ESWL would have a more favorable financial result for the hospital.

5.10 Artificial Insemination for a Single Woman

A thirty-eight-year-old Belgian woman visited a gynecologist and requested artificial insemination. She was a history professor at a local university and had never been married. During a relationship with a previous boyfriend, she had seen a physician because of infertility. She had been diagnosed as having endometriosis,[49] which was believed to be the cause of the infertility. However, after receiving treatment for the endometriosis, she continued to be infertile. More recently she had developed a relationship with a man who was separated from his wife and had a teenage son. After a few months she became pregnant but subsequently miscarried. Learning that she could conceive encouraged her to try to get pregnant again. However, her boyfriend did not desire additional children and had recently broken off the relationship, an event that had been traumatic for her.

Currently she was not romantically involved, but she desired to have a child. Her financial situation appeared sound. She earned a moderate salary as a professor and owned her own home. She lived alone, with relatives living in Belgium.

The patient also revealed that she was currently seeing a psychiatrist. For a number of years she had been suffering from pronounced mood swings and anxiety attacks, and she was taking medications for her condition. These included daily doses of lithium to reduce the mood swings and alprazolam to reduce anxiety. In the evenings she was also using triazolam, a sleep-inducing agent. She said that if she became pregnant she would temporarily stop taking these drugs in order to protect her fetus. The physician said that he would like to consult with her psychiatrist before making a decision about artificial insemination, and the patient agreed to this.

Several aspects of the woman's behavior during the office visit were disturbing to the physician. Before seeing him, she told the nurse that she would kill herself if she did not obtain artificial insemination. She also told the physician that she had requested artificial insemination from a gynecologist in another city who turned down her request, and she was now suing him because of his refusal. The physician perceived these remarks as threats aimed at influencing him to carry out her request.

The physician and the patient agreed to meet again after the psychiatric consultation. Discussion with the psychiatrist provided additional information about the patient. Professionally, she was quite accomplished as a scholar. She had published numerous articles and traveled frequently to give invited lectures. The psychiatric problems, however, had been present for about twenty years and had two distinct features. One was an affective disorder involving depression. The other was a panic anxiety disorder. There did not appear to be any perceptual or thought disorder. She had a history of minor and major depressive episodes lasting up to three weeks, sometimes requiring hospitalization. The episodes usually followed some type of rejection, such as rejection of an article by a journal or separation from a boyfriend. Even when depression was not severe enough to require hospitalization, it interfered with her work by causing an inability to concentrate. When relationships ended, there was usually severe anxiety, sometimes reaching a panic state with severe psychomotor agitation. The anxiety was also quite disruptive to her daily life. The psychiatrist believed that she was still suffering from the breakup of her most recent relationship. The patient sometimes experienced rapid mood shifts, from a normal mood to anxiety to depression. At times she rapidly developed severe suicidal moods. In fact, the psychiatrist had first seen her during such an emergency. Over the years various drugs were unsuccessful in controlling her illness. The lithium treatment had recently begun, and the patient reported that although she continued to have mood swings and anxiety, their severity was diminished.

Upon receiving this information, the gynecologist was faced with the decision of whether to carry out the patient's request. Some have claimed that artificial insemination for single women should never be performed, based on concern for the well-being of the potential offspring. It has been suggested that children raised by single women experience serious disadvantages compared to children raised in traditional two-parent households. Several specific concerns might be raised. First, the absence of a father might be detrimental. It might be claimed that such absence would adversely affect a boy's acquisition of appropriate sex-role behavior and traits—for example, a boy might tend to become less "masculine." A second concern is the problem of time. A single woman who is trying to earn a living, raise a child, and have at least some social life may have limited time to spend with the child. This might adversely affect a child's cognitive and social development.

The physician was aware of several responses that might be made to these concerns. First, it could be argued that the supposed disadvantages are not present, or at least are not as great as the critics seem to think. Consider the concern about sex-role behavior. Although there are empirical studies concluding that boys from father-absent homes are less "masculine" than boys raised with fathers, the differences are only moderate.[50] Moreover, the concepts of "masculine" and "feminine" are value-laden, and the conclusion that a boy who becomes less "masculine" is thereby harmed can be challenged. Second, it might be argued that potential disadvantages can be diminished by appropriate counseling and compensatory actions. Consider the problem of time. Although studies have indicated that absence of a father tends to have a detrimental effect on a child's cognitive development,[51] other studies have suggested that other forms of child-adult interaction can help remedy such deficits.[52] Such sources might include relatives or teaching-oriented child-care services. Thus, the single woman could be counseled about the importance of providing sufficient child-adult interaction. Third, even if there are disadvantages in comparison to children raised in two-parent households, it does not follow that it is contrary to the interests of a child of a single woman to be brought into existence. Taking into account the benefits to the child of being alive as well as supposed disadvantages, one might hold that if the life is beneficial on balance, then coming into being is in the child's interests. Although life might not be beneficial on balance in some cases, such as children with seriously debilitating or painful genetic diseases, such a conclusion could not typically be drawn concerning children raised by single women. Thus, these various responses suggest that concern for the well-being of offspring does not require that requests for artificial insemination by single women always be refused.

A second type of objection to performing artificial insemination for single women concerns the well-being of society. The practice may contribute to a breakdown of the traditional pattern of two-parent heterosexual families and decay of traditional values of family life. However, replies can be made to these concerns as well. First, it is reasonable to believe that most people will continue to choose heterosexual marriage as the basis of family life. Second, if there were greater diversity of family arrangements, any supposed harms would have to be balanced against the enhanced autonomy of individuals in pursuing alternative living arrangements.

In addition, there are positive reasons that support carrying out the requests of single women for artificial insemination. Doing so promotes the autonomy and well-being of the women who make such requests; they are given the opportunity to experience the benefits of parenthood.

Additional considerations arose from the specific features of this case. Concern for the well-being of the offspring suggested several reasons against performing artificial insemination. First, if the patient had a child and later committed suicide, not only would the child be left without a caretaker, but the death

Physicians, Third Parties, and Society 217

could be highly traumatic for the child. Second, the debilitating effects of the patient's anxiety attacks and depressive episodes might seriously impair her ability to care for the child. Third, there is evidence that each of the drugs she was taking is capable of causing birth defects. Although she was willing to discontinue the drugs during early pregnancy, there might be a need to resume them if she had an anxiety attack during that period. Fourth, with no family members living near who could help care for the child, it was unclear who would provide care if the patient became ill or when she traveled to give lectures.

If one holds that it is permissible to perform artificial insemination for single women, then the question arises about whether it should be performed in this case even though the woman had a psychiatric illness. On one hand, her psychiatric problems seemed likely to compromise the quality of care a child would receive. On the other hand, it might be argued that in spite of the woman's problems, the child's life would probably be, on balance, a benefit to the child.

Commentary

The responsibilities of physicians toward their patients form the cornerstone of medical ethics. However, conflicts between the interests of patients and others sometimes raise questions about how—and even whether—the physician ought to fulfill those responsibilities. Such conflicts have become more common in recent years as a result of social changes affecting American medicine. For example, increased litigation about bad medical outcomes has strongly influenced physicians to consider the medicolegal implications of their clinical decisions. Concern to prevent a lawsuit or acquire evidence to defend a potential suit sometimes provides a reason to perform additional diagnostic tests or to alter therapy provided. In view of such legal considerations, physicians are sometimes faced with balancing the interests of patients against their own legal interests. Another social development has been the enunciation by courts of legal duties of physicians toward third parties. For example, physicians with knowledge that a patient intends to harm a third party may have a legal obligation to warn the threatened individual if possible.[53] Other conflicts have arisen from public pressures to control the costs of health care. Third-party reimbursement based on fees for services rendered, which encourages physicians to order procedures without regard to costs, has been replaced in many settings by payment methods that provide physicians incentives to contain costs. Thus, physicians must sometimes weigh the patient's need for a procedure against the hospital's interest in controlling costs. Because of the influence of various social forces, conflicts between the interests of patients and others have emerged as a pervasive ethical issue in contemporary medicine.

In discussing conflicts between patient and family in chapter 2, we outlined a moral framework that is relevant to the value conflicts considered here. According to a traditional principle of medical ethics, which we refer to as the principle of patient advocacy, the physician's primary obligations are owed to the patient. However, there is controversy about the limits of the physician's obligations, because the principle can be interpreted in at least two ways. Some hold it to mean that the duties to patient should always take precedence. According to this view, serving patients is so central to the role of the physician that permitting other interests to have priority is a failure to fulfill that role. We refer to this as the strict-advocacy view.[54] Others interpret the principle to state that duties to patients are prima facie ones that normally take priority over the interests of others but in some circumstances can be overridden by them. We refer to this as the modified-advocacy view.

In order to better understand and evaluate these two views, it is helpful to consider their implications in a variety of circumstances. First, we consider their implications for conflicts between the interests of the patient and those of the physician. Second, we apply them to conflicts between the patient and specific third parties. Finally, we deal with conflicts between duties to patients and the interests of the public.

Patients and Physicians

The first type of value conflict involves tension between the interests of the physician and those of the patient. Various moral interests of the physician can be involved in such conflicts, but physician well-being and autonomy are commonly at stake. Although both interests can be involved, it will facilitate discussion if we begin with cases in which the predominant focus is on the physician's autonomy.

There are at least two types of situations in which the autonomy of the physician conflicts with patient interests. In one type, the patient requests a procedure that the physician does not want to perform. An example is case 5.1, involving a pregnant woman with a history of genital herpes. During active phases, genital herpes is transmissible by physical contact. The patient was concerned because her fetus could acquire herpes if vaginal delivery occurred during an active phase. If infected, there would be a high risk of serious handicap or death. Although the risk to the fetus could be avoided by cesarean section, surgical delivery would involve maternal risks of hemorrhage, wound infection, and other complications. In selecting a method of delivery in cases of maternal herpes, the obstetrician used a widely followed approach of ascertaining whether active infection is present at the time of delivery. If cultures are positive or there are other signs of infection, a cesarean section is recommended. If not, vaginal delivery is recommended. Although the physician recommended this approach, the patient rejected it because it is not ''100 percent certain'' to protect the fetus. She insisted on having a cesarean section. The physician, on the other hand, did not want to perform a cesarean section unless the patient's subsequent clinical course made it medically indicated.

In the second type of situation involving physician autonomy, the interests of patients conflict with the liberty of physicians to conduct their medical practices in accordance with sound business principles. One important issue concerns the liberty of physicians to withhold services when patients are unable to pay for care. In case 5.2, a pediatrician had provided care for several years to J.D., a six-year-old boy. Initially J.D.'s parents had paid their bills promptly. After their separation, however, the bills were paid only after long delays. At one point, the account had been in arrears for sixteen months when J.D.'s mother phoned the pediatrician to report that a member of her household had contracted hepatitis B. The pediatrician could significantly reduce J.D.'s risk of acquiring hepatitis B by injections of hepatitis B immune globulin. The mother did not currently have the money to cover the cost of the drug, which was $165, and she did not think she could get the money from J.D.'s father. Thus, the physician faced the question of whether to purchase the drug and administer it with little likelihood of payment.

In other cases the predominant value in conflict with patient interests is the well-being of the physician. An example is case 5.3, involving a twenty-eight-year-old woman in labor at term with frank breech presentation. During the past several decades, prompt cesarean section had become the widely preferred method of delivering the term frank breech fetus, despite increased maternal complications associated with cesarean section compared to vaginal delivery. Cesarean delivery was preferred because it was believed that there are increased risks for the term breech fetus associated with vaginal delivery. Injured-baby suits related to complications of vaginal delivery had also become common, with large settlements sometimes awarded to plaintiffs. More recently, several studies had provided evidence that the risk of fetal handicap or death caused by trial of labor is quite low in selected cases. Because the clinical criteria for trial of labor were met in this case, concern for the well-being of the woman suggested that it should be recommended. On the other hand, the possibility of fetal complications resulting in a lawsuit suggested that prompt cesarean section should be recommended.

In these cases physicians must decide whether to permit a risk or loss to their own interests in order to promote the interests of their patients. There is an ethical principle concerning our obligations to protect others that appears to be especially relevant to this type of decision. This principle, which we shall refer to as the *aid principle,* can be stated as follows: we all have obligations to prevent harm to others, provided that doing so does not involve substantial sacrifice of, or risk to, our own interests.[55]

The proviso in this principle suggests that the duties of physicians to protect the interests of their patients might be overridden if carrying out the duty would require a significant sacrifice. However, the matter is not so straightforward. The aid principle stated above describes *general* obligations that each of us has toward all other persons. In addition to having these general obligations, physicians stand in a relationship to their patients that creates *special* obligations to promote the patient's interests. The relationship may also increase the degree of sacrifice they ought to make in providing assistance. Thus, a central issue raised by these cases concerns how much personal risk or sacrifice there must be in order for physicians to be justified in giving priority to their own interests. According to one view, the degree of sacrifice that a physician should undertake on behalf of patients is substantially higher than that required in the absence of such a special relationship.[56] A second view holds that the limits of sacrifice can exceed—but are not always substantially higher than—the limits required by the general duty we all have to assist others. Following our usual terminology, we shall refer to these two positions as the strict- and modified-advocacy views, respectively.

Several considerations support the strict-advocacy view. First, physicians generally present themselves as putting the interests of patients first. Thus, it is usually implicit in the agreement between physician and patient that the physician will not allow personal interests to interfere with the task of promoting the health-related interests of the patient, despite the inconvenience, fatigue, or risk that may be involved. Second, because patients are often highly dependent on their physicians, the role of physician is properly considered a fiduciary one. A fiduciary role requires acting in the best interests of another. Thus, it can be argued that physicians who put their own interests above those of patients violate their fiduciary obligations. Third, when physicians place their own interests first, indirect negative consequences can occur such as loss of trust in physicians. Diminished trust might cause potential patients to be less willing to seek needed medical care. Also, to the extent that trust promotes the aims of the therapeutic relationship, therapy might be less effective in some cases.

In favor of the modified-advocacy view, on the other hand, several considerations suggest that the limits of sacrifice by physicians should not always be substantially higher than those required by the aid principle. First, the implicit agreement between physicians and patients is interpreted by supporters of the modified-advocacy view to mean that physicians should *normally* put the interests of patients first. This interpretation does not require physicians to always undergo substantial degrees of self-sacrifice on behalf of patients. Second, the degree of harm to the patient's interests resulting from a relaxation of the physician's commitment may be, on balance, relatively low in some cases. In case 5.1, for example, damage to the patient's interest in autonomy in refusing her request for a cesarean section would be partly offset by avoiding the risk to her well-being associated with cesarean delivery. If harm to patients' interests is low enough, it may be outweighed by other considerations. Third, physician interests sacrificed in giving priority to patients are sometimes quite substantial. In case 5.1, for example, performing the cesarean section would require the physician to violate his firmly held conviction about what is necessary to provide high-quality care. Similarly, in case 5.3 a decision not to perform cesarean section might expose the physician to serious emotional and financial strains associated with a lawsuit. Fourth, giving priority to patients sometimes has negative consequences in addition to harms to the physician's interests. For example, because standards of medical practice are typically based on a concern to maximize the ratio of patient benefits to harms, violations might weaken practices that protect patients and decrease overall confidence in the quality of care.

The strict- and modified-advocacy views lead to different patterns of reasoning about the cases being considered. According to the strict-advocacy view, the role of the physician involves sacrifice substantially beyond what would be required of one not in a special relationship to the patient. Thus, barring extreme circumstances, decisions should assign priority to the patient's interests. In case 5.1 the physician should give priority to the patient's request for cesarean section rather than his own preference to not perform the surgical procedure. In case 5.2 the financial cost and loss of physician liberty in providing free care appears above the limit of what is ordinarily required by the aid principle. However, because the strict-advocacy view holds that the limits of required sacrifice are substantially higher for those in special relationships, it would conclude that the physician should purchase and administer the hepatitis vaccine. Similarly, the obstetrician in case 5.3 should set aside concerns about possible litigation in deciding how to discuss the options concerning delivery. If trial of labor is the safer method of delivery for mother and fetus, then it should be recommended.

The modified-advocacy view holds that decisions should be made by weighing several considerations, including the degree of sacrifice to the physician's interests, the degree to which the patient's interests would be damaged, and the broader consequences of compromising the patient's interests. If the physician's sacrifice would be beyond the limit of what is generally required by the aid principle, then the physician may sometimes decline to make that sacrifice when damage to the patient's interests would be minor, or broader negative consequences would be avoided. In case 5.1, carrying out the patient's request would involve a significant sacrifice of the obstetrician's autonomy, because he does not wish to violate a widely accepted standard of professional practice. Moreover, because refusing her request might avoid risks of cesarean section, the degree to which her interests would be harmed by refusal is relatively low. Thus, the modified-advocacy view might lead to the conclusion that her request should be refused. In case 5.3 the physician's legal risks would be significant if vaginal delivery were attempted. Furthermore, the maternal risks of cesarean section would be partially offset by reduction of risk to the fetus. Thus, it might be concluded that the physician's legal risks tip the balance in favor of cesarean delivery. By contrast, in case 5.2 the degree of potential harm to the patient in acquiring hepatitis is great. Although the pediatrician's loss of liberty and financial cost in providing free care would exceed the limits required by the aid principle, a proponent of the modified-advocacy view might conclude that the patient's interests outweigh those of the physician.

Patients and Specific Third Parties

The second type of value conflict involves opposition between the interests of the patient and those of a specific third party.[57] In these situations, the physician has the opportunity to protect or promote the welfare of the third party. However, this will compromise the patient's interests, especially those related to autonomy or personal welfare.

A common species of this conflict involves the interests of the patient and other specific persons. Often, the conflict arises as a result of information disclosed confidentially within the therapeutic relationship. When the information suggests that another person may be seriously harmed by the patient, protecting the interests of the person at risk might require violation of confidentiality. For example, in case 5.5 a forty-two-year-old man had been referred by his lawyer for psychological evaluation before trial on charges of having sexual relations with adolescent boys. During the interview the patient revealed that he was currently involved in a "love relationship" with a thirteen-year-old boy. The patient also revealed the boy's name and where he lived. When pressed by the psychiatrist, he flatly rejected suggestions that he should break off the relationship. Thus, the psychiatrist was faced with the question of whether he should violate confidentiality and attempt to protect the boy by notifying his parents, the child welfare agency, or legal authorities.

Another species of the conflict between the interests of patients and those of specific third parties involves health-care institutions. Frequently, the interests of patients related to the provision of treatment do not square with organizational goals or patterns of service delivery utilized by health-care institutions. For example, in case 5.6 an eighty-two-year-old man had multiple myeloma, a cancer of the bone marrow. The cancer cells release a large amount of protein that sometimes causes life-threatening kidney failure, as happened in this case. A consulting nephrologist recommended dialysis treatment. However, the attending physician decided not to accept this recommendation. In his view, the patient would survive only a few months. Death from kidney failure would involve significantly less pain and suffering than death from cancer. Moreover, dialysis is not always effective and can interfere with the patient's quality of life. The nephrology consultant believed that the attending physician was violating the patient's right to make an informed decision, as well as choosing a course of action that might not promote the patient's well-being. On the other hand, speaking directly with the patient would violate the established system for providing consultations, which assigned to the attending physician the obligation to assess and interpret consultative advice for the patient. This might result in open conflict with the attending physician and leave the patient confused, anxious, and mistrustful of the staff. As a result, the interest of the institution in smooth and efficient provision of services could be adversely affected.

The strict- and modified-advocacy views yield distinctively different approaches to these situations. Proponents of the strict-advocacy view maintain that there are good reasons for not permitting the interests of specific third parties to override the commitment to serve the patient's interests.[58] First, alteration of the physician's commitment may seriously compromise moral interests of the patient. One is the patient's exercise of personal autonomy. An important component of personal autonomy is the ability to control the dissemination of personal information about oneself. Failure to meet a patient's expectation of confidentiality undermines his or her control over highly sensitive information. For example, in case 5.5 protection of the young man at risk requires violation of an explicit promise not to disclose highly sensitive information. Similarly, efforts by physicians to serve institutional interests may undercut the patient's control over his or her treatment. For example, in case 5.6 the nephrologist's adherence to the established protocol for providing consultation is likely to result in the patient being uninformed about important alternative treatments.

Another endangered moral interest of the patient involves his or her well-being. In many situations, the physician cannot protect the interests of a specific third party without compromising the patient's welfare. In case 5.5 contact with child welfare or legal authorities may place the patient at risk of additional legal charges, as well as making it less likely that he will initiate psychiatric therapy. Similarly, in case 5.6 adherence by the nephrologist to institutional rules for providing consultation may result in the patient's acceptance of a decision that significantly shortens his life and prevents him from receiving treatment in a manner he considers compatible with his welfare.

A second consideration supporting the strict-advocacy view is the frequent uncertainty about the potential effectiveness of the physician in protecting the interests of the third party.[59] For example, the psychiatrist in case 5.5 did not know beforehand whether reporting the case to child welfare authorities would lead to expeditious intervention on behalf of the adolescent boy. Child welfare agencies are typically overwhelmed with such reports and, consequently, may react slowly and ineffectively in investigating and processing complaints. Similarly, failure of the nephrologist to intervene in case 5.6 may serve the immediate interests of the institution but could result in serious legal liability for the hospital, if the patient or next of kin later suspect that the quality of care has been inadequate.

A third factor favoring the strict-advocacy view is that options are often available for protecting third-party interests that do not require physicians to compromise their commitment to the patient. The psychiatrist in case 5.5 might have successfully enlisted the aid of the patient's criminal lawyer in convincing him to end his relationship with the adolescent boy, without violating confidentiality. Similarly, the nephrologist in case 5.6 might have tried to secure review of the case in a regular clinical conference designed to assess case management.

Finally, proponents of the strict-advocacy view often point to negative consequences of altering the commitment to the patient that outweigh its intended positive result. For example, confidentiality encourages patients to reveal information needed to provide effective treatment. When medical care involves sensitive matters such as sexual behavior or mental illness, patients are unlikely to share important but potentially damaging information if they believe that the physician may violate their confidence. Moreover, if mistrust causes patients to avoid needed treatment, the general well-being of society may be compromised. In case 5.5 violation of the patient's confidentiality may discourage other sex offenders from seeking treatment at the sexual treatment unit. The result may be a substantial increment of harm to both persons needing treatment and their potential victims, which outweighs the harm to the adolescent boy.

Proponents of the modified-advocacy view maintain that considerations identified by supporters of the strict-advocacy approach provide a basis for claiming only that the physician should *normally* assign priority to the patient's interests.

They argue that there are also good reasons for holding that in some situations this commitment should be altered to enhance the interests of specific third parties. First, circumstances occur in which failure to alter the commitment to the patient may result in serious and irreversible harm to other specific parties.[60] For example, in case 5.5 it is probable that continuation of the abusive sexual relationship would seriously disrupt the adolescent boy's psychosexual development, resulting in lifelong impairment of his ability to engage in loving personal relationships.

Second, it is claimed that in many situations the physician can effectively protect the interests of specific third parties by altering the commitment to the patient. For example, it is highly likely that further harm to the adolescent in case 5.5 would be prevented if the child welfare agency or the legal authorities were informed about the ongoing relationship with the patient. Moreover, it is possible that counseling for the young man could be provided in the psychiatrist's unit, because victims are also regularly seen in the clinic.

Third, defenders of a modified-advocacy view point out that there is frequently no viable option to altering the commitment to the patient if the welfare of a specific third party is not to be seriously and irreparably compromised. In case 5.5 the psychiatrist might try further to persuade the patient to discontinue the relationship. However, the patient had indicated that he saw nothing wrong with his actions. As a result, it is unlikely that the young man could be protected unless the physician disclosed the information to public authorities.

Finally, proponents of the modified-advocacy view claim that often the indirect negative consequences of altering the commitment to the patient are not sufficient to outweigh its positive results. On one hand, the interests of the specific third party to be protected are often much more important than the compromised interests of the patient. For example, irreversible impairment of the adolescent boy's psychosexual development in case 5.5 might be considered much weightier than the added legal risk to which the patient would be subjected by violation of confidentiality. On the other hand, indirect negative consequences of altering the physician's commitment to the patient may often be of minimal significance. For example, the need to violate patient confidentiality to protect substantial third-party interests does not often occur. It is unlikely that isolated violations to prevent serious and irreversible harms to other parties will cause a general erosion of trust in physicians sufficient to discourage many persons from seeking treatment.

Application of these contrasting positions yields differing moral assessments of the physician's options in cases 5.5 and 5.6. According to the strict-advocacy view, the psychiatrist in case 5.5 should not report the patient's current relationship with an adolescent boy to social welfare or legal authorities. Reporting the patient would exhibit disrespect for the patient's autonomy, because highly sensitive information about the patient would be disclosed without his consent. Moreover, disclosure of the information would be likely to impair the patient's well-being, because it would increase his legal jeopardy and make him less likely to accept treatment. Similarly, in case 5.6 the consulting nephrologist should speak directly with the patient regarding treatment alternatives. This course of action would provide the patient with the opportunity to make an informed decision about treatment options and might result in determination that dialysis would better serve his welfare interests.

However, the modified-advocacy view would require weighing the relevant moral considerations in each case to determine whether the interests of the patient should take priority. For example, in case 5.5 it might be argued that the constellation of moral factors clearly favored violation of the patient's confidentiality. The adolescent boy was at risk of suffering serious and irreversible harm. Reporting the situation to public authorities would likely result in discontinuation of the relationship. Moreover, there were no viable options available to the physician for protecting the interests of both his patient and the young man. However, a very different conclusion might be drawn in case 5.6. The nephrologist might effectively protect the interests of the institution in the smooth and efficient provision of medical services, but failure to discuss the medical options with the patient might expose the hospital to later legal liability. In addition, it might be argued that the interests of the patient clearly possessed greater moral weight than the interests of the institution. Failure to consult with the patient may result in a treatment contrary to his preferences and welfare interests. By comparison, the institution may only suffer a temporary disruption in cordial relationships among staff members. As a result, a proponent of the modified-advocacy view might claim that the consultant's commitment to serve the patient's interests should not be altered.

Patient Care and Public Interests

The obligations of the physician to protect the moral interests of the patient may also conflict with interests of the general public. Public interests involve states of affairs that support the activities of most or all members of the community.[61] They may be acknowledged in varying degrees by social policies that constrain the physician's behavior in the therapeutic relationship. In some cases, public interests are embodied in laws setting specific constraints on the physician's behavior. For example, there is a public interest in gathering basic demographic data about the frequency and pattern of births and deaths, because this information is needed in planning social programs. Thus, physicians are required by law to file birth and death certificates.

Other public interests are formalized in statutory law but result in only indirect constraints on the physician's behavior. For example, there is a public interest in controlling government health-care expenditures. By 1986, health-care expenditures consumed 10.8 percent of the gross national product, double the percentage expended in 1960.[62] More than 40 percent of these expenditures were covered with federal dollars. Hospital costs account for a substantial portion of federal health-care expenditures, and cost-containment efforts have focused on this sector. Until recently, the federal government reimbursed hospitals for individual procedures, thus providing little incentive for limiting interventions. A new policy involves reimbursing hospitals with a fixed payment based on each patient's specific diagnosis. If the cost of services outruns the per-case reimbursement, hospitals must absorb the losses. Thus, hospitals must limit their expenditures.

One approach involves influencing the clinical practice of physicians by using computerized systems for monitoring the frequency with which physicians order procedures compared to their colleagues. Restriction or removal of staff privileges might be threatened for those who substantially exceed norms of practice established by these analyses. Thus, the public interest in cost containment has led to indirect constraints on clinical practice.[63]

Finally, there are public interests that are not embodied in statutory law, even though they may be affected by the physician's clinical decisions. For example, there is a public interest in ensuring that children become productive members of society and are not dependent on society for their basic welfare needs. Moreover, raising children in the traditional family is viewed as the most effective means for achieving their personal development.

Noncoital reproductive technologies allow persons to circumvent a variety of problems preventing pregnancy.[64] Their availability to married persons expands their reproductive options and promotes nurturance of children in the traditional family. However, physicians are not prohibited from providing noncoital reproductive services to unmarried persons.[65] Thus, despite the public interest in the upbringing of children in the traditional family, specific restrictions have not been set on the use of these technologies.

Problems arise because actions of the physician in fulfilling therapeutic obligations may compromise public interests. One type of conflict occurs when statutory law prohibits actions that enhance the patient's moral interests. In case 5.7 the patient was a thirty-eight-year-old woman undergoing an abortion because the fetus had a serious genetic abnormality. When the abortion was performed, a male infant weighing nine and a half ounces was delivered alive and briefly survived. Later, a hospital clerk brought a birth certificate to the physician which he declined to sign because its presentation to his patient for signing might be emotionally traumatic. Relabeling the event as a birth rather than an abortion might cause severe guilt or remorse about the infant's death.

Another type of conflict is posed by the indirect pressures placed on physicians to consider cost factors in clinical decisions. The focus here is not medical procedures considered useless; eliminating them is not contrary to the patient's moral interests. Rather, the question is whether physicians should ever withhold potentially beneficial treatment based on cost considerations. In case 5.8 the patient was terminally ill with cancer of the uterus. A blockage caused by the tumor had developed in her intestines, and nourishment was being provided through a central venous catheter (parenteral hyperalimentation).[66] The physician questioned whether the potential benefits of hyperalimentation justified its costs to the state. Its use might briefly prolong the woman's life, but it might also permit additional pain and suffering from progression of the tumor. Provision of this marginal benefit would cost the government $175 per day. In case 5.9 an indigent patient required treatment for a kidney stone. The patient's welfare would be best served by lithotripsy. This would involve much less pain and suffering and a less lengthy hospitalization than surgery. However, at a recent meeting staff physicians had been told that the public hospital was losing more than eight hundred thousand dollars per month. The patient's physician knew that the hospital received more adequate reimbursement from the federal government when surgery was performed. Thus, the procedure involving less pain and suffering was likely to be less profitable for the hospital.

Dilemmas in patient care also involve public interests not embodied in statutory law. Although there is a public interest in the nurturance of children in the traditional family, noncoital techniques permit men and women to beget and rear their own genetic offspring as single parents. For example, in case 5.10 a single woman requested artificial insemination. She was a successful scholar, and her financial status appeared quite satisfactory. However, she had no family to assist in caring for the child. She also had suffered from recurrent episodes of serious depression, for which treatment had not been effective. The physician knew there were no legal restrictions on the use of artificial insemination. On the other hand, he recognized the difficult problems in raising a child as a single parent, which might be compounded by the patient's psychiatric problems.

The strict-advocacy view and the modified-advocacy position represent fundamentally different approaches to circumstances in which the moral interests of the patient conflict with public interests. Proponents of the strict-advocacy view maintain that the physician should assign priority to the patient's moral interests, because these interests will be seriously undermined if the physician is assigned a role in balancing them against public interests. When public interests are assigned greater moral importance, social mechanisms for their protection should be utilized that do not rely on the physician.

Proponents of this view maintain that several key moral interests of the patient will otherwise be endangered. One involves the patient's well-being. First, if physicians must consider public interests, they are likely to be less aggressive in securing all resources needed to provide optimal care.[67] For example, the physician pressured to reduce costs may fail to vigorously seek intensive care for a patient who may profit from close monitoring. Similarly, a physician who is expected to protect the public interest in the proper nurturance of children may be less likely to suggest services that could assist a single person in overcoming fertility problems. Second, physicians are likely to take account of public interests by using rules of thumb that are often not sensitive to the special needs or circumstances of specific patients.[68] For example, a clinical rule for cost containment may limit a procedure whose use is generally of marginal benefit, such as "no hyperalimentation for terminally ill cancer patients." Nevertheless, the procedure may substantially benefit a patient whose quality of life remains quite good except for nutritional problems. Again, a rule of thumb for allocating noncoital reproductive services, such as "no artificial insemination for single women," may ignore the excellent resources particular single women may possess for nurturing a child.[69]

Another key moral interest endangered, according to the strict-advocacy view, is the personal autonomy of patients. The doctrine of informed consent requires that patients be apprised of alternative treatments that may be compatible with their interests or preferences. However, when available medical procedures are withheld by the physician to reduce public expenditures, patients are denied treatment they may desire and whose use is not foreclosed by law. For example, a decision to reduce costs by offering surgery rather than lithotripsy for treatment of kidney stones denies the patient the opportunity to consider a treatment whose use is not legally prohibited. Likewise, denial of noncoital reproductive services to a single person, despite the absence of legal restrictions, may frustrate an interest occupying a central place in that individual's life plans. Moreover, unless patients are familiar with treatment alternatives, they may not even know when a service has been denied based on public interests.[70]

A third important moral interest undermined, according to proponents of the strict-advocacy view, is the patient's interest in fair treatment. One concern is that individual physicians acting as guardians of public interests may make very different decisions regarding similarly situated patients. For example, some physicians may routinely decline to offer hyperalimentation to terminally ill cancer patients as a cost-reduction measure, whereas others might provide the treatment if it offers some benefit. Again, some physicians, but not others, may decline the request of single women for artificial insemination based on the public interest in proper nurturance of children. A second problem is that societal biases against specific groups may be reflected in clinical decisions designed to protect public interests. Cost-containment strategies, for example, may compromise more severely the welfare of elderly persons than those in other age groups.[71] Likewise, negative social attitudes toward lesbians may lead physicians to deny them noncoital reproductive services more frequently than other single women.

Moreover, proponents of the strict-advocacy view maintain that there are usually alternative mechanisms for protecting public interests that do not require the physician to compromise the interests of the patient. For example, reliance on physicians may not be necessary to control costs. Some commentators maintain that cost containment can be effectively achieved only by requiring careful cost/benefit assessment of expensive new technologies before their widespread use is permitted.[72] In addition, regulatory agencies or individual hospitals might develop protocols specifying the clinical circumstances in which particular diagnostic or therapeutic modalities may or may not be used.[73] Similarly, there are public policy options for promoting the interest of society in the nurturance of children in the traditional family. Laws might restrict access to noncoital reproductive services to married couples. This approach would enhance the optimal development of children while not relying on the physician to assess the suitability of particular unmarried persons for parenting.

By contrast, proponents of the modified-advocacy view hold that the physician should sometimes serve as a guardian of public interests. The argument involves

Physicians, Third Parties, and Society   229

at least three points. First, it is claimed that some public interests assume moral priority over the interests of individual patients. For example, there is a weighty public interest in effective cost containment. The rate of increase in hospital costs continues to outstrip the cost of living index, further impairing the capacity of government to provide minimally adequate health care for indigent and elderly persons. Steep increases also reduce the funds available for non-health-related social programs. Likewise, the well-being of the community is substantially enhanced by the development of children into productive and independent members of society. Given the importance of these factors in promoting the interests of society, they may be assigned priority over the conflicting interests of particular persons.

A second factor supporting the physician's role as a guardian of public interests is evidence that the physician may be the most effective agent for protecting or promoting these interests. A useful illustration relates to cost containment. Numerous regulatory efforts have failed to stem rapidly rising expenditures. These have included development of alternative delivery systems (e.g., health maintenance organizations), certificate-of-need programs designed to restrict duplication of costly facilities and equipment, and utilization review programs to identify overuse of resources and procedures.[74] However, because physicians initiate almost 80 percent of hospital expenses, altering their clinical practice may substantially reduce expenditures. Again, it might be argued that the individual physician is the most effective guardian of the public interest in selective provision of noncoital reproductive services. Proper nurturance of children depends on a variety of resources that individual patients may not possess, such as adequate financial means, maturity of attitudes about child rearing, and availability of social supports to assist in child care. It might be claimed that the physician is best situated to assess whether these resources are possessed by persons requesting reproductive services.

A third factor in a modified-advocacy view is the claim that assigning the physician a role in safeguarding public interests may be the best means for limiting the damage to the moral interests of patients. For example, it might be maintained that the individual physician is able to implement cost-containment practices without compromising the quality of patient care. Systemwide rules or hospital protocols restricting the availability of resources may be too inflexible to take account of special circumstances of specific patients. By contrast, the physician has the knowledge of the patient's situation to determine whether specific procedures are useless, marginally beneficial, or clearly necessary for adequate care.[75] Likewise, assignment of a gatekeeping role to physicians may be the most sensitive way to distribute noncoital reproductive services. Legislative or regulatory attempts to classify ineligible persons would necessarily define general properties that do not correlate uniformly with inability to provide adequate nurturance for a child. By contrast, the physician can ferret out through careful clinical assessment persons who are grossly deficient in the resources needed to provide adequate nurturance for a child while not denying services to others.[76] Thus, proponents of the modified-advocacy view maintain that the physician may sometimes serve as a guardian of public interests.

The strict-advocacy view and modified-advocacy position yield different conclusions regarding the cases discussed. According to the strict-advocacy approach, the physician in case 5.7 should decline to prepare a birth certificate, even though the action violates a legal obligation, if securing his patient's signature is likely to cause serious emotional distress. In cases 5.8 and 5.9 cost containment should be secondary in the choice of treatment. The terminally ill cancer patient in case 5.8 should continue to receive hyperalimentation if sensitive and open discussion indicates that this will best satisfy her current needs and preferences. Lithotripsy rather than surgery should be offered to the patient in case 5.9, because it constitutes an effective treatment involving less pain and discomfort than surgery. In case 5.10 the gynecologist should provide artificial insemination to the single woman unless careful assessment reveals decisive reasons why it is contrary to her own moral interests.

The modified-advocacy view, however, leads to different results. This position requires the physician to weigh the moral interests of the patient against public interests. For example, in case 5.7 the importance of the public interest in collection of basic demographic information is reflected in the legal obligation to file a birth certificate. In addition, there is a more general public interest in law-abiding behavior. By contrast, the primary interest of the patient involves freedom from emotional distress. It might be possible to reduce the impact of signing the certificate through sensitive interaction with the patient. Thus, it might be argued that the physician should act in accord with his legal obligation.

In cases 5.8 and 5.9 the public interest in cost containment must be weighed against the patient's interests. In case 5.8 provision of hyperalimentation to the terminally ill cancer patient will cost the government about five thousand dollars if she survives one month. On the other hand, the physician believes that continued use of the procedure will be only marginally beneficial—allowing brief prolongation of life while permitting additional pain and suffering from spread of the cancer. Thus, on the modified-advocacy view it might be appropriate to recommend discontinuation of the procedure. By contrast, in case 5.9 lithotripsy will provide the patient with an effective treatment for his kidney stones with much less pain, suffering, and convalescence than surgery. Moreover, the average saving to the hospital in performing surgery is only about one thousand dollars per case. As a result, the weight of the respective interests seems to fall clearly on the side of the patient.

Finally, in case 5.10 the interest of the patient in the experience of raising a child must be weighed against the public interest in ensuring the adequate nurturance of children. Both sets of interests possess substantial importance. However, the opportunity to reproduce is usually considered a basic moral interest, because raising children plays a central role in the life plans of many individuals. Thus, a proponent of the modified-advocacy view might claim that the physician should refuse to provide artificial insemination only if the evidence strongly suggests that she will be unable to provide minimally adequate nurturance for a child.

A Framework for Weighing Competing Interests

The discussion has focused on whether it is sometimes morally appropriate for the physician to compromise the interests of the patient in order to protect or enhance the interests of other parties. The initial presumption was that the physician should give priority to the patient's interests. However, this presumption must be assessed in light of several moral considerations that may either sustain or override it in specific circumstances.

Several factors requiring consideration have emerged from the discussion. First, the importance of the affected moral interests of the patient must be assessed, as well as the likelihood of injury to those interests if the physician acts to further the interests of others. Second, role-related duties of the other party, which may require some sacrifice for the sake of the patient, must be clarified. Third, the probability and magnitude of the risk to the interests of the other party must be established. Fourth, it must be determined whether alteration of the physician's commitment to the patient will effectively mitigate the risk to the other party. Fifth, even if the alteration of this commitment will promote the interests of the other party, the indirect negative consequences must be weighed against its positive results. Finally, it must be determined whether there is an alternative approach to protecting the interests of the other party, which is as effective and has as favorable a balance of overall consequences, without requiring compromise of the physician's commitment to serve the patient.

The strength of the strict- and modified-advocacy views depends on the assessment of these factors in specific types of situations. Situations in which reasons supporting the strict-advocacy view have substantial weight have certain characteristic features. One is that the interests of the patient endangered by alteration of the physician's commitment are especially weighty or important. Another is that the other party may have some special role obligation to accept attenuation of his or her interests for the sake of the patient. A third feature is that there may be important negative consequences, such as loss of public trust in physicians, which outweigh the positive results sought through alteration of the physician's commitment to the patient. Finally, there are usually viable alternatives for protecting the interests of the other party requiring less severe compromise of the physician's commitment to the patient. By contrast, situations in which arguments for the modified-advocacy view carry substantial weight have a different set of characteristics. It is usually the case that the probability and/or magnitude of the risk to the other party is substantial. In addition, alteration of the physician's commitment to the patient will effectively reduce the risk to the other party. Finally, there may be no useful alternatives for protecting the interests of the other party less disruptive of the therapeutic relationship.

Attention to these various considerations permits some general conclusions about the comparative strengths of the strict- and modified-advocacy views in dealing with the types of conflicts of interest examined in this chapter. First, defense of the strict-advocacy view is easiest to mount when the party whose interests conflict with those of the patient has special role-related obligations to protect the patient's interests. For example, we have reviewed situations in which the interests of physicians conflict with the patient's moral interests. Because physicians have fiduciary responsibilities to protect the interests of patients, it can be argued that they should accept substantial attenuation of their own interests for the sake of the patient. Nevertheless, the strict-advocacy view may not be justified for all situations in which physicians' interests conflict with those of the patient. Role-related duties possess special stringency, but they may also have clear limits. Thus, their existence creates only a presumption in favor of the strict-advocacy view.

Second, the strongest case for the modified-advocacy view involves situations that have three main features. First, a specific third party is at high risk of suffering a serious and irreversible harm. Second, the physician is able to effectively reduce or eliminate this risk by altering the commitment to serve the patient's interests. Third, there are no decisive negative consequences of altering the physician's commitment that outweigh the benefits accruing to the third party. The classical situation satisfying these conditions occurs when information provided under the protection of confidentiality suggests that another person may be seriously harmed by the patient. Nevertheless, fulfillment of these conditions is not sufficient to establish the modified-advocacy view in these situations. There must also be no effective alternative for protecting the interests of the third party that permits less severe compromise of the commitment to serve the patient's moral interests.

Third, arguments for the strict- and modified-advocacy views are more evenly balanced in regard to public interests that conflict with the interests of the patient. On one hand, there are significant public interests that may be effectively enhanced by the physician through alteration of the commitment to the patient. These include public health goals, such as the gathering of important demographic data as represented in case 5.7, as well as the goal of implementing effective cost containment as examined in cases 5.8 and 5.9. On the other hand, a difficult obstacle facing proposals to alter the physician's role duties for the sake of public interests involves establishing that there are no effective policy alternatives requiring less severe compromise of the physician's commitment to the patient. For example, many commentators maintain that effective cost containment must focus on controlling the introduction of expensive new technologies that accelerate the cost spiral. Another difficult problem is establishing that the negative consequences for the interests of patients will not outweigh the positive results of altering the physician's commitment. In particular, there is a serious risk that different physicians will unevenly execute public responsibilities, resulting in unfair distribution of the burdens of protecting these interests among similarly situated patients.

Although these various themes emerge from an analysis of the comparative strength of arguments for the strict- and modified-advocacy views in the context of specific conflicts of interests, it is clear that they indicate only general trends in the strength of arguments for or against each view. This review has also stressed the fact that these general trends may not always hold sway. Thus, assessment of the relative merits of the strict- and modified-advocacy views requires painstaking analysis of the moral considerations identified for each kind of situation in which conflicts of interest challenge the presumption that the physician should assign priority to the patient's interests.

Notes

1. A. J. Nahmias et al., "Perinatal Risk Associated with Maternal Genital Herpes Simplex Virus Infection," *American Journal of Obstetrics and Gynecology* 110 (1971): 825.
2. A. J. Nahmias and A. Visintine, "Herpes Simplex," in J. S. Remington and J. O. Klein, eds., *Infectious Diseases of the Fetus and Newborn Infant* (Philadelphia: W. B. Saunders, 1976), pp. 156–90.
3. J. A. Pritchard and P. C. MacDonald, *Williams Obstetrics*, 16th ed. (New York: Appleton-Century-Crofts, 1976), pp. 1082–83; J. R. Evrard and E. M. Gold, "Cesarean Section and Maternal Mortality in Rhode Island," *Obstetrics and Gynecology* 50 (1977): 594–97; G. L. Rubin et al., "Maternal Death after Cesarean Section in Georgia," *American Journal of Obstetrics and Gynecology* 139 (1981): 681–85.
4. J. H. Grossman III, W. C. Wallen, and J. L. Sever, "Management of Genital Herpes Simplex Virus Infection during Pregnancy," *Obstetrics and Gynecology* 58 (1981): 1–4.
5. J. H. Harger et al., "Characteristics and Management of Pregnancy in Women with Genital Herpes Simplex Virus Infection," *American Journal of Obstetrics and Gynecology* 145 (1983): 784–91.
6. L. A. Vontver et al., "Recurrent Genital Herpes Simplex Virus Infection in Pregnancy: Infant Outcome and Frequency of Asymptomatic Recurrences," *American Journal of Obstetrics and Gynecology* 143 (1982): 75–84.
7. F. H. Boehm et al., "Management of Genital Herpes Simplex Virus Infection Occurring during Pregnancy," *American Journal of Obstetrics and Gynecology* 141 (1981): 735–40.
8. An antigen is a substance capable of producing a specific immune response, such as the production of antibodies. An antigen can be a bacterium, a toxin, a protein, or almost any other kind of large molecule and is usually material foreign to the body. Because different viruses have unique antigenic materials, the presence of antigens in the bloodstream can be used to identify these viruses. In hepatitis B, the presence of surface antigen and e antigen correlates with high infectivity of the viral strain.
9. Jaundice or icterus involves an abnormal coloration of the skin, whites of the eyes, and the urine as well as other body tissues. It is caused by excess bilirubin circulating in the blood. The latter substance is normally processed in the liver and converted into

bile. However, when many liver cells have been damaged or destroyed by infection, excess bilirubin is liberated into the general circulation and causes yellowish discoloration of the skin.
10. Presentation is the part of the fetus presenting itself at the cervical opening. Normally, the top of the head presents, referred to as vertex presentation. In breech presentation, as described earlier, the feet or buttocks present.
11. In *frank* breech presentation, both legs are flexed at the hips and extended at the knees.
12. Ultrasound can provide measurements of body parts such as head diameter and abdominal circumference. Given such measurements, various formulas can be used to estimate fetal weight.
13. In attempting external version, the obstetrician places hands on the woman's abdomen, exerting gentle pressure against the fetus in order to rotate it.
14. Fetal distress refers to insufficient oxygenation of the fetus. A standard method of detecting fetal distress is monitoring of the fetal heart rate. Certain patterns of deceleration of heart rate are associated with fetal distress. Serious distress is an indication for emergency cesarean section in order to prevent fetal harm.
15. Although the abdomen of a term fetus can be larger than the head, the abdomen is more compressible and can assume a smaller diameter during birth.
16. A prolapsed cord is one that emerges through the cervical opening before delivery of the fetus.
17. Cesarean Birth Task Force, National Institute of Child Health and Development, "The National Institutes of Health Consensus Development Statement on Cesarean Childbirth: A Summary," *Journal of Reproductive Medicine* 26 (1981): 107.
18. Joseph V. Collea, Connie Chein, and Edward J. Quilligan, "The Randomized Management of Term Frank Breech Presentation: A Study of 208 Cases," *American Journal of Obstetrics and Gynecology* 137 (1980): 235–42.
19. The degree of impairment varies. In some cases, wrist and finger movement is intact, but there is weakness of the shoulder and elbow. In other cases there is paralysis of the whole arm. The degree of recovery also varies. Some recover completely within a few days; recovery might take months for others. In extreme cases, there is permanent paralysis of the entire arm.
20. Similar conclusions are stated by, among others, Tracy A. Flanagan et al., "Management of Term Breech Presentation," *American Journal of Obstetrics and Gynecology* 156 (1987): 1492–99.
21. In *complete* breech presentation, both legs are flexed at the hips, and at least one is flexed at the knee. In *footling* breech, one or both legs are not flexed at the hips, and one or both feet present.
22. An X ray could also further confirm that the presentation was frank.
23. A maternal death rate of 30.9 per 100,000 cesarean sections, compared to 2.7 per 100,000 vaginal deliveries, was reported by Evrard and Gold, "Cesarean Section and Maternal Mortality." A mortality rate for cesarean section of 59.3 per 100,000 in contrast to 9.7 deaths per 100,000 vaginal deliveries was found by Rubin et al., "Maternal Death after Cesarean Section."
24. The doll's-eye movement, or oculocephalic reflex, is tested by holding the eyelids open and quickly turning the head to one side, then to the other. In a comatose patient with an intact brain stem, the eyes move in the opposite direction as if still gazing ahead in their initial position.

25. The ciliospinal reflex is a dilatation of the pupils following stimulation of the skin of the neck by pinching or scratching.
26. D. L. Breo, D. Lefton, and M. E. Rust, "MDs Face Unprecedented Murder Charge," *American Medical News*, September 16, 1983, p. 1.
27. "MD Charged with Murder in Abortion Case," *American Medical News*, October 26, 1984, p. 8.
28. B. D. Blumberg, M. S. Golbus, and K. H. Hanson, "The Psychological Sequelae of Abortion Performed for a Genetic Indication," *American Journal of Obstetrics and Gynecology* 122 (1975); 799–808.
29. D. A. Grimes and W. Cates, Jr., "The Comparative Efficacy and Safety of Intraamniotic Prostaglandin F_2 and Hypertonic Saline for Second-Trimester Abortion," *Journal of Reproductive Medicine* 22 (1979): 248.
30. A dilatation and curettage (D&C) is a procedure in which the cervix is dilated using a graduated series of blunt metal rods and the lining of the uterus is scraped with a curet (a spoonlike instrument). In a fractional D&C, the cervical canal is scraped first, and the material that is removed is analyzed separately from the uterine scrapings.
31. Adenocarcinoma of the uterus is the most common type of uterine cancer and originates in the glandular tissue lining the interior of the uterus.
32. Staging is the classification of the extent of the spread of a cancer at diagnosis. The stage of the patient's tumor is useful in determining prognosis and appropriate treatment. In stage II adenocarcinoma of the uterus, the tumor is confined to the uterus and cervix.
33. Treatment by intracavitary radiation consists of temporary placement of radium capsules inside the uterus. In external treatment the radiation source is outside the body.
34. A nasoenteric-decompression tube is a plastic tube inserted nasally and passed through the stomach into the intestinal tract.
35. Creatinine and urea nitrogen are waste products cleared from the body by the kidneys.
36. Hydronephrosis, as defined earlier, is the accumulation of urine within the kidney caused by obstructed outflow. It causes distension and damage to the kidney.
37. Septicemia is a systemic disease characterized by the presence of microorganisms, or toxic chemicals produced by them, in the blood. The entry site of the catheter is a potential source of invasion of the bloodstream by microorganisms. Thus, care must be taken to keep the entry site and tube sterile. When septicemia occurs, the catheter is considered a likely source of the infection and is removed.
38. In a loop jejunostomy, a small loop of jejunum (upper part of the small intestine) is pulled outside the body through a surgical incision in the abdominal wall. The loop is sutured in place, and an opening (stoma) is created in the apex of the loop to allow egress of its contents.
39. A pneumothorax is an accumulation of air in the space surrounding a lung, resulting in collapse of the lung. Air can enter through a needle hole during attempts to puncture a vein. Air embolus refers to introduction of air into a vein.
40. Ronald Bayer et al., "The Care of the Terminally Ill: Morality and Economics," *New England Journal of Medicine* 309 (1983): 1490–94.
41. Robert Riehle et al., "Extracorporeal Shock-Wave Lithotripsy for Upper Urinary Tract Calculi," *Journal of the American Medical Association* 255 (1986): 2043–48.

42. For example, see Joseph Segura et al., "Percutaneous Removal of Kidney Stones: Review of 1,000 Cases," *Journal of Urology* 134 (1985): 1077–81.
43. Regarding ESWL, see George Drach et al., "Report of the United States Cooperative Study of Extracorporeal Shock Wave Lithotripsy," *Journal of Urology* 135 (1986): 1127–33. Secondary procedure rates for PN are examined by Segura et al., "Percutaneous Removal of Kidney Stones," pp. 1078–79.
44. Jan-Peter Jantzen et al., "Management of Urolithiasis: An Analysis of 1,293 Lithotriptor Procedures," *Texas Medicine* 82 (1986): 37–43.
45. Drach et al., "Report of the United States Cooperative Study," p. 1130.
46. George Branner and William Bush, "Percutaneous Ultrasonic versus Surgical Removal of Kidney Stones," *Surgery, Gynecology and Obstetrics* 161 (1985): 473–78.
47. See Robert Riehle et al., "Impact of Shockwave Lithotripsy on Upper Urinary Tract Calculi," *Urology* 28 (1986): 261–69; and Segura et al., "Percutaneous Removal of Kidney Stones," p. 1078.
48. For example, see E. L. Palfrey et al., "Report on the First 1000 Patients Treated at St. Thomas' Hospital by Extracorporeal Shock-wave Lithotripsy," *British Journal of Urology* 58 (1986): 573–77; and Michael Brown et al., "Comparison of the Costs and Morbidity of Percutaneous and Open Flank Procedures," *Journal of Urology* 135 (1986): 1150–52. However, R. V. Clayman et al. report postdischarge convalescence after PN of only two to five days. See "Percutaneous Nephrolithotomy: Extraction of Renal and Ureteral Calculi from 100 Patients," *Journal of Urology* 131 (1984): 868–71.
49. Endometriosis is a condition in which tissue resembling the endometrium (the inner layer of the uterus) proliferates outside the uterus. The tissue is usually responsive to the changing hormone levels of the menstrual cycle and, like the endometrium, produces periodic bleeding in response to those changes. Endometriosis can cause pain, abnormal vaginal bleeding, and infertility.
50. A review of such empirical studies is found in E. Herzog and C. E. Sudia, "Fatherless Homes: A Review of Research," *Children* 15 (1968): 177–82.
51. A review of these studies is provided by M. Shinn, "Father Absence and Children's Cognitive Development," *Psychological Bulletin* 85 (1978): 295–324.
52. S. M. Crossman and G. N. Adams, "Divorce, Single Parenting, and Child Development," *Journal of Psychology* 106 (1980): 205–17.
53. The seminal case setting forth this legal obligation was *Tarasoff* v. *Regents of the University of California*, 529 P.2d 553 (1974).
54. Statements that appear to express the strict-advocacy view are cited in chapter 2, notes 8, 9, and 10. Another example is Abrams, "Patient Advocate," p. 1784.
55. Harm is an adverse effect on any of a person's moral interests. For example, harms prevented or incurred in fulfilling one's obligations under the aid principle can include diminution of liberty. Thus, we must distinguish the concept of harm as used here from its usual meaning in statements of the general duty of beneficence. The latter incorporates a narrower concept of harm, referring exclusively to adverse effects on one's well-being. Because there does not appear to be good reason to exclude other moral interests in formulating the moral obligation to assist persons, the aid principle appears to be more appropriate to the present discussion than a principle employing the more restricted concept of harm.
56. The view in question does not maintain that there are no limits to the sacrifice required by physicians. Such an extreme view would have serious problems. Con-

sider, for example, a psychiatric patient who attempts to harm his therapist and can be stopped only by harmful force. The implication would be that the therapist does not have the usual right of self-defense. To consider another example, some patient requests conceivably could require violations of conscience by physicians. Our usual strong regard for freedom of conscience would have to be set aside. Thus, the view that physicians must make unlimited sacrifice is untenable.

57. Here we consider third parties who are not members of the patient's family. Conflicts between patient and family are considered in chapter 2.

58. In defining the scope of the strict-advocacy view, we set aside cases in which there is a clear statutory obligation to report medical information to public authorities and a general expectation among patients that physicians will comply with these requirements. Clinical decision making takes place within a legal framework that sometimes requires such reporting, as in the case of venereal and other communicable diseases, gunshot wounds, child abuse, abortion, and other matters involving public interests. Moreover, patients generally know about and expect physicians to fulfill these legal responsibilities. As a result, both physicians and patients enter the therapeutic relationship with an implicit understanding that these limits on confidentiality will be observed. Few would argue—nor does it seem justifiable to claim—that the physician should serve as a strict advocate by declining to make the required reports whenever it would compromise the patient's interests. Thus, in distinguishing the strict- and modified-advocacy views, we set aside this category of situations.

59. See Michael Kottow, "Medical Confidentiality: An Intransigent and Absolute Obligation," *Journal of Medical Ethics* 12 (1986): 117–22.

60. See, e.g., *Tarasoff,* esp. p. 568.

61. See Joel Feinberg, *Harm to Others* (New York: Oxford University Press, 1984), pp. 221–25.

62. See Eli Ginzberg, "A Hard Look at Cost Containment," *New England Journal of Medicine* 316 (1987): 1151–54.

63. Cost containment can be implemented in numerous ways, with somewhat different consequences for the moral interests of the patient. At the systems level, efforts might include limiting the introduction of expensive technologies, developing less costly delivery systems, establishing professional review committees to control overuse of services, and altering insurance coverage and reimbursement policies. In the individual hospital, programs whose costs exceed government reimbursement might be reduced or eliminated, whereas profitable services might be expanded. Fewer personnel might be retained to provide specific services. Efforts might also be made to alter the clinical practice of physicians. Finally, physician behavior might be influenced in several ways. Committees might develop protocols specifying treatments that cannot be used for patients with specific diagnoses or prognoses. Another approach involves positive financial incentives, such as profit sharing and bonuses for physicians who limit their use of procedures. A third strategy involves a monitoring program as described above. We examine only the latter cost-containment strategy, because it is the most common approach to influencing physician behavior.

64. Two important noncoital reproductive procedures are artificial insemination and in vitro fertilization. The former utilizes the sperm of either a woman's husband or some other donor. It was developed to overcome medical problems of the male partner, such as impotence, infertility, or possession of a transmissible genetic defect. In vitro

fertilization involves fertilization of the female egg in the laboratory, followed by its insertion into the womb. It can be used to circumvent abnormalities of the female reproductive tract that prevent conception, as well as to achieve fertilization when the male partner has a low sperm count impeding in vivo fertilization.

65. There are laws regulating the use of in vitro fertilization and artificial insemination, as well as laws delineating legal relationships between the involved parties (donors, recipients, spouses, etc.). However, no laws specifically address the rights of unmarried persons to utilize these services. See Ethics Committee of the American Fertility Society, "Ethical Considerations of the New Reproductive Technologies," *Fertility and Sterility* 46 (1986): 7S–15S.
66. The procedures used in providing hyperalimentation, as well as the risks and benefits of this treatment, are described in case 5.8.
67. See Norman Levinsky, "The Doctor's Master," *New England Journal of Medicine* 31 (1984): 1573–75.
68. Ibid.
69. See Michael Bayles, *Reproductive Ethics* (Englewood Cliffs, N.J.: Prentice-Hall, 1984), pp. 17–18.
70. See Haavi Morreim, "Cost Containment: Issues of Moral Conflict and Justice," *Theoretical Medicine* 6 (1985): 257–79.
71. Levinsky, "The Doctor's Master," p. 1574.
72. See William Schwartz, "The Inevitable Failure of Current Cost-Containment Strategies," *Journal of the American Medical Association* 257 (1987): 220–24.
73. See Robert Veatch, "DRGs and the Ethical Reallocation of Resources," *Hastings Center Report* 16 (June 1986): 32–40.
74. See Ginzberg, "A Hard Look at Cost Containment," pp. 1152–53.
75. See Lester Thurow, "Learning to Say 'No,'" *New England Journal of Medicine* 311 (1984): 1569–71.
76. See Carson Strong and Jay Schinfeld, "The Single Woman and Artificial Insemination by Donor," *Journal of Reproductive Medicine* 29 (1984): 293–99.

Topical Index to Cases

Abortion	2.7, 5.7
Adolescents	
Confidentiality	2.5, 2.6
Informed consent	2.3, 2.5, 2.6, 3.7, 4.3
Allocation of scarce resources	3.2, 5.8, 5.9
Allowing to die (*see* Withholding treatment)	
Alternative treatment modalities, risk/benefit assessment	3.6, 3.8, 3.10, 4.8, 5.1, 5.3, 5.6
Artificial insemination	5.10
Behavior control (*see* Electroconvulsive therapy; Involuntary commitment; Suicide)	
Competence, determination of	1.1, 1.2, 1.3, 1.6, 3.9
Confidentiality	2.5, 2.6, 5.5
Contraception	2.6, 2.8, 3.9
Cost containment	5.8, 5.9
Electroconvulsive therapy	1.1
Euthanasia, passive (*see* Withholding treatment)	
Experimentation (*see* Research involving human subjects)	
Incompetence (*see* Competence, determination of)	
Informed consent (*see also* Adolescents; Research involving human subjects)	
Affective factors	1.1, 1.2, 1.3, 1.4, 1.5, 1.6, 1.8, 1.9, 2.1, 2.3, 2.4, 3.1, 3.7, 4.3, 4.4, 4.8, 5.1, 5.3
Comprehension	1.2, 1.5, 1.6, 1.9, 2.1, 2.4, 4.4, 5.3, 5.6

240   A Casebook of Medical Ethics

Persuasion and voluntariness	1.4, 1.5, 3.1, 3.2, 3.7, 4.5, 4.9, 5.1, 5.3, 5.8
Intraprofessional issues	
Consultation relationships	5.6
Standards of customary care	5.1, 5.4
Involuntary commitment	1.1, 1.3, 1.8
Legal constraints on clinical decisions	2.7, 2.8, 2.10, 3.8, 3.9, 5.3, 5.5, 5.7
Maternal-fetal conflict	2.7, 2.9, 2.10, 4.8, 5.3
Mentally retarded patients, rights of	2.7, 2.8, 3.5, 3.8, 3.9, 3.10
Ordinary/extraordinary means distinction (*see* Withholding treatment)	
Parental authority, limits of	2.2, 2.3, 2.4, 2.5, 2.6, 2.7, 2.8, 3.7, 3.10, 4.9, 5.1
Randomized clinical trials (*see* Research involving human subjects)	
Refusal of treatment	
Adult patients	1.1, 1.2, 1.3, 1.4, 1.6, 1.8, 2.1, 3.3
Family	1.7, 2.2, 2.4, 2.9, 4.9, 5.4
Pregnant women	2.10
Reproductive issues (*see* Abortion; Adolescents; Artificial insemination; Contraception; Sex reassignment; Sterilization)	
Research involving human subjects	
Children	2.2, 4.3, 4.6, 4.9
Compensation for injuries	4.10
Deception	4.1
Informed consent	4.1, 4.2, 4.3, 4.4, 4.5, 4.7, 4.8, 4.9, 4.10
Nontherapeutic procedures	4.6, 4.7
Randomized clinical trials	4.2, 4.8
Risk/benefit assessment	4.7, 4.8
Undue inducement	4.5
Right to health care	2.7, 5.2, 5.8, 5.9, 5.10
Sex reassignment	1.9
Sterilization	2.8, 3.8, 3.9
Suicide	1.8, 5.4
Truth telling	1.10, 2.1, 2.3, 2.5, 3.2, 4.1, 5.7, 5.9
Withholding treatment	
Do-not-resuscitate orders	3.4, 3.5, 5.6
General	2.3
Handicapped newborns	1.10, 2.4, 3.4, 3.5
Incompetent adults	1.6, 1.7, 2.1, 3.1, 3.2, 3.3, 5.4
Nutrition and hydration	1.2, 3.3, 3.5, 5.8